LIFE'S GOOD

IT'S THE DISEASE THAT'S THE PROBLEM

peace life good
Hazel

An inspirational true story about living well with a terminal disease

by Hazel Carter

Proceeds to MND Association, Marie Curie and The Myton Hospices

COMMENTS ABOUT THIS BOOK

"I have had the pleasure of reading the draft manuscript of Hazel's book. It is a candid, completely honest and heart-rending account of both what it is like to live with MND but also to be the carer of a loved one. It doesn't just deal with the medical issues and practicalities, but also the emotional impact and the effect it has on close relationships and the ripple effect of that. It sets out how it felt to live through something that you can barely imagine and raised my knowledge of the disease, and my already huge respect for carers, who in my opinion, are unsung heroes and should be celebrated. Although this book is about a devastating disease, it is also about deep love and the human spirit, which I found deeply uplifting. This is what I take away from reading this book - an awareness of MND and the need to help find a solution to it, and that love, and a beautiful human spirit, makes the world go round - even in times like this."
Rachel Hardy

"I was unaware of this disease until it affected the lives of my friends Alan and Hazel. Hazel has lovingly and eloquently compiled this book to navigate us through a journey of experiences which greatly affected her life and eventually deprived Alan of his life. The book will be an eye opener to family and friends as well as informative to the medical and caring professions. 10/10 Hazel for compiling an honest and frank account of yours and Alan's experience with this Mean Nasty Disease."
Julie Turney

"This book manages to do the impossible - it is very easily read whilst also being highly informative. It is in the form of a diary so can be put down and picked up easily, but the information contained therein is invaluable to anyone involved in the care of someone with a terminal illness. So often, health professionals only get to see things from their own perspective or skillset. This book provides the full holistic, warts and all, across-the-board, viewpoint so is crucial for both carers and medical professionals alike. Uniquely, it is written by the wife of someone with MND, who maintained a comprehensive diary through her husband's diagnosis, treatment, care and decline."
Richard Todd

"The book gives a clear understanding of living with and caring for someone with MND. It takes you on a heart-wrenching journey and is told through 'true love' for one another. It shows how strength and determination can help someone with MND live the best possible life. I've learnt so much about MND by reading the in-depth daily journal, showing the difficulties experienced, the professional support needed, the physical and emotional effects and much more. I feel the book could help professionals/carers/friends have a greater insight from first being diagnosed with this cruel disease to 'End of Life'!"

Carol Harvey

Written and first published by Hazel Carter in 2023

lifesgoodbook.co.uk

Copyright © Hazel Carter 2023

Cover design by Peter McNougher of Candoo Web Design

ISBN - 978-1-9196122-3-2

Printed in UK by
Vauxhall Printing Co Ltd
76 Wordsworth Road,
B10 0EE

Information provided by MND Association, Marie Curie and The Myton Hospices is current at the time of publication.

This book does not provide medical advice. No content is intended to be a substitute for professional medical advice, diagnosis, or treatment. The views expressed in this book are purely the views of the author. The author is not a medical expert and recommends readers affected by MND always consult their GP, MND specialist and other medical specialists appropriately.

This book is dedicated to my husband.

The finest man I have ever known.

Alan Carter

21st June 1954 - 5th June 2019

Also, to the invisible heroes - family members and friends,

who selflessly give of themselves every day,

caring for a loved one they cannot save.

Poem by Daren Stanley
Person living with motor neurone disease

I'm holding onto every breath,
I've got MND, the slow death,
But why the slow death they say,
As I watch myself waste away.

Every second of every minute of every hour of every day,
Stay strong, you got this, fight it, they say,
As a tear rolls down my face, I close my eyes and pray.

The researchers are close to a breakthrough, they say,
Another tear rolls down my face, I close my eyes and pray,
My arms I cannot move, my legs they cannot walk,
It won't be long before I cannot talk.

So much frustration, anger, and pain,
How much I would give to be me once again.

The breakthrough is what we want,
To find that magic pill,
To help stop the thousands from being so ill,
So how close are they, how soon will it be,
I hope and pray it's in time for me.

Life's Good

It's the disease that's the problem

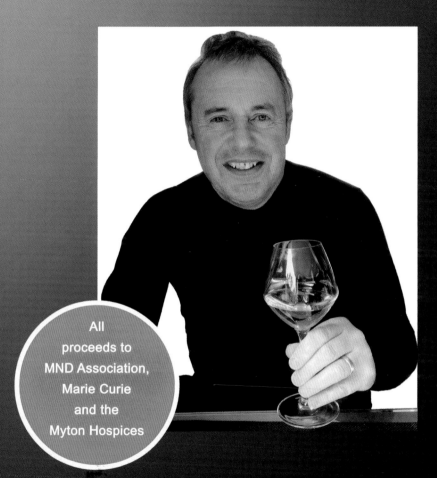

All proceeds to MND Association, Marie Curie and the Myton Hospices

An inspirational true story about living well with a terminal disease by Hazel Carter

Foreword by Dame Pamela Shaw
Professor of Neurology, University of Sheffield

Caring for a loved one who suddenly receives a terminal diagnosis is a massive challenge, but with the right mindset, anything is possible.

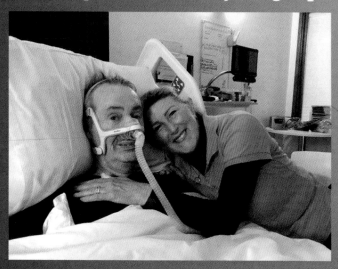

When Hazel's husband, Alan, was diagnosed with amyotrophic lateral sclerosis (ALS), the most common form of motor neurone disease (MND), it was devastating, but the disease did not stop the couple in their tracks.

A prognosis of six months to two years to live, and no hope of a cure, spurred them on to take a holiday of a lifetime overseas, have four UK breaks and enjoy countless social events, while Alan became gradually locked into a failing body, and dependent on a ventilator to breathe.

In this book Hazel describes the ups and downs of their adventures, the challenges of providing care in their home and how their deep love for each other kept them strong. She also shares her private thoughts and feelings, and tips she hopes readers will find useful.

Buy this book if:
- You know someone with a terminal disease, in particular MND
- You work in the health sector or for a care company
- You make decisions affecting people with life limiting diseases

MND affects people of all ages, gender, and backgrounds. Professor Stephen Hawking, David Niven, Ronnie Corbett and Doddie Weir OBE died from it. Sportsmen, Rob Burrow MBE, Stephen Darby, Ed Slater and musician Roberta Flack have also been struck by the disease.

SCAN ME

Order at: lifesgoodbook.co.uk

Price £12.99

Contact: hazel@lifesgoodbook.co.uk   ISBN: 978-1-9196122-3-2

CONTENTS

FAMILY MEMBERS MENTIONED IN THIS BOOK

Alan's relatives

Joan - Alan's mum
Freda - Alan's aunt
Pauline Beard - Alan's elder sister. Simon Beard - Pauline's husband
Helen Bowden - Pauline and Simon's daughter. Richard Bowden - Helen's husband
William and Thomas, Helen and Richard's sons
Matthew Beard - Alan's nephew. Suzanne Beard - Matthew's wife
Viv Cuthbertson - Alan's younger sister. John Cuthbertson - Viv's husband
Ben Cuthbertson - Viv and John's son. Claire - Ben's fiancée. Mia Alana, their daughter
Tom Cuthbertson - Viv and John's youngest son
Kathleen - cousin, and her husband, Michael
Christine - cousin, and her husband, Dennis
Eric – cousin
Renee - 2nd cousin
Joni - 2nd cousin, and her husband, Jim
Lindsey - 2nd cousin
Gillian - 2nd cousin

Hazel's relatives

Yvonne - Hazel's mum
Rowena (Ro) King - sister.
Steve King - Rowena's husband
Darren King - Rowena and Steve's son. Suzanne King - Darren's wife
Millie and Ollie - Darren and Suzanne's twins
Melissa King - Rowena and Steve's daughter
Kevin Essery - Hazel's brother
Sue Essery - Kevin's wife
Martyn - Kevin and Sue's son. Katie - Martyn's partner
Tyler - Martyn and Katie's son
Alex - Kevin and Sue's youngest son. Kayleigh - Alex's wife
Clare Golder - Sister
David Golder - Clare's husband
Andrew Golder - Clare and David's eldest son. Lauren - Andrew's wife

INTRODUCTION

Can you imagine how you would feel if you or someone you loved were told, that within a year, you will become completely paralysed, become dependent on a machine to help you breathe, lose your ability to speak, to swallow and maybe lose your mental capacity too?

When my husband, Alan, was diagnosed with motor neurone disease (MND) in November 2017, our world turned upside down. Every aspect of our lives was changed dramatically. The future we planned together was destroyed and we fell into a void of unpredictability with no hope of a positive outcome. There was also a massive ripple effect across our respective families and our circle of friends.

Once the shock subsided, I became thirsty for knowledge, but due to the nature of the disease, there were no simple answers. "MND affects everyone differently" was what I was told. It's true, everyone's physical journey with the condition is unique. However, anyone facing a terminal diagnosis has a massive mental battle on their hands. In our case, sometimes, the psychological challenges turned out to be as great, if not greater, than the physical ones.

Even after hours of frantic research, I struggled to find detailed information, from the perspective of a family member carer. I wanted to know what to expect or, at least, have some idea what the future might be like. I wanted tips on how to be an effective carer and how to provide strong moral support to my dying husband. **This book aims to fill that void.**

In recent years the media has increased awareness of MND. Until ITV included a story line about MND in Coronation Street, news stories were mainly about people in the world of sport. Such news was slightly misleading. MND can affect anyone. It is as indiscriminate as it is devastating. Anyone from any background, age or gender can get it. It leaves people locked into a failing body, unable to move, swallow, talk and eventually breathe. A third of those diagnosed die within twelve months - over half die within two years. In the meantime, their families care for them in their own homes. No one hears about them in the media. So, on their behalf, here is the story my husband gave me permission to share.

This book is an open and full account of the physical and psychological ups and downs we tackled during Alan's time with the disease. It details how we coped at his various milestones - the loss of use of arms, legs, torso muscles, breathing, swallowing and speech muscles. I have shared details of our daily routines, our coping strategies and the lessons I learned. Importantly I have tried to show how the positive mindset we adopted helped us deal with our situation. Also, how the resources we drew upon enabled us to live as full and normal a life as possible, even though the challenges of the disease were ever present and often unpredictable.

I have written this book to raise awareness and also to raise funds for the charities that supported us. All proceeds will be donated to them. I will not receive any revenue.

Three groups of people will benefit from reading this book:

Friends and family members who are caring for a loved one with a terminal illness, especially MND.

Medical professionals, and healthcare workers, because it provides a far wider perspective than they can gain during their brief interactions with people affected by neurological, degenerative diseases. This book should be read by **GPs, neurologists, physiotherapists, occupational therapists, alternative therapists, complementary therapists, respiratory nurses, hospice staff, dieticians, speech and language therapists, social workers, communications technicians, wheelchair technicians, psychologists and those in adult care services.**

MPs and policy makers who, hopefully, by reading this book, will be better informed when they are called upon to make decisions that affect families living with MND and other neurological degenerative conditions.

This book has been produced using extracts from the journals and notes I kept every day during Alan's illness.

I am not a professional writer. This is my first, and probably only, book. Several people have read through the drafts, but there may still be the odd typing error, spelling mistake or grammatical error. Please try to ignore them.

I have tried to recall everything accurately, but due to my emotions at the time, my perspective and clarity of certain events may not be exactly as others experienced them.

Also included in this book are:

- Unedited extracts from the audio biography Alan made in the months before he died,
- Poems which randomly formed in my head during Alan's illness,

- Practical tips and guidance based on my experience and the benefit of hindsight.

Finally, we know permanent sleep comes to us all eventually. Some welcome it because they have lived a long life or, they believe in an afterlife. Others dread it.

Alan did not fear dying, but he did not want to die.

He did not want to leave me, his family and friends.

He had lived a full life, but was only sixty-two. He had so much planned for his future when MND struck him out of the blue.

With no surgery to cut out the offending cells and only one old, ineffective drug available for MND, the only weapon he had to help him keep going, was his will to live.

Before he fell into his permanent sleep, I made it my mission to help him love his life with his terminal condition, as much as he had loved his life before MND came along.

I hope you will agree with me, when you have finished this book, life is for living - don't put off the things you have been thinking about doing. Also, take nothing for granted, because none of us will live forever.

Hazel

FOREWORD

Hazel Carter has written a very moving and vivid account of the remarkable journey she and her husband Alan made, as a couple, through the distressing and difficult months from receiving his diagnosis of motor neurone disease (MND) in November 2017, to the end of Alan's life in 2019. Hazel's courageous intentions in writing this manuscript have been to provide information, practical advice and support to people living with MND and their families and friends; to provide a detailed perspective on MND for the whole range of health care professionals involved in the care of MND patients; and to inform government, policy makers and funding bodies about MND and the huge unmet need for more effective neuroprotective therapies to slow down disease progression.

Hazel presents a graphic daily journal of what life was like for them, as a devoted couple, throughout this 18 month journey. She has succeeded very well in filling a void in the understanding of anyone who has not been through this experience – giving examples of how to be an effective carer and moral supporter of her husband and detailing the daily routines, coping strategies and lessons learned along the way. She has taught me, as an experienced MND neurologist, things I didn't know, such as the existence of radar keys for access to public disability toilets and tilt-in-space shower chairs.

Alan was clearly a wonderful, inspirational person who loved life and adored his wife. He was very fit and athletic, enjoying cycling, running, fell walking and skiing. Clearly he was loved and admired by family, colleagues and a huge network of friends. Through these pages his remarkable human spirit and stoicism emerges, coping with the devastating effects of rapidly progressive MND with great courage and determination and without losing his sense of humour. His grace and dignity in the face of adversity, including the support needed with the most personal of daily activities, is very clear.

The emotional impact and fears when confronted by the rapid deterioration of Alan's condition are vividly described, as is his constant concern for the impact of his illness on Hazel. This portrayal of Alan reinforces my view that MND tends to happen to the nicest of people, often very active and sporty, and who somehow can face this devastating disease with a huge amount of stoicism and dignity.

Hazel is a real heroine. Alan was the love of her life and she made it her mission to help her husband enjoy his life and bring him hope, fun and every possible support both physically and psychologically, despite the impact of disease. She put great thought into creating special times for them both including embracing Sunderland football club events and magical holidays! She achieved all this despite the constant fear for the future and emotional pain, which at times made her physically unwell. A vivid picture of the impact of MND emerges from her descriptions of daily life – the sleepless nights, the loss of a successful career which she enjoyed, the times feeling more like a nurse than a wife, the conversion of their lovely home, Carter Castle, into a house filled with constant comings and goings and medical equipment, the feeling at times that the burden of all that needed to be done was overwhelming.

Alan and Hazel, a popular and very special couple, received wonderful support from their family and network of friends. Visitors came almost every day to offer comfort, support and practical help. Their difficult situation brought out the very best in people, including at times the kindness of strangers. With this support, Hazel wisely sometimes found time to "recharge her batteries" with occasional games of golf, a few days of skiing and meetings with friends. The input from health care professionals and carers was in general excellent, but Hazel was a tigress on behalf of her husband when an occasional person did not provide the right level of caring support.

MND is a devastating condition, which varies in terms of its speed of progression. When progression is rapid, as in Alan's case, it is both extremely frightening for all involved and, in his case, meant that he could not be included in the clinical trial participation he was hoping for. No sooner does one disabling symptom arise, when another problem rapidly follows. Progress has been made in recent years, both in terms of symptom management and neuroprotective therapy developments, though the pace of medicine and science seems frustratingly slow for those impacted by MND. I and other specialists in this field of medicine, regard MND in 2023 as a neurodegenerative condition poised for the emergence of more effective treatments in the near future (Nature Reviews Drug Discovery Dec 21;2022:1-28 PMID:36543887).

The UK Government recently pledged £50M of research funding over 5 years to create a national MND Research Institute, persuaded by people living with MND, including famous sports personalities, as well as neurologists and neuroscientists. We believe that this will create a "step-change" in the way that effective therapies can be developed and allow greater access for MND patients to clinical trials. I very much hope the politicians and research funders who can make this national institute a reality, will read the heart-rending account of this devastating disease, with a life-time risk of 1 in 300 people, and provide the funding to make this step-change a reality. For Alan's sake, and the many other patients who will face this journey in the future, I sincerely hope this compelling and excellent account will contribute to realising the urgent need to accelerate and fund our efforts to find effective treatments for MND.

Professor Dame Pamela Shaw

Professor Dame Pamela Shaw DBE MBBS MD FRCP FMedSci FAAN FANA FAAAS
Professor of Neurology
Honorary Consultant Neurologist, Sheffield Teaching Hospitals NHS Foundation Trust
Director of the Sheffield Institute for Translational Neuroscience (SITraN)
Director Sheffield NIHR Biomedical Research Centre for Translational Neuroscience
Director of the cross-faculty Neuroscience Research Institute University of Sheffield

THE LAST ROOM

Within an hour of me reaching Warwick Hospital, where Alan had spent the last week, an ambulance crew arrived to move him to the Marie Curie Hospice, Solihull.

A week ago, I thought Alan was going to die. For the second time in 2019 he had been rushed into hospital with a raging temperature, racing heart and low oxygen saturation levels. He had developed aspiration pneumonia because MND had weakened his swallowing muscles.

As I followed the ambulance in my car, tears poured down my cheeks.

At the hospice, three nurses rallied around Alan and wheeled him into room number nine. Through the two wide, full-length windows to the left of the bed, I could see a lovely garden. I knew Alan would never walk in it, but I was told the bed could be wheeled outside on sunny days.

A heavy, high back, pale blue chair rested by the left side of the modern, high specification bed.

The bed had buttons on its side so nurses could raise and lower Alan's head and knees. The whole bed could be lowered or raised so he could be washed or hoisted out into a chair.

Opposite the bed was a recessed wash basin, with one of those special taps with a big paddle so it could be operated with your elbow or forearm. On the wall above the basin, there was a TV.

Next to the door into the room from the corridor, on the right of the bed, was a small grey, round table with two matching chairs. It sat under a window with venetian blinds to provide privacy from the corridor.

On the back wall, to the right of the bed, was a whiteboard. Attached to it was a bright green pot containing coloured marker pens. On the full-length maroon glass panel behind the headboard of the bed, were call buttons, gadgets and lights - none of which Alan could access because, for many months, he had been completely paralysed.

From this day onwards, this clinical, but smart, twelve-foot by twelve-foot room would be the centre of our world and the last room in which Alan would live.

PART 1 - ALAN AND HAZEL

Alan

(Transcription from Alan's audio biography, made 1st Feb 2019)

"I was born in Sunderland in 1954. My childhood was good. I went to Barns School. Gran lived over the road, so I spent a lot of time there - it was nice and handy for the school. I then went on to Bede Grammar School. I started well, but I turned out to be an academic failure, so I left school at seventeen. I got a job with a local painting and decorating company as a trainee surveyor. The people I worked with were a mixed bag - some had fought their way through the 2nd World War. I aspired to become somebody with a profession, so after four years I went to work in Hartlepool. I was there for a couple of years and then went to work for another building company in Burnley. I was determined to become a quantity surveyor - all these moves were helping me along the way.

I enjoyed my time in Sunderland. Your hometown is where you grow up, find your friends, and discover your football team, which I have been following ever since, with all the heartache that brings.

I saw all the changes in Sunderland. Once upon a time it was the biggest shipbuilding town in the world so there were lots of allied trades. Then shipbuilding fell into decline. Coalmining was the next big industry. It was almost a truism that you either went into the shipyards or down the mines. Fortunately, I escaped both.

At the age of twenty-six, yet another recession was gripping the country. In 1980/81 I went out to work in Saudi Arabia for eighteen months. When I came back to the UK, I continued working in the construction industry. In 1983 I went to work in Leeds - it was the second big move of my life. I lived in the outskirts of Leeds where I met and married a local girl.

In 1996, I was offered some work in the Midlands, so I moved down there temporarily. Eventually my wife and I split up, so I made a permanent move down to the Midlands. Workwise, I was still in the construction industry but had moved into project management work. It was a good change.

In due course I met a couple of lads around about my age who were doing similar work. We formed our own company called ABC Solutions, which we incorporated in 1998. The name came from the surnames of the three of us who founded the business - Addis, Beacham, Carter.

The "A" did not last too long, because he could not fit into a small corporate business, so he left. Simon Beacham and I carried on running the company until I received my diagnosis. Simon was fully understanding of my predicament. My life expectancy at that time was six months to two years. If it was only going to be six months, there was no way I was going to carry on working. So just shy of the 20th anniversary of forming ABC Solutions, I retired.

I'd been a relatively fit bloke. I enjoyed sports - in particular, running. When I was in Leeds, I used to enjoy squash and tennis. In my early thirties I took up skiing and loved it. Pretty much every year ever since I went on at least one skiing holiday per season.

When I started to have problems with my legs (not because of MND but just age catching up with me), I took up cycling.

Hazel and I met in 2006 on 14th June. We were internet daters. I saw her profile on the dating site and fell in love with her straight away, so I pursued her. We got off to a slow start. I wrote out what I thought was a wonderful introduction. All I got back was a "Do you think we have potential?" That was one of the sites standard responses. I didn't realise at the time she had not actually activated her profile with that website, so that was all she could reply.

Anyway, I felt a bit deflated after that, but I thought I would kick myself if I did not try again. So, I thought I would have another go. After pursuing her for about six weeks, we met in Broadway. It was a nice evening. She was a skier, but she was also a golfer.

On our third date she talked about golf. It was clear to me that if I was going to keep this relationship, I needed to take up golf, so I got some lessons and bought some clubs and started playing golf. I played golf in the summer, went skiing in the winter, and went cycling any time I could.

The next couple of years were pretty much idyllic. I had a house in Long Marston on the other side of Stratford-upon-Avon. I sold that in 2008/9 and moved in with Hazel. We had a lot of good times. We enjoyed our holidays. We did road trips to the United States and South Africa. We continued with our skiing holidays, either with each other, or with friends.

I proposed to Hazel in Rome, at twelve minutes past twelve on 12th of the 12th, 2012. I didn't plan it that way, it was just a quirk that was possible.

We got married on 14th June 2014 - that was eight years to the day since we had our first date in Broadway. We had about sixty guests in the day, plus another forty on the evening.

The room in which the ceremony was held was on the ground floor and opened out into the gardens. I remember standing there waiting for Hazel to arrive and when she did, I was in tears. She just looked so beautiful."

Hazel

I was born in North Devon in 1957 but my parents moved our family to the Midlands in 1962.

The eldest of five children, I left school at age sixteen because my parents needed me to bring some income into the household. The careers I fancied pursuing needed more qualifications than the eight O-levels I achieved, so I resigned myself to the idea of becoming a secretary, getting married and having a family.

My first job was in an employment agency. After a few years I moved to an administration job in a life insurance company. When I wanted a more demanding job I moved to another life insurance company where, during my ten years, I became the first woman to be promoted into a sales management position. My whole working life was spent in the Financial Services sector, eventually achieving senior management and leadership roles in sales, marketing and acquisitions.

In 1977 I met David. We married in 1982. In 1987 he secured an opportunity to move to Australia where his family lived. It was neither practical, nor desirable for me to emigrate, so we separated for two years and divorced amicably in 1989.

In 2005 I had a total hysterectomy following two years of severe pain with fibroids and endometriosis. Facing life with no husband and knowing I would never be a mum left me feeling depressed. I found some solace in volunteering, in particular with children in care and children and adults with disabilities.

In 2006, I reluctantly tried internet dating. I was beginning to lose heart when a handsome skier called Alan Carter found my profile and contacted me.

After a few weeks of chatting, by email and phone, we arranged a blind date for 14th June. We took a long walk and spent hours discussing our skiing experiences over dinner. When Alan asked to see me again the following Wednesday because it was his birthday, I was a bit concerned that he had no friends. Months later he told me he fell in love with me as soon as he saw my internet dating profile and did not want to spend his birthday with anyone else.

Alan was tall – five foot ten inches. He looked after himself, ate sensibly, drank moderately and enjoyed pushing himself physically through individual pursuits like running and cycling. He had a toned, athletic eleven stone body, dark hair, tanned face, warm eyes and full lips that I could not resist. He took pride in his appearance but was not a prima donna. Self-confident but not arrogant. For a long time after meeting him, I could not believe he was real.

Very quickly we agreed not to date anyone else. We also decided to have a date night every month to celebrate our meeting. We took it in turns to come up with novel ideas to surprise each other and to avoid going to the same place twice. The romance began!

Before the end of 2006 Alan had joined Shirley Golf Club, where I had been a member since 1992. I knew then he was a keeper. We spent our first Christmas together skiing in Italy. The first of many fantastic alpine holidays. By 2009 he had moved in with me.

Alan and I were compatible on every level. Between us we arranged some wonderful holidays, playing golf, skiing and driving thousands of miles on road trips. We enjoyed get-togethers with friends, family parties, entering golf competitions, going to the theatre, concerts and movies. After unsuccessful past relationships and some tough times in life, we were both ready to throw ourselves headlong into a fully committed, loyal and rewarding relationship. There were no doubts in my mind, this was it.

The engagement of two of our friends in 2012 made me realise I was ready to be married again. I began dropping what I thought were obvious hints to Alan about my feelings.

After struggling for five hours to reach to the top of Ben Nevis in June 2012, I hoped Alan would propose to me. At the top of the mountain, I asked, "Have you got anything you would like to say to me?" He replied with "Well done." I was so disappointed I hardly spoke to him during the four-hour descent down to the car park!

When I eventually plucked up the courage to tell Alan how I felt, to my great surprise, he announced, "We will marry one day!" A few weeks later Alan and I went shopping for a ring, ready for Alan to propose when the time was right.

On a stroll one sunny December morning on holiday in Rome, Alan purchased a bunch of roses and suddenly started walking very quickly. We eventually arrived at a palace where he got down on one knee and started to propose! There was a political rally taking place, so before he finished his speech, I said, "Oh no, not here."

We walked a little further to the Pantheon where Alan finished his proposal. Over a champagne lunch to celebrate our engagement, he told me the rush earlier was because he wanted to propose at twelve minutes past twelve on the 12th of the 12th, 2012. How unique!

14th June 2014

We immortalised our blind date by marrying on 14th June at The Welcombe Hotel in Stratford-upon-Avon, where we had once had a date. The sun shone all day.

Our bridesmaids were my two sisters, Rowena and Clare, plus my sister-in-law, Sue. Alan's nephew Matthew was our best man and his other nephews, Ben and Tom, were our groomsmen. Alan's niece, Helen, and my godson and nephew Andrew, were our witnesses.

My brother Kevin walked me down the aisle to the Bob Dylan song *Make You Feel My Love* sung by Adele. Alan shed a tear (or three!).

During the ceremony we all chuckled when Alan had to remind Tyler, my three-year-old great nephew, how we had rehearsed him bringing the wedding rings down the aisle to Alan. Our wedding rings were made from a gold bracelet Alan had been given when he worked abroad. Inscribed inside were our names and "14.06 and forever."

Alan and I walked into the Wedding Breakfast room from two separate doors to the song *How do you like your eggs in the morning?* We were wearing black satin bride and groom robes over our wedding clothes. We met in the middle of the room and sexily took off each other's robes. It was great fun doing something different.

Speeches

The 'Father of the Bride' speech was given by brother, Kevin.

In my speech, I presented Alan with a list of all the things I loved about him. Then I read a poem I had composed.

When we met you blew me away,
How I bless that special day.
It's my honour to become your wife,
To commit to you for the rest of my life.
You make me laugh day after day,
You're the finest man I know, in every way.
You bring me sunshine with your smile,
When I'm with you, I'm happy all the while.
You are my rock, and more besides,
You are my buddy, and my prize.
My life is joyous because you came along,

If I could, I'd write you a song.
I love you more each day,
In many more ways than I can say.
You mean the world to me.
By your side, for the rest of my life
Is where I want to be.

As I handed over the microphone to him, Alan said, "Wow"!

Extracts from Alan's wedding speech

"Good afternoon everyone, and welcome! Please may I start by introducing you to my stunning wife, the beautiful Mrs Hazel Elaine Carter!! (Alan's speech continued with thanking people for travelling so far to be with us and remembering our dads who had passed away. Alan made various toasts, thanking our best man, the bridesmaids, groomsmen, witnesses and our mums) "Hazel and I met later in life than we would have wanted to. Knowing that we'd never rack up the years together and enjoy annual anniversaries, we decided to celebrate on a monthly basis. We've celebrated in restaurants, at Birmingham's Christmas market, picnics and even on a cross channel ferry! Today is our 96th anniversary and what a way to celebrate!

Over the last eight years, people have asked me how I met Hazel. It was through an internet dating site. I took one look at Hazel's profile and, if it is possible to fall in love with someone by looking at their photographs and reading their profile description, I most certainly did. I wrote to her via the website, a letter which I was sure would generate some interest but all I eventually got back was a standard response, "Do you think we have potential?" It wasn't encouraging.

And I was a disappointed man!

But undeterred, I sat down and wrote again, and I received a very, very positive reply!

And I was a delighted man!

We arranged our first date, in Broadway, on 14th June 2006. A cool evening (comment on today's weather). We got on well and only talked about skiing. A second date was arranged for the following week and then a third, a Friday night, here, at the Welcombe Hotel, for 8pm. And by 8:25 Hazel was a no-show.

And I was a despondent man.

But then she arrived, drove into the car park in her blue Renault Meganne, top down…. that's the car, not Hazel, blonde hair blowing in the breeze. And I was once again, a happy man!

For the past eighteen months, Hazel's hard work has created the wedding we are all enjoying today. From having the picture in her mind, to making just about all the many items that decorate these tables and this room. Every evening, just doing a little bit more but still finding time to arrange family parties, hen parties, helping disadvantaged children, including a trip to three orphanages in Botswana, working full time and of course, playing golf!

Hazel, in the early days I referred to you as my Pink Princess and today more than ever you look just like a very beautiful princess. You are my best friend and my soulmate, and I love you so much. The last eight years have been brilliant but today we are starting the rest of our lives together as a married couple, with so much to look forward to.

And today, I am an ecstatic man!

Ladies and gentlemen, will you please raise your glasses and toast The Bride, Mrs Carter… To Hazel. Thank you"

Married Life
Alan's 60th birthday took place while we were on honeymoon in Mauritius. I planned a surprise romantic dinner on the beach. Just as the main courses were being served, the heavens opened so we had to abandon the white chiffon draped table surrounded by uplighters. It didn't matter, we were in love and in paradise.

Married life was just as wonderful as pre-married life, with the added bonus of feeling secure and contented all the time.

One day I asked, "How do you feel now we are married?" Alan admitted we probably should have done it earlier.

In January 2017, we celebrated my 60th birthday in Obergurgl - one of our favourite ski resorts - with several skiing friends from the UK.

During the spring of 2017, Alan and I created a bucket list of trips we wanted to do leading up to our retirement, and long distance, long duration holidays to go on after retirement. We planned to stop work when Alan reached sixty-five, downsize to a smaller home, and start working through the bucket list.

Life however had a different plan for us.

PART 2 – DIAGNOSIS

2017

May (Transcription from Alan's audio biography made 1st Feb 2019)
"In about May 2017, I noticed my right arm was not lifting as heavy a weight as my left arm was when I was at the gym. I started to lose dexterity in the fingers of my right hand. I would pick things up and drop them.

Then I started to get muscle twitches (fasciculations) in my right arm. I didn't think anything of it at first. I thought maybe it was a trapped nerve, or something equally minor."

September - "I've got a problem with my right arm"
After a golf game on holiday in Turkey, Alan shocked me. "I'm having issues with my right arm. I might have pulled a muscle, or at worst had a mild stroke."

Following a visit to his GP, Alan reported, "The doctor said the twitching and loss of grip in my right hand, might be Parkinson's, Multiple Sclerosis (MS) or MND. He's referred me to a neurosurgeon."

When I regained some composure, I did what no doctor wants to you to do - I opened the internet. I had some knowledge of Parkinson's and MS but knew nothing about MND. What I learned was deeply distressing. I immediately urged Alan to call his medical insurance company to see if he was eligible to see a neurosurgeon privately.

First meeting with Neurosurgeon
A private meeting was arranged with, Dr El-Maghraby (Dr El for short), a neurosurgeon at the BMI clinic near Coventry Hospital.

After tapping at some trigger points and sticking some pins into Alan's limbs, Dr El asked Alan to walk in a straight line with his eyes closed. Dr El kept giving him encouraging praise, but my heart sank as I watched my lovely, strong, healthy, husband struggle with the walk. I hoped and prayed Alan was not too aware of how badly he had done.

Dr El said, "You are showing signs of MND." In that moment, my world shifted. Suddenly everything felt slightly out of kilter. Terror began to loom deep inside me. I tried to stay calm as Dr El explained the next step was an MRI scan of Alan's brain and spine.

Second meeting with Neurosurgeon

"Good news," declared Dr El, "The MRI shows there is no cancer in the spine or brain." He then proposed Alan go for electrical conductivity tests. (My earlier research informed me such tests measured how fast impulses move down the nerves from the brain to the muscles).

5th November - Final meeting with Neurosurgeon

Dr El declared, "There is inflammation of the muscles," swiftly followed by, "I am referring you to a neurologist, Dr Thomas, who can discuss medication," and finally, "There is nothing I can do as a neurosurgeon."

Alan pressed Dr El for more information. The doctor chose his words carefully. "What you have is affecting your nerves in the spinal cord and that affects the muscles." My heart felt heavy as I sensed the tension in Alan's voice, "What caused it and what's the prognosis?" I could see Dr El was struggling to help Alan satisfy his need for answers, so I stepped in as gently as I could. "Alan, maybe we should address such questions to Dr Thomas who sounds like a specialist."

Neither of us spoke as we returned to our car. Two statements echoed around in my mind. "You are showing signs of MND" ... "There is nothing I can do for you as a surgeon."

On the drive home we talked about what to tell family. Our nephew's fortieth birthday party was coming up. All Alan's family would be there. We agreed it was best to be vague about the results. We did not want to ruin the celebrations. The message was to be, "There is inflammation of the nerves and the next step is to see a neurologist." Alan asked me "Isn't this what Stephen Hawking had?" I knew it was, but to save his feelings, I said, "I believe it may have been."

We ate dinner in silence. Everything felt odd.

We went to bed earlier than normal and held each other tightly. I could feel Alan's arm twitching. It also felt unusually cold, something he had been complaining of on and off for weeks.

"Are you alright?" Alan asked. I lied, "I am okay." He probably knew I wasn't by my uneven breathing and constant swallowing as I fought back my tears.

Alan drifted off to sleep, but I could not settle. I started thinking about the research I had done about MND and the survival rate. Eventually I moved to the spare bedroom with my iPhone.

That's when I broke down. Deep despair consumed me. I sobbed uncontrollably. Thoughts raced around my mind. My head throbbed. I grabbed a box of tissues and fired up the iPhone. I found Lou Gehrig's biography. He was an American baseball player, who, at the top of his career, was forced to retire at age thirty-six. He died three years later. His condition was a form of MND called Amyotrophic (meaning no nourishment) Lateral Sclerosis (ALS). In America, MND is known as ALS or Lou Gehrig's disease.

The page said: "ALS is a fatal neurodegenerative disease that paralyses its victims. Movement initiating nerve cells in the brain and muscle controlling nerve cells in the spinal cord die. The condition leaves people 'locked in' but fully conscious. In many cases swallowing muscles are affected, so there is a need to be fed through a tube in the tummy, or an affected person will die. Breathing muscles can also be affected so a person with ALS may need a machine to help them breathe, or they will die. In rare cases, they go on to develop a form of dementia, leaving them without mental capacity but still able to feel emotions." NO!

Watching the trailer of the film *A Brief History of Everything* reminded me about Stephen Hawking's symptoms. I felt sick. After I checked the MND Association website, I emailed my friend, Jill Duffin, asking if I could call her in the morning. I had known Jill since 2005 and had always found her to be balanced whenever I needed a sounding board. Eventually I fell asleep and was awakened the next morning by a kiss from Alan.

Tuesday 7th November – Tears

While getting ready for work I bumped into Alan on the landing. "This is not how it was meant to be," he said as we held each other. Unusually he cried as I hugged him. I felt so much love for him. This hug was extra special because we both knew one day his arms would stop working so returning my hugs would be impossible. I felt like my love for him was overflowing.

When Alan arrived home from work that evening, we spoke about his thoughts and feelings. He told me he felt it was not fair because of all the things we would not be able to do. He also said, "It's not fair on you because you are going to end up as my carer." I tried to reassure him, but he was tearful. We discussed how his work colleagues might react to the news and how we might tell friends and family.

Wednesday 8th November - Everything I thought of unsettled me

Before work, Alan and I had a brief conversation about practical matters. Things like the need to sell the MGB he had owned for thirty-seven years and

14

replacing the hall and lounge carpets with hard surfaces on the assumption that one day he would end up living downstairs and using a wheelchair.

During the morning, I spoke with Jill. She helped me get my thoughts straight, even though my heart was breaking. I also phoned Andy, the husband of another good, long-term friend, Jo. He was a wheelchair specialist. Jo answered Andy's phone, so I brought her up to date. She was very sympathetic and promised to ask Andy to call Alan.

When Alan arrived home from work I asked how he had been. He admitted that "negative thoughts" had plagued him at work, but he had "fought them off." Later when I asked what the thoughts were, all I got was "I don't remember." I suspected he did remember but didn't want to share. He did admit he had to turn the radio off when they played *How do you like your eggs in the morning?* - our Wedding Breakfast song and *We can rule the world* by Take That - the tune we had for signing of the Wedding register. Oddly that day I had heard *I was born to love you* by Queen - the song we walked up the aisle to after saying our vows. How spooky!

All day I felt weird, numb and unsettled. When I was not doing work, all I thought about was the challenges ahead.

Thursday 9th November - The truth was too hard to face
While cuddling in bed Alan divulged, "My left arm and legs are tingling." That was a new symptom. Alan agreed to be proactive about getting an appointment with Dr Thomas.

I started a list - well, a couple of lists. List one, which we worked on together, was all the things we could still do, even when Alan became less able. We agreed to prioritise the bucket list and start going on some of the trips before it was too late.

List two, I worked on in private. While my mind was relatively clear I felt the need to capture ideas of what I could do with my time if I were on my own and not working - in case things moved quickly. After just a few minutes I gave up. It was far too distressing thinking of life without Alan.

During the day, the new bed we had ordered arrived. I decided not to ring Alan, hoping it would be a nice surprise when he got home. As the delivery men struggled to get the bed upstairs, I accidently opened a letter addressed to Alan. It was a copy letter to Dr Thomas from Dr El-Maghraby. 'There is evidence of motor neurone disease' he wrote. 'Please would Dr Thomas see Alan with regard to the MND.'

For a long time, I glared at the letter, stunned. Surely Dr El would not put statements like that in black and white if there was any doubt. The words of the song I walked down the aisle to sprang into my head. "There is nothing I wouldn't do, to make you feel my love." I took the difficult decision not to show this stark letter to Alan until I had to.

Friday 10th November - Trying to forget

We set off for Strudford Luxury Lodges in North Yorkshire to meet Alan's family and celebrate the fortieth birthday of our nephew, Richard.

Having decided we were not going to be telling the family everything, we didn't talk much about Alan's health on the journey. Instead, we listened to the radio and sang along to happy tunes. On arrival at the lodges there was a typical warm welcome from all the family.

Saturday 11th November - Thinking about telling people

For the first time in ages, I went for a short run. It felt good to be away from everyone and in touch with nature for a while. I decided I needed to start keeping a journal of how Alan's condition progressed and any meetings we had with medical professionals, as I found it hard to think straight some days.

After a brief soak in the hot tub with Alan, we had breakfast. Alan and I were sharing a lodge with his sister, Viv and her husband, John. Before we popped over to Richard's lodge for cake, Viv asked, "How's your arm?" Alan explained his symptoms and the next steps. As agreed he avoided mentioning MND.

During a walk, I found myself taking pictures and making videos of Alan as he ambled along with his family. It was a glorious day with stunning views across green fields and a wide blue sky. It felt good to be away from home. When I reached Alan's side, I could sense he was deep in thought.

"What's on your mind, Al?"

"I'm thinking of telling the family in age order, starting with Pauline, ending with Tom."

"Do you want me with you when the time comes?"

Without hesitation he confirmed, "Yes."

We discussed the practical steps of Alan working part time or retiring early from ABC Solutions. He had set up the company over twenty years earlier with his good friend, Simon Beacham. Various questions stumbled out of me. "Should I only work part time? Would keeping up normal life help us? We're planning to retire in two years - should we stop immediately instead?" The only thing we agreed on was we should catch up with long lost old friends, and make sure we spent time wisely.

Sunday 12th November - Some plans of which you can no longer be a part
Alan and I woke early. Although it was a cold morning, we decided to use the hot tub again. In the bubbling water, I gazed through the trees at the low winter sun. My mind soon began to wander. "Are you okay, babe?" Alan asked. I couldn't answer. He held me and the tears began to fall.

At dinner, I found the conversations difficult. There was talk of doing something like this weekend again in 2020 when there were three significant birthdays. No one mentioned Alan would be sixty-five in June 2019. Then a chilling thought caught me. Alan may not survive that long!

Monday 13th November - The *Peace of Mind* list
After breakfast we all met for a last walk around the outskirts of the lodges site. Alan and I walked hand in hand, in total silence. I wondered if he was thinking the same thoughts as me - how much longer will we be able to walk together, like this? I could feel a knot building in my throat and despair stirring in me.

As we locked up the door on the lodge, I felt the urge to tell everyone what we were dealing with. Instead, I mentioned to Viv, "These lodges are not wheelchair accessible." As we all hugged and said our goodbyes, I felt myself welling up. Viv noticed, "Are you okay Hazel?" All I could manage was, "I don't like goodbyes."

On the way home, we stopped at Thirsk, for a stroll and coffee. I confessed "I accidentally opened something addressed to you the other day. It was a copy of a letter from Dr El to Dr Thomas. I chose to keep it from you. I didn't want it to spoil this weekend." Alan didn't ask what was in the letter, but said he appreciated my thoughtfulness.

Back at the car, I was filled with a compelling desire to run away together with Alan. "Should we resign from our jobs immediately and just do this sort of thing all the time?" We resisted the urge to make a bid for freedom. Instead, we compiled a list of questions to ask Dr Thomas on 21st November, then continued home.

In our kitchen we hugged in silence for a long time. Will Alan always be able to feel my hugs, I wondered? Although I had done a lot of secret research since MND had been suggested, there was still so much I didn't know.

17

While watching TV later that evening, it was clear Alan's mind was elsewhere. Eventually, he asked to see the letter from Dr El. For a long time after he read it there was silence. With an unhappy face he whispered, "None of this is fair on you." "Please don't say that Al. We met for a reason. I am not afraid of looking after you. I gained a lot of experience of helping people with disabilities through my volunteer work. We will be okay."

Alan talked a lot about the loss of our planned future together. I couldn't respond. Thinking about letting go of our dreams was too painful. We agreed it was a good idea to get in touch with the MND Association. We would also watch films and read books about people who had gone through life with physical challenges, so we could get tips and be inspired. We also talked about how our news would shock and affect our circle of friends and family.

We concluded we should be open with everyone, rather than try to pretend everything was okay. Privately, perhaps selfishly, I thought once this news is public, everyone will want a piece of Alan. Very soon our lovely, private bubble would burst, and our lives would never be the same again.

We talked a lot about practical things. The idea of moving to a flat in sheltered housing was discussed, as potentially a better choice than adapting our home, Carter Castle, as it was affectionately known. Several times Alan mentioned getting wills sorted out. We decided to create a *To Do* list which later became known as the *Peace of Mind* list. Alan's motivation came from his desire not to leave 'loose ends' for me to deal with after he died.

During this long conversation I kept feeling like a hole was opening up inside me. November felt like an unlucky month. My father had been taken ill in November 2000 and died from liver cancer, two months later. My mind wandered to what Christmas would be like with this huge burden looming over us.

The thought that we wouldn't know when our last walk would be, or our last anything would be - until it was too late – troubled me. I considered, do you make the day you do something nice for the last time an extra special day, even though it will feel sorrowful? I decided, every day should be made special - and special days would be made incredible. Isn't that the sort of advice any of us would give someone else facing this sort of thing? Live life to the full. Enjoy life while you can. Make the most of every day. How easy would that be, I wondered, with a death sentence hanging over us?

AUTHOR'S NOTE

Over time MND proved to be an unpredictable beast. Changes came suddenly which meant many times we didn't realise we were doing something for the last time.

It turned out 'going public' was a good decision. The huge amount of love and support we received made the whole terrible situation easier to cope with. It did however create the problem of needing to keep a lot of people informed as to progress.

Tuesday 14th November - Blissful ignorance

On Facebook I noticed Alan's second cousin in America, Renee, had been posting a lot about fundraising for ALS (the name used for MND in America). A brief message to her revealed, "I was diagnosed with the condition in 2006." I was shocked. There were no signs of it when we visited her in 2007. It was encouraging to think Alan could have eleven years, or more, of life!

At my GP practice I enquired which doctor knew the most about MND. It was confirmed that the practice would only provide secondary care for Alan. The specialists at the hospital would provide primary care.

At this stage I was blissfully ignorant about how much medical intervention would be needed. I also had no concept of the range of health professionals that would become part of Alan's journey.

Wednesday 15th November - Suggestions from friends

Alan appeared lighter in spirit over breakfast - more like his old self. A telephone call with a physiotherapist friend in London was useful. One piece of advice she gave was to access emotional support from trained professionals. "You may not always be able to say how you really feel to family, friends, or Alan." It was also suggested we get a referral to a private neuro-physio who could start work on Alan's joint mobility as early as possible. Finally, "Your role will be to encourage Alan to keep pushing himself and to help him stay emotionally strong."

I drove to the house of my friend Teresa Meredith to give her a birthday card. I could not conceal that something was wrong from her and her husband, Phil. They were shocked and saddened when I revealed our news, and extremely loving and supportive when my tears fell. Phil knew of a successful cyclist who had developed MND and had lived for thirty years. This was encouraging news.

At the annual Ladies Prize Presentation Dinner at the Shirley Golf Club, a brief chat with the wife of our golf pro, sparked a mental note to encourage Alan to see the pro as soon as possible. Continuing to play golf could be positive for Alan, even if he had to adapt his golf swing. When I got home, it was good to see that Alan was still in a light mood.

Friday 17th November - Another person's experience of MND

My morning was spent at my mum's flat while an occupational therapist (OT) assessed mum following a series of falls. While I walked the therapist to her car, I explained my situation. She confided her uncle had been diagnosed with MND two years ago at age fifty-nine.

Initially her uncle and his wife travelled abroad a lot, but he was already experiencing breathing difficulties limiting his ability to fly. This information made me more determined that Alan and I should press on with our foreign travel plans as soon as possible. She promised to take my situation into account when putting together her recommendations for mum's care.

Saturday 18th November - Assisted suicide ruled out, for now

As always at weekends, Alan cooked poached eggs on muffins for us. It made me unhappy to think this wonderful weekend ritual would come to an end one day. After eating I told Alan, "I sometimes feel what's happening to us is unreal." To which he replied, "I know it's real - I feel it."

We discussed my fears of being alone and heartbroken after Alan died. Also, I shared how my work had always been my stabiliser during difficult times in the past, but how I now wanted to spend all my time with him. We concluded if I stopped work to care for him, I could always return to it later, to help me through the loneliness.

Alan said he could not bear the idea of having to breathe via a machine but agreed he would review his thinking about using a ventilator when the illness reached that stage. We agreed we could not predict how we might feel as things progressed. I made Alan promise he would not make decisions based just on my needs.

I gingerly raised the subject of Noel Farrelly - a person with MND forced to go to Switzerland because he wanted assisted suicide. We felt there was some merit in campaigning for it to be allowed in the UK.

At one point Alan looked at me intently, "From the minute I saw your internet dating photo back in 2006 I knew you were the one. You are perfect." My heart broke. We hugged and cried together.

While I was out shopping, I was squeezed in for a haircut at my usual salon. My stylist could tell I was not my usual self, so I shared our news. She told me an amazing but shocking story. "While I was washing a client's hair some months ago, I noticed a change in the lady's hair texture. I suggested she see her GP. The lady was eventually diagnosed with MND and four months later she died. Her lungs collapsed."

A chill ran over me. Could it happen that quickly?

During the afternoon, whilst watching the Scotland versus New Zealand rugby match, an ex-Scottish team player called Doddie Weir was interviewed. He was diagnosed with MND in December 2016. His walking looked good, but I could see his hands were stiff.

Doddie was doing lots of fundraising and had a great mindset. I particularly liked it when instead of saying he had MND he said, "This condition that has got hold of me at the moment...." I thought it must be so weird for Alan seeing another person with the same condition. It occurred to me I could not put myself in Alan's shoes, but I could help him remember all the great things we had done and help him enjoy the life he had left.

As I was preparing a meal for our expected dinner party guests, Alan asked, "Can we have a night off talking about MND? We had a fun evening with our friends, Carol and Graham Harvey, with no mention of Alan's health. I took photographs of the three of them - the beginning of the memory making.

Sunday 19th November - Worries creeping in
In bed while hugging I could feel twitches all over Alan's body. The twitches that told him this was real, now made his MND real to me too.

When my eyes opened, I felt sad as I looked at my arm resting on Alan's chest. One day, there would be no Alan to hug. The tears quietly built as I listened to Alan's rhythmic breathing and thought about how bleak life would be without him. Then I began to fret. Might his lungs collapse before we had 'put his house in order', before we made the most of his remaining life and before we had created all the memories that would sustain me after he died? It became too depressing lying next to Alan, so I got up.

AUTHOR'S NOTE
In these early weeks, it gave Alan comfort to behave as if everything was normal, even though sometimes simple tasks, like washing up, became a high-risk as his grip weakened.

For me, 'normal' was a thing of the past. I constantly ached with emotional pain and my mind would not be still.

Monday 20th November - Our job is to love Alan and keep everything happy for him

Once more I found it hard to stay in bed for long after I woke up. Feeling Alan's muscles twitching involuntarily all over his body was an uncomfortable reminder he was ill. In the morning, I visited mum in readiness for her meeting with a psychologist. Mum was diagnosed with vascular dementia with Lewy Bodies in 2015. Since then, she had depended on me as her principal carer.

To enable her to understand the reasons why Alan and I might have to move to a new house, or she might have to move to a care home, I explained more about Alan's condition. She was, as I expected, downcast. She was mostly worried about the impact on her if we moved far away. I assured her nothing would change in the short term. I told her it was her job to help me love Alan and keep everything fun and happy for him. She liked that idea.

Later in the day I visited a client in Peterborough and afterwards I had a drink with my friend Jane, who lived in the area. She told me she knew a lady called Ann in Colchester whose husband had died from MND. She said Ann was campaigning on behalf of MND Association and would be able to give me more insight. Jane promised to connect me up with Ann. She also mentioned an MND drug available from USA which Ann would know more about. Being with Jane calmed me. She was both practical and empathetic.

Gradually I discovered that talking to friends about Alan and finding out how other people had lived with terminal diseases, gave me some strength.

Tuesday 21st November - 'D' Day

My mind was spinning out of control and my emotions were all over the place when I woke up. Unusually, a poem started to form in my head, so I wrote it down.

CRUEL WORLD

Cruel world,
What have we done to deserve this?
What pain, what injustice.
You bring this beauty of a man into my life,
Then you deal us this blow.

You take my heart and twist it,

You dig a hole in my being,
You make me face my deepest fears,
And what do you give me in return?

You make a man so pure and strong,
And you break him with a cruel disease.
You take his spirit and screw it up,
Like wastepaper.

What is the purpose of this?
What is the plan?
What can we do?
How will we cope?

I don't have words to express how I feel,
I don't know how I will face this challenge.
I don't want to have to deal with this,
And yet I must.

Tell me what I can do,
What can I say?
Tell me why us? Why now?
It's too cruel, too hard, too sad.

We don't know how long we have,
Or what it will be like.
We just know,
It hurts like hell.

If there is such a thing as the worst day of your life, this was to be mine.
I felt odd and off balance, in anticipation of our meeting with Dr Thomas. The
thought of what he might say made me feel sick.

The sky was grey. The red autumn leaves that had adorned the tree opposite
our house were almost all gone. It was eerily quiet in our lounge apart from
the gentle whirr of my PC, the faint ticking of the clock on the mantelpiece, the
hum of the central heating and the occasional sound of the builders working
on the house next door.

Is this the calm before the storm I thought to myself? It would be the last day
we would be in our private bubble of uncertainty. If MND was confirmed, our
lives would change irrevocably. Life would not gently bump along without care

or concern as it had done before this month. Life would become chaotic and full of uncertainty.

This was diagnosis day, and I was dreading it.

Alan was unusually cheerful. I couldn't decide if he'd somehow managed to forget all of this, or if he was putting on a brave face. How was he feeling deep down? He had told his business partner, Simon, what was going on and had booked to see his financial planner. Suddenly he proudly announced, "I've found a new way to do up the cuffs on my shirt." I flinched, caught by the thought of all the small things he would struggle with as his arms became paralysed. A tear fell as I realised how much I loved watching him dress himself each morning. I knew I would miss seeing that in in the future.

Intending to be comforting, Dr Thomas explained, "I am one of the top men in the region for people with MND." Alongside physically examining Alan, Dr Thomas spent a long time listening to Alan's account of his symptoms - poor grip in right hand and loss of dexterity, twitching, mild dull ache in right forearm, tingles in left arm, legs and feet, the occasional difficulty in swallowing (the last one was a surprise to me).

When the doctor told us one of the sure signs of MND was a wasting of one of the muscles on the back of the hand, at the base of the thumb (which is fed by a deep branch of a nerve), I felt angry that Alan had gone through so much to get a definite diagnosis.

Dr Thomas took time to explain about the tough journey ahead and the importance of being positive. "You should focus on the fact that you have led a good, long life and have a loving wife." He finished with, "Sometimes I have to tell people in their mid-twenties they have this condition."

To be sure we understood, Alan asked the questions we had prepared:

What is it?

Dr Thomas answered, "Clinically, it looks like MND."

What are the different levels?

Answer: "ALS is the most common form, where the whole body is affected."

What is likely to happen in the short, medium, long-term?

Answer: "I have not known anyone live more than five years with the condition." He added, "Given the level of progression and the results of the scans, you should think in terms of six months to two years."

I felt a shockwave come off Alan, bounce off me and whizz around the room. Everything we had read pointed to life expectancy of two to five years. Time stood still. The moment frozen. Alan took a breath. With a shaky voice he continued.

What are the effects of the disease?

Answer: "No two people are the same. Progression varies and can include paralysis, loss of speech, loss of swallowing and an inability to breathe unaided, but not necessarily all of those things, and in no particular order."

Can I carry on as normal, or are things like exercise to be avoided?

Answer: "Yes, do whatever makes you happy."

Is there anything I should stop doing or start doing?

Answer: "Carry on living life."

Can I still travel - fly?

Answer: "Yes."

What medicines are available?

Answer: "There is no cure."

Any suggestions regarding diet?

Answer: "Eat everything you like."

Is it okay to drink alcohol?

Answer: "Yes."

What kind of care/support network is available and how do we access it?

Answer: "I will refer you on."

And the final question, "Are there any other tests to be done to provide further clarity?"

Answer: "There is no point in running other tests because it's clear, you have MND."

I felt as if the ground had opened up and swallowed me whole. I dared not breathe as I tried to process what I had just heard.

Dr Thomas explained, "I may not be your consultant going forward." (That was a shame - he was excellent). "I will connect you up with the specialist team based at the Queen Elizabeth Hospital in Birmingham."

He gave Alan a three-month prescription of Riluzole. An internet check on the drug later told me that it was used to treat Amyotrophic Lateral Sclerosis (ALS), delaying the onset of ventilator dependence, or the need for tracheostomy, for about two to three months.

We drove home in silence. Shell shocked. We had both prepared for this news, but still it was hard to take in.

Immediately we were home, Alan began the daunting task of telling his family the news in age order. First to be telephoned was his elder sister, Pauline. Her reaction said it all. "God, Alan," followed by lots of questions. Neither of them could decide on the best way of telling his niece, Helen and nephew, Matthew.

Then we rang Alan's younger sister, Viv. Her reactions were much the same, but she asked fewer questions. (I sensed she was hurting).

Alan sent a text to Simon, his business partner, confirming the diagnosis. Alan and I were sure Simon would be a great support through this. Alan and I agreed we both wanted to stop work as soon as possible. Six months to two years was no time at all, especially if much of it would involve life in a wheelchair.

Dinner was washed down with a bottle of Chateauneuf du Pape before we watched TV, doing our best to stay calm. Out of the blue Alan said, "I feel sad. We have not had enough time together." I held my breath as he finished with, "The last eleven years have been the best of my life." Tears rolling down my face I managed,m "I never knew true love until I met you."

Thursday 23rd November - The power of hope
Alan went to Solihull hospital for a pre-med blood test and then to his office for half a day.

My boss and I had a telephone chat. By the end we had agreed a plan for him to update my team and my colleagues. It was kind of him to say, "You are a strong woman, Hazel." I felt like a wreck of a woman.

My sister, Clare, had been emotional on receiving our news last evening, so I checked in with her by text. "I didn't sleep well," she replied. I suddenly realised, all the people we were telling needed support. I hoped we had enough strength to go around.

Also, I was worried about Viv, so I called her. We agreed a plan for Alan and I telling her two sons, Ben and Tom. We also talked about going to the Lake District to see her and Alan's mum, and finally, the plans for Viv's 60th. "You are marvellous, Hazel." It was a kind comment but I felt numb and empty.

Outside, I spotted two of our neighbours, chatting near our house. I darted out and gave them our news. Baz was stunned and asked more questions than Alex. I thought Alan might appreciate some male company and invited them to spend more time with him.

I called my friend Christine Cooper and updated her. She asked lots of questions and offered practical tips. My friend, Teresa, was with her. Later, Teresa sent me a text. "There is a lot of love flying around for you and Alan."

During lunch at home, Alan revealed "I found out today, there is a guy in the IT department who was wrongly diagnosed with MND." Then with a tear in his eye, he added, "I don't think there is any doubt in my case though."

Listening to Alan shuffling papers in his office, while the autumn wind blew down the chimney, was strangely comforting, even though I knew Alan was starting to get his affairs in order.

I asked Alan, "What's on your mind?" His response was, "How you are going to cope after I die?" That had been on my mind too. I spent my time worrying what his thoughts and feelings were. Today I realised he spent his time worrying about mine! Every little bit of him - his feel, his smell, his breathing, his movement, his thinking, his speaking - were all massively important and precious to me.

While the workmen removed our glass conservatory roof and changed it to a solid one, Alan and I agreed turning the dining room into his bedroom would be a good idea. It had a lovely view through the conservatory to the back garden.

At about 2:30pm we went for a walk and chatted mostly about when we would stop work and what we would do in our enforced early retirement. On the way home we bumped into John, another neighbour from our cul-de-sac, so we broke our news to him. "Oh," he said, "my sister has been living with MND for thirty years." I began to question exactly how rare this disease was.

Next, we spotted, Andy, who lived in the house to our left, so told him and his wife Ann. They were sympathetic and offered to help in any way. We were blessed having these wonderful people living near us - a good reason not to move house.

Back inside our house, there was a knock at the door. Sue, wife of neighbour Alex, told us, "I have knowledge of MND" and encouraged our plans for living life to the full while planning for difficult times ahead.

The MND Association helpline lady gave us useful phone numbers and promised to send leaflets about drug trials, etc. Our GP phoned and, much to our relief, confirmed liver and blood tests were fine so he had released a prescription for Riluzole (the only drug that might buy us a few precious months).

Out of desperation I commenced a search for a suitable drug trial. Tirasemtiv came up but did not look hopeful. Stem cell therapy was also in early trials. The Sheffield hospital Interleukin-2 drug trial looked like a possibility. Considering joining a drug trial gave Alan a little hope but mostly it gave him the chance he wanted, to do something, no matter how small, to help others.

Secretly I hoped that being on a trial would give Alan pole position for any new drug if the trial were successful. I felt we were grasping at straws, the chances of a cure coming in Alan's lifetime was minuscule, but we had to give it a try. While there was hope we had something, no matter how flimsy, to hold on to.

I felt low and had a lot on my mind by the time bedtime came. Before turning the lights out Alan and I had briefly chatted about the strangeness of waiting for the next part of his body to stop working. It was clear to me, we both feared that suddenly he was going to decline.

AUTHOR'S NOTE
The helpline number can be found on *mndassociation.org/support-and-information/our-services/mnd-connect*

Friday 24th November - What to do with offers of help
During the night a million thoughts whirred around my mind. Everyone we had spoken with to date had said lovely things and very kindly offered help. I was at a loss to think what helpers could do but knew we needed to harness offers of support somehow, even though at this stage we were coping.

Alan would need a purpose once he stopped work. He had never done fundraising and was not a 'front and centre' sort of chap so, certainly, things might not be easy for him. We found out that Solihull Council had not yet signed up to the MND Charter, but I was not sure he had the strength or passion for that type of campaigning. Most days Alan spent time in his home office sorting out his papers. I imagined he felt powerless and hopeless. I decided he needed daily tasks - things to keep him engaged and busy.

I sent a long email to my good friend, Jo, sharing some of my fears and concerns. I found it helped me to get such thoughts off my mind. I don't know exactly what time I eventually went to sleep but I got up at 7am and prepared for a day of meetings in London.

Before I set off to catch the train, I suggested to Alan he tackle three tasks:

- Contact the MND support organiser
- Contact the MND care organiser
- Contact the benefits department at MND

During the day I called John Biggs, my ex-boss from my days in an executive search firm. He said, "I like Alan. Had we lived closer I am sure we would have become friends." He promised to pass on the news to the rest of my old work colleagues. They kindly sent me texts and emails afterwards.

On hearing my news, one of my current team said, "Even though you have not been in the company a long time you have touched a lot of people and are warmly regarded by many." My HR Director called me. "I nursed my dad before he died from MND, so I know what you are heading into." Until I received this call, I had no idea someone I knew had first-hand experience of the disease.

"The company are offering for you to take December off on full pay." I felt blessed to work for such an understanding business.

Spending the day at work was a great tonic for me. Should I maybe stay on for a few months? On my way home from the office I briefly popped in to see mum. She was clearly getting anxious about the potential changes so I took time to provide as much reassurance as I could. Alan's nephew, Ben, gradually became upset as the news we shared over the phone sank in. He agreed with us we would only call Tom, his younger brother, when Ben could be present.

Alan and I had a long chat about the conflict between doing the fun things on the pre-retirement bucket list and sorting out domestic things. Against my instincts we agreed to prioritise practical things ahead of enjoying ourselves, as Alan wanted to tick off things he felt 'he should have done,' to ease his mind.

Saturday 25th November - Support arrives from friends and strangers

Our morning was spent in bed listening to the Ashes commentary from Australia. Afterwards Alan cooked our traditional weekend breakfast of poached eggs on muffins.

In the golf club car park, I felt nervous and out of kilter. It was Lady Captain's Drive In day. Most of the lady members would be there. I got agitated trying to assemble the golf trolley I needed to borrow from Alan as mine had been stolen some weeks beforehand.

As I entered the locker room, I could hear laughter and voices and had to take a deep breath before I could enter. The first person to speak to me was a lady I was due to play in a knockout competition. She was keen to agree a date for our match. I told her I was going to concede the match. She wanted to know why but I could not tell her.

Then I saw my friend Dawn. Straight away she could sense something was wrong. She took me away from the crowd. We hugged as I broke the news. At one point another friend, Carol O'Hare, came into the locker room but left quickly when she realised something was wrong.

Dawn was brilliant - supportive, practical, thoughtful. She came up with several ideas of things Alan could do with limited mobility. We also discussed financial things such as lasting powers of attorney which she said could be done online.

In the golf club lounge, several ladies hugged me without knowing why I was tearful. I spotted Karen Johnson, a lady with a senior non-clinical role at the QE Hospital. She suggested we find out who was leading the study in Sheffield and go and see them urgently. She said she would check which of the neurologists at the QE were experts in MND. Her message was clear, we needed to get professional support, and quickly.

In Solihull, on my way to meet Alan, I saw some fundraisers collecting donations for MND. When I spoke with the lady volunteer, she kindly gave me the contact details for local support. I gave her a big donation and a long hug. This stranger helped me feel less alone. Alan and I did some Christmas shopping. While we were in one store, we bumped into Andy and Dawn from the golf club. Alan told them about his diagnosis. Andy told Alan about a footballer who had MND.

AUTHOR'S NOTE

I read one of Alan's diaries three years after he died. In there, on this day, he wrote: "Got the worst possible news on Tuesday and that is, I have motor neurone disease. Shit. Bollocks. Fuck."

Monday 27th November - Talking to those who know
Karen, who worked at the QE, met me at the club and confirmed most of Alan's care would be at our home. Any in-patient care would most likely be at the Marie Curie Hospice. I felt scared - I was uncertain where medical assistance would come from if I needed it at home. Finally, she said the multidisciplinary team at Solihull were highly regarded. We were lucky to live in an area that appeared to be well geared up for this rare disease. Karen also gave me the number for Caroline Davis - the regional MND Nurse at the QE hospital. When I called Caroline, she agreed to visit us on Thursday.

On my way home I spoke to Angela and David, our skiing and golfing friends from Wokingham. "You can call me any time, day or night Hazel." I cried when she said, "You know we love you."

Alan was in good spirits after gaining useful information at his meeting with the regional care coordinator for people with MND. She told him she would connect us to Caroline Davis (with whom I had already spoken) and other specialist support people.

Over dinner, Alan told me, "The mother of someone at work has just been diagnosed with MND" and "A lady at work had an ex-boyfriend whose mother had it." We both questioned whether this disease was rare. We agreed Alan would investigate the drugs trials at Sheffield and Oxford and contact the person who runs local support group meetings at the Marie Curie Hospice in Solihull.

While relaxing in the lounge Alan suddenly said, "I love you." I immediately hugged him. I realised that all day I had been thinking of him, worrying about his lungs and how much time we had left.

It was just one week since we had seen Dr Thomas. So much had happened in that time.

Tuesday 28th November - Template for a living will
I felt weird most of the day while working in our Amersham office. My motivation was low. One of the regional managers who had heard my news produced a template for a living will which he highly recommended Alan put in place.

On my way home I called some friends. First, an ex-golf club friend, Iris. Normally a chatty woman, she fell silent on hearing our news. When the shock subsided, she went into action mode. "Come to us," she said, "I will cook."

Another friend, Val, asked me to pop in on her before I went home, so I did. I had lodged with her and her husband Richard when I was between homes in 2004. Val always made me feel very protected - she treated me like a daughter. We had a long, tearful chat. As I left, she gave me a huge hug saying, "I love you to bits," over and over. I cried some more.

When I got home, Alan was cooking a chicken hotpot. He had seen his financial planner and had decided to transfer his affairs to my financial adviser. On the kitchen table was a huge bouquet of flowers from my boss. A lump came to my throat. I struggled not to cry in front of Alan.

Wednesday 29th November - is MND rare or not?
My boss gave me a hug and we talked about Alan's condition before getting down to work business. At the senior management team meeting, I received hugs from several work colleagues. My boss's PA held my hand as she told me, "You are valued by the company. They don't want you to leave."

During the afternoon I spoke with another work colleague. He had heard the news and mentioned the captain at his golf club had been recently diagnosed with MND.

When I called my brother Kevin to arrange a meeting, I withheld the news. Ironically, he said he could not chat for long - he was on his way to attend to one of his clients who had MND! Kevin was fond of Alan. He regarded Alan more as a brother, than a brother-in-law.

Alan was not in the house when I arrived home. I instantly started worrying. Had he had a fall or crashed the car because of his weak leg? I decided to research gadgets that send an alert if the wearer fell.

Alan got a longer than normal hug from me when he arrived home. He'd been at the gym after work. He told me, "The mother-in-law of a lady at work died from MND."

I told him, "The son of a woman who lives in mum's retirement home, also has it." Again, we questioned if MND is rare or not.

We decided to put up the Christmas tree. Instead of it being the upsetting task I had dreaded, we had lots of fun and laughter. It felt good to be doing normal things and forgetting for a moment what loomed over us.

Thursday 30th November - Meeting the MND nurse

My work email inbox included some lovely supportive emails from my boss's secretary and other work colleagues. At a coffee meeting with my friend Jo, she said she would ask her husband, Andy to send us some information. He worked at a company which provided wheelchairs.

At home Alan and I spoke to my financial adviser. He confirmed he could help us sort out the wills and guide us regarding lasting powers of attorney. He would also crunch the numbers regarding moving to a new house. His calculations would consider Alan's income ceasing and my income halving, at the same time as us spending more on travelling while Alan was well enough. He would also factor in that we were already committed to an upstairs bathroom renovation, a new solid roof on the conservatory and the financial gifts Alan wanted to make to his family. He understood our situation having lost his wife when she was only fifty-two.

After lunch, Caroline Davis arrived. She was the specialist MND based at the QE Hospital. We discussed the importance of us still going on holidays, doing fundraising if we wished, Alan trying to get on drug trials and the neurologist Alan would come under at QE. She told us about Fiona, the occupational therapist (OT) at the Marie Curie Hospice, who would be key to us. She advised that Alan should keep his weight up, but we should watch out for choking on food or saliva. She also explained that if Alan kept waking at night it would be a sign that his body was not expelling CO_2 effectively. I was feeling scared at this point - was I to become a nurse?

Caroline gave us a comprehensive MND pack (which I found overwhelming) and provided helpful contact numbers. She also said she would arrange lung function tests - to establish a baseline - and a meeting with the neurologist. The benefits of the drug Riluzole were discussed. They appeared minimal and there were side-effects, so liver function would need monitoring.

The main thing we learned was a prognosis of six months to two years was usual for people who start MND in the Bulbar (throat) region. Alan had the ALS type of MND, so could live longer. "The problem with ALS," Caroline explained, "is it's unpredictable. Anything could go wrong next. There is no way of knowing if progression will be slow or fast."

We were shocked when we learned that Caroline alone looked after 310 people in the Midlands area. How did she cope? How much of her time would we get? As she left, I told Caroline, "Today started as a grey day, but you have bought some sunshine with you."

Alan and I packed up the car and set off to visit Viv and her husband John, in Cumbria. Alan was cheerful on the journey. We chatted and sang songs. He ate four muffins - to keep his weight up he said!

Viv and I had a long hug in her kitchen and had a brief chat before returning to the hall where Alan and John were chatting. I thought is this how it's going to be when we meet people - me talking to the women while Alan talks to the men? Probably.

Over drinks and dinner we gave Viv and John all the information we had. We told them about a blog we had found called 'Pain in the ALS' and our plan for posting an announcement on Facebook. It occurred to me we could keep most people updated via Facebook. I didn't fancy creating a blog on top of everything else I was handling.

Before I fell asleep that night a short poem popped into my head.

SMILING
When I think of you,
It's your face I see,
Lying on the pillow,
smiling back at me.

Friday 1st December - Creating advance notes for loved ones, just in case

During the night I kept waking up - my mind full of random thoughts - so I got up around 5am and did some paperwork. I returned to bed at 6:45am and slept till 8am.

After a leisurely breakfast, Alan and I composed a note to his mum (to give to her as a backup in case Alan found it hard to get the right messages across to her). Creating the note seemed to help Alan get his thoughts in order. Afterwards we drove to Kendal and had a leisurely lunch, followed by shopping for Christmas gifts.

Back at Viv's, we hugged Alan's mum and had a short chat about her journey, before delivering the worst news a son should have to give to his mother.

"I need to have a chat with you, Mam." Alan said.

She replied, "It must be important."

"It is."

And so, it began - the slow, carefully worded, softened message about his diagnosis.

At one point, it looked like his ninety-six-year-old mum might cry, but mostly she wanted answers to questions to help her to believe he was okay. She was aware that David Niven had died from MND. It was useful being able to say Alan's 2nd cousin in America had been living with the condition since 2006.

Late into the morning hours I read the information MND Association had sent us.

Saturday 2nd December - You're not dead yet

On our way back to our home we took a planned detour via Great Barr to see my brother Kevin and his wife Sue. We gave them our news. Sue looked relieved but I don't think she realised the full implications of MND at that time. She had been worried that we might be emigrating, or that one of us had cancer. Kevin was more concerned. He had a client who had MND. The gentleman had lost the use of his hands initially and then had fallen down the stairs due to weakening of his legs. It was a very sharp reminder of the sort of thing that could happen to Alan. Kevin strongly recommended we get on with enjoying life while Alan was still able. Going on a cruise was suggested because cruise companies were used to wheelchair users.

After meeting Kevin, Alan and I finalised the wording of the Facebook announcement. I was keen to go public as soon as possible, but first we needed to tell the rest of my family members and our friends.

After collecting my mum from her flat in our village, and buying some fish and chips, the three of us watched *Strictly Come Dancing*. It was always fun trying to pre-empt the judges' comments and guess the judges' scores. Alan had learned to ballroom dance before I met him. We tried a few ballroom classes together, but we had far more fun learning the modern style of jive dancing, called Ceroc.

After I had taken mum home, Alan and I started to prepare for the next day's Sunday brunch party for a group of our friends known as *The Ski Gang*. Tomorrow eight more people would receive our shocking news.

Before retiring to bed, I checked emails. There were messages from some of my ex-work colleagues. One, from Vicky, announced she was doing the Swansea half marathon in the summer. It finished with, "I am going to raise funds for MND now, because you are the most dedicated couple I know." For the first time in days, the floodgates opened, and I cried uncontrollably. It had probably been building for a while. The grief was overwhelming. The brightness that Caroline had brought with her on Thursday disappeared.

Late into the night I wrote to friends from the days when I was involved with a charity called *More to Life* and to my cousins in Devon. I wanted them to hear the news directly from me. I felt like taking Angela up on her offer to call at any time of the night. Instead, I ate loads of chocolates. I also sent a message to Carol, who had recently been to dinner at ours, asking to meet. I wanted to give her the news in person.

AUTHOR'S NOTE
In these early months after diagnosis, I occasionally felt like life had come to an end. Then I would find some energy and positivity from goodness knows where. We knew Alan's condition would take his life, but while he was still alive there was still life to live.

The phrase 'You are not dead yet' became something that would motivate us. And 'Where there is a will, there is a way' would help us try things some people might think were beyond our range. I don't know where we got the strength from some days, but somehow, we managed to rise above our situation and make the most of our days/weeks/months. My brother Kevin's advice turned out to be key in what happened over the following twelve months. During that time, despite various practical challenges, we had a holiday in Vietnam, two breaks to Wales, a road trip around Scotland and a holiday in Whitby.

I found out about *More to Life* (MTL) when I was receiving counselling after my hysterectomy in 2005. From those dark days I had made lifelong friends through MTL. The feelings of loss I was currently going through were similar to those I experienced when I was told I would never be a mother. Indeed, as Alan's MND progressed, I often drew on some of the coping strategies I used back in 2005/6 - looking hard for the positives in a negative situation.

AUTHOR'S NOTE
More to Life, is a support organisation for people who are involuntarily childless - *fertilitynetworkuk.org/life-without-children/faqs*

Sunday 3rd December - How much love
After breakfast, Alan spoke with his cousin Christine and her husband Dennis in Cumbria. We also had a chat with his sister, Viv, who confirmed she had felt better after seeing Alan. We spent the rest of the morning preparing for *The Ski Gang* Sunday brunch. At one point Alan and I became distraught. We hugged and cried. It felt like sadness had its arms around us, squeezing us and forcing tears out of our eyes.

As we prepared the food, I realised there would come a time when Alan would not be able to help me prepare for these types of parties. We always worked as a team at such events - sharing the job of creating the food and making the house nice. It was a dismal thought - we loved home entertaining.

Bev and John Hadley, and Phil arrived first. Then Malcolm and his son Tristan and Tristan's girlfriend, Sarah. We could not wait for Nina and Robert to arrive, so I gave everyone a Buck's Fizz and then made our announcement. Bev looked startled. She said she knew four people that had MND. Her view was that it was not rare as people thought. Malcolm used humour to defuse the tense situation. Nina and Robert arrived and did not say much on hearing the news. I felt sorry for these friends who had known Alan for many more years than I had.

After eating brunch, we moved into the lounge for coffee/tea. I surprised Robert with a birthday cake. A conversation took place about our plans. Most people thought I should keep on working, as work would give me relief from the stress of caring. Some understood my fear of being alone in our home after Alan died. Later in the day Julie called to say Phil would sit with Alan anytime I needed a break. This kind offer gave me strength.

Before bed, Alan mentioned that he didn't feel sad or angry. I was pleased as I regarded anger as a destructive, negative emotion that would hold him back. I didn't tell him I was feeling tired and hollow inside.

AUTHOR'S NOTE
Whilst it was draining telling all our friends our news, it quickly became

apparent how much we were loved and who we might be able to rely on in the months ahead. I started to keep a list of all the people who had offered help, ready for the days I might need it.

Taking photos of our friends together with Alan became a regular habit for me. None of us knew when the last time they would see Alan would be. Alan's lungs could fail or, he could have a fatal fall, at any time. Capturing these happy times became important to me. We would be able to look at them when Alan was fully paralysed and I would have them to reflect upon, for the rest of my life.

Monday 4th December - Pretending I was okay, was not okay

This was the first day I appreciated my company's generous offer to take this month off. It was nice waking up on what would normally be a busy working day and being able to spend some quiet time with Alan.

While we ate the leftovers from the Sunday party, I asked Alan if he was still worried about me. "I'm worried about how you are going to cope caring for me and your mum at the same time." Also, "I'm worried about how you will cope afterwards." The word 'afterwards' used in isolation, became popular instead of 'after I die' or 'when I am dead.'

I told him, I have already started a list of things I could do to fill my life and feel as fulfilled as possible when the time came. We both started to cry. To ease his pain, I told him, "The love I have received from you so far, and will receive in the time we have left, will keep me going." There was no reply. "Al, what we have between us is rare and extremely special. I feel blessed to have finally found someone with whom I could have this kind of deep and meaningful relationship." I did not tell him I felt heartbroken that one day it would be over.

Later, we checked the *To Do* list and Alan called his cousin Eric to update him. In the afternoon, we did some decorating of the master bedroom, the sort of task we had always enjoyed doing together. Alan was very keen to get this room finished so we could move into it. I was concerned how exhausted this work would make him and how much longer he would be able to climb the stairs to sleep upstairs.

After Alan went to bed, I sent some emails to Alan's cousins in America. Also, I started posting our latest photographs on Facebook. I listened to some songs on YouTube, 'The Rose' by Bette Midler and 'Into the West' by Annie Lennox kicked off my tears.

Then another poem came to me:

I CANNOT SAVE YOU
I cannot save you from the world you inhabit,
I cannot spare you from the torture you will endure.
I cannot make this awful thing disappear,
I cannot hold you enough to take away your fear.
I can only tell you how,
You've changed my life,
In so many ways.
And I can love you,
With all my heart,
Till the end of your days.

By 2am I was feeling wretched. Staying up late after Alan went to bed and drowning in my sorrow had become a pattern. During the day there were light moments, black humour, jokes and laughter. Sometimes we discussed finding an open space and just screaming. We never did it - neither of us had the energy.

Most of the time I felt empty. I had heard about the dark days of depression being called 'The Black Dog'. It scared me to feel like that. I worried friends would get fed up with me if I could not pull myself together. Also, I knew bottling up my emotions and pretending I was okay, was not okay.

AUTHOR'S NOTE
Having spent all our relationship being open and honest with each other, it was a shock to me that occasionally now I found it hard to tell Alan how I felt. In my mind it was not right to add to his troubles by making him feel unhappy or guilty.

Tuesday 5th December - Still breaking the sad news
After just a few hours' sleep it was time to get up. I felt rough. During the night I sent texts to some of my friends saying I needed help. Angela was in Austria but called me anyway. She and her husband Dave were due to join us at our ski holiday in Saalbach in January - assuming Alan was well enough to travel. I poured my heart out to her.

Alan went to work but came home at lunchtime. In the afternoon he painted more of the master bedroom. Alan's American cousin replied to my email saying it was important to, "Do what brings you peace and strength." Great advice for all of us anytime, I thought.

At 5:30pm I left to meet my friend Carol who had recently been to dinner at our house. We found a quiet corner at The Belfry and I broke the news. She was angry, saying, "It's not fair that bad people are spared this kind of thing." We chatted and hugged. Carol still had a bit of a cold. Suddenly, I started to worry about germ transfer.

I arrived home at 7pm, in time for dinner with our golf club friends Carol and John. We had nibbles and red wine and I showed Carol around the house. On the landing, Carol confided, "Alan often speaks highly of you. The strong love you two have will get you through." (Interestingly, the other Carol had said the same sort of thing at the Belfry, adding that Alan could not be in better hands).

Before Carol and John left, Carol gave me a ceramic angel inscribed with, "Wherever you go, whatever you do, may your guardian angel watch over you." Later in the month I would put it on our Christmas tree. Alan and I managed to get an early night. I fell straight to sleep.

AUTHOR'S NOTE
Creating a list of 'Things to do after Alan dies' was extremely difficult. I felt sick imagining a future without Alan. One of the downsides of being so incredibly close was the huge hole his death would leave in my life. However, instinctively, I knew having a list tucked away somewhere, ready for when I needed it, would be useful in the days of grief when I would not be able to think straight.

Friday 8th December - Hoping for a drug trial
We spent the 6th and 7th of December decorating the master bedroom. For a change, everything felt normal, like the old days - before 'D' (Diagnosis) Day.

While I was in London on business, Alan wrote to Professor Dame Pamela Shaw at Sheffield, asking if he could be considered for the drug trial. She replied immediately asking to meet him. It was a ray of sunshine in our world of darkness. Alan celebrated by putting up some decorative lights in the kitchen. Seeing them, and him smiling, was a delight when I got home.

Later that evening Alan said, "You are my rock. I can anchor myself through you." He was normally a man of few words but, when he spoke about his feelings, there was never any doubt about their meaning.

"Do you feel depressed Al?"

Straightaway, he said, "No."

I was pleased.

Saturday 9th December - Surrounded by love

Over breakfast I asked, "When do you feel most down, Al?"

"It's worse when I am alone, because that's when I think about missing seeing my great nephews grow up and how the lives of my three nephews and my niece will develop."

I had no helpful response but decided he should not be left alone for too long.

After a relaxing day, we packed an overnight bag and set off for Alan's Christmas office party - a masked ball - at a hotel in Earlswood. Alan's company shared the event with Aggora, a business owned by Simon Pointon.

Simon Beacham, Alan's business partner, arrived first for pre-dinner drinks in our room with his wife Rachel and daughter Maddie. They were followed by Christina Wooley, the office manager, and her husband Chris.

The mood was light as we drank champagne and ate nibbles. At one point we all started singing the theme tune from *Strictly Come Dancing*. I captured the memories in videos and photos. The party was brilliant. We were sat on table number fourteen - our favourite number. Alan won a TV in the raffle. The reindeer racing was good fun. We tried our hand at blackjack and roulette using the imitation money we had all been given. I placed a bet on number fourteen while Alan was at the bar and 'miraculously' I won! I hoped it was a lucky sign.

Watching Alan dance and sing on the dancefloor was bittersweet. He looked full of life and energy but, I worried he was doing too much, and wondered how long he would be able to dance. At various times there were circles of people around Alan and me. Love was literally surrounding us.

As we were about to retire to bed, Simon Pointon insisted we returned to the dancefloor. The next song was *Spirit in the Sky*. The lyrics, "When I die and they lay me to rest," made me cry. Alan's work colleagues, Paul and Jo, quickly hugged me, as did Simon Pointon's wife.

Rachel started to sob late into the evening. While I hugged her she said, "I wish I could take the disease away from Alan." I held her and tried hard to hold back my own tears.

Sunday 10th December - Snow arriving but losing the sparkle in my life

Overnight a foot of snow had fallen so plans for lunch with my friend Jo were abandoned. Simon, Rachel and Maddie helped us clear the snow off our car and I carefully drove us home. After Alan and I had unpacked in the spare room

I suggested we lie down for a while on the single bed. We quickly fell asleep - waking two hours later.

On the *Strictly Come Dancing* results show, one of the judges said a dancer had lost her sparkle. Spontaneously I shared my thoughts with Alan. "You have bought massive sparkle to my life. I'm not looking forward to losing it."

Monday 11th December - What can I do

With snow still thick on the ground, I did some office work in morning. I could not bring myself to do any decorating in the afternoon, so sent out the agreed announcement on Facebook and LinkedIn instead. Before long responses to my post were flooding in. Judith, a work colleague from the 1990's asked me for my email address.

A breakthrough drug for Huntington's Disease was announced on the news. I felt hopeful about a cure for MND in Alan's lifetime, until I remembered MND is a complex disease, caused by multiple factors. It occurred to me I should do some fundraising to help the MND community but I was not fit enough for any long runs, walks, swims or cycle rides. I did not have enough knowledge to be a campaigner, or spare time to do volunteering. My helplessness felt frustrating.

We looked forward to seeing Alan's GP to collect a referral letter to Professor Dame Pamela Shaw, regarding the Sheffield drug trial. Once we had the letter, we would be able to organise a trip to Sheffield.
Just before I went to sleep, I wrote a couple of poems.

WHO KNOWS WHAT'S AHEAD
You don't know what's ahead of you,
Only what's behind.
You cannot predict the future,
Only try to calm your mind.

The worry never leaves you,
Despite your best endeavours.
It's always looming over you,
Like forthcoming gloomy weather.

It's hard to forget the words he used,
The expert who knows your fate.
You need to fill your time up
Before it gets too late.

But you cannot think beyond today,
Because the future's full of fear.
It's not possible to plan ahead,
When you don't know if you'll be here.

I AM NO USE EITHER
The comments came in thick and fast,
To our Facebook post last night.
Comforting and supportive, you should be glad
But deep inside you don't feel right.

It's no use fighting this invisible foe,
You have to accept what's coming your way.
You have to try to keep cheerful,
Even when you know there's no use.
You're just counting time,
And hoping for miracles that may never come.

Silently it's coming, it's moving closer each day,
It cannot be reasoned with,
It has control.
You cannot command it to go away,
It has the power.

It will claim you, no matter what I do.
I have to give you up to it,
But I don't want you to go.
I want to stop it, and stop it now,
Before too much of you goes.
But I can't.
I'm no use either.

AUTHOR'S NOTE
Huntington's disease is an illness caused by a faulty gene in a person's DNA. It affects the network of nerve tissues in the brain and spinal cord that co-ordinate your body's activities. It can cause changes with movement, learning, thinking and emotions.

Tuesday 12th December - Celebrating the good times

On this day in 2012, Alan proposed to me in Rome. How different life had become to the one we imagined.

Although I did not want Alan to know my anguish, I had never kept any secrets or feelings from him, so I read him my latest poems. Afterwards, I asked, "Is my love for you enough?" Once again he confirmed, "You are my rock." I posted a note on Facebook about it being the 5th anniversary of our engagement then had to leave for a business meeting.

When I arrived home, I saw an email from Judith, an ex-work colleague. Her firm had July 2018 free as a month for supporting a charity. She asked me to send her information so she could put a case forward for the MND Association. Dinner was washed down with a bottle of prosecco while we reminisced about this day in 2012.

Wednesday 13th December - Drawing on my coping strategies

I woke up with a prosecco induced headache. I felt out of sorts and stressed most of the day. Luckily, I was working from home. Alan came home at lunchtime. We drove to a local health centre where I had a much-needed neck massage from my ex-lodger, Jaki.

Alan and I went to the Marie Curie Hospice for our first monthly MND support group meeting. There was no one involved with MND at the hospice. We had got our dates mixed up - the meeting was the next day! However, one of the nurses gave us useful information about the various MND sessions available and organised a hot drink for us. She explained that there was a 'man shed' available for all male patients facing personal loss, either through their own illness or because they were bereaved. How unfortunate, I thought, that there was not a 'Girls' Grotto' too.

At home I prepared a supper for Teresa, Christine, Frankie and Jenny - my girlfriends from the *More to Life* support group. We had known each other since 2005 and had catch up meetings every four or five months. Jenny had to leave before dessert and our short meditation session. It was hard to concentrate on conscious breathing as I could hear Alan chatting to Christine's husband, John, in the next room. Before leaving, Christine suggested Alan and I joined them on their cruise in March. It was a nice idea, but we could not commit to anything until we knew if Alan had been accepted on the drug trial or not.

Thursday 14ᵗʰ December - Website searches

Scouring the MND Association website shop I found plenty of useful items. I ordered, wristbands, collection boxes, bunting, pin badges and posters. While reading stories about people, who had not lived long with the disease on the MND Association website, Alan became tearful. I went to bed thinking, today was our three and a half year wedding anniversary, and eleven and a half years since we met. Normally, we would have celebrated such an event. We did not even discuss it.

We had always been close but, I was beginning to fear this dreadful disease was taking something away from us.

Friday 15ᵗʰ December - Conflicting emotions

Alan needed a lift to work so he did not have to drive after his firm's Christmas lunch. At his office we went to see Matthew Wheeler and Rob Oliver. These two men, who worked at Aggora, had decided to cycle from Lands' End to John O'Groats, fundraising for the MND Association, together with another man who would be raising funds for the Parkinson's UK charity. It was very moving listening to Matt and Rob saying that knowing Alan had the disease was a motivator for them. Neither of them had done anything like this before, so it was going to be a major challenge. Later Alan and I talked of surprising them as they cycled through the Midlands and following them in our car through the final stages of their journey. We felt they deserved our moral support and we fancied a trip to Scotland. We didn't stop to think how limited Alan's mobility might be by April.

For some days I had been hiding my feelings from Alan, but once at home, my emotions overflowed. We had agreed in the early days of Alan's MND journey not to get angry, or ask questions that had no answer, such as, "Why me?" and not do self-pity. But I was beginning to feel anger and self-pity.

Outside the noisy pub in Warwick, I sat in the car for a while, filled with dread at the idea of going inside to collect Alan and seeing all the happy partygoers. I felt like an outsider - not part of the typical December party scene. I wanted to go in and shout, "I cannot be happy - my husband is dying!"

Later in the evening I started writing out Christmas cards. It was depressing realising there were still a lot of people who needed to be informed of Alan's illness. On my phone, there was a voice message from mum. "A lady called Elaine, who lives in my retirement block, wants to talk with you. Her son has been going strong with MND for several years." My spirits lifted. Alan was a fit, healthy man, I thought surely, he would live longer than the two-year prognosis.

My friend, Teresa sent me a note about the Huntington Disease drug breakthrough. She was hopeful it might lead to an effective MND drug. I sent an abrupt message back saying that the diseases were quite different. Later, I reflected on what I had written and feared it was too rude. The underlying anger I was feeling had got the better of me and I felt awful about being so rude to a dear friend.

Saturday 16ᵗʰ December - Being more than a carer

Alan and I had an honest chat before getting up. I told him, "I'm worried your frustration with yourself might make it hard for both of us to cope." I also confided, "It was hard coming into the pub last night." Ever the wise, unselfish one, Alan responded with, "You should ensure you get some time to yourself instead of spending all your time as my carer."

For the first time in three months, I went for a three-mile run. Getting out in the fresh air, away from everything, even for a short time, felt good and I suddenly thought I should challenge myself to do my first ever 10k run in 2018. Lunch with Jo and her husband, Andy, lifted my mood further.

When I arrived home a Fortnum and Mason hamper had been delivered - a surprise gift from my company. The thought of giving up a job I loved and was good at, and leaving work colleagues I liked and who respected me, was unsettling. I had worked full time since I was sixteen and had built up a good reputation in my industry. Work had been my rock through my life's ups and downs. It was hard to imagine returning to the commercial world after Alan died. Effectively, I was facing early retirement without achieving my full potential and with no celebration after over forty years of dedicated service.

Earlier that evening, Dawn, from the golf club, and her husband Tony, came round to watch the *Strictly Come Dancing* final with us. As Dawn helped me wash up in the kitchen we hugged when I began to weep for no reason, other than just sheer sadness. A plan was made for us to join them to watch some international rugby at their house in the coming weeks. It was always good to have nice things to look forward to.

Sunday 17ᵗʰ December - Setting targets for myself

With mum safely in my car I drove to Tamworth to drop off Christmas gifts for my sister, Rowena (Ro), and her husband, Steve. Ro became melancholy when talking about Alan and her own husband's ill health. I felt surprisingly calm as

I hugged her. Listening to other people's difficulties and challenges was easier than thinking about my own. I was reminded that Buddhists look upon our own suffering as part of a much bigger picture, where others are suffering too.

Alan, mum and I attended a Carols by Candlelight service at the church of my friend Alison. I wished I had the sort of faith Alison and others had. Before going to bed I entered the Stratford-upon-Avon 10k race due to be held in September 2018 and set what I felt would be a challenging fundraising target.

Tuesday 19th December - Dealing with the world outside

At a garden centre I had another meeting with my friend Carol. Her small, energetic grandson was with her which made conversation difficult. Normally Carol and I had uplifting chats, but after this one, I felt low. My old downcast feelings about not being a mother had bubbled up, this time in the context of being a widow with no children or grandchildren to bring joy and give me a reason to carry on living.

On my way home I visited Elaine, the lady in mum's retirement block. She explained how her thirty-year-old son in Ireland, was diagnosed with MND eight years ago. He had lived a full life since diagnosis, including getting married and having a son! It was moving and inspirational talking to Elaine. I admired how she was handling things, especially as she had her own personal medical challenges.

Later that evening I wrote a new poem:

BEING TOGETHER
We want to be together,
No matter what the weather,
Or the world outside.

We like to walk and cuddle,
And snuggle in a huddle,
Forget the world outside.

We talk and laugh and cry,
With no thoughts of last goodbyes,
No thoughts of the world outside.

We want peace and calm and love,
And help from up above,
No need for the world outside.

We need to be together,
In tune, in love, forever,
Free from the world outside.

Wednesday 20th December - What I will miss

The team of three people I was responsible for at work were based in Plymouth. They made kind comments during my conference call with them. Later in the day a lovely, personalised Christmas card arrived from them.

All the time I had known Alan he had been good at giving me cards and leaving romantic notes for me around the house. He also showed his love for me in lots of acts of service. Before I went to bed this short verse came to me:

THE THINGS YOU DO
All the lovely things you do,
I will miss them.
I will miss you.

Friday 22nd December - Am I prepared?

I woke up feeling off kilter. My calves were twitching - something that had only recently started to happen. I was worried about mum as she was having some very odd hallucinations. I also started thinking about how ill-prepared I felt for Alan's deterioration. Negative projection was something I was generally able to avoid but, when my mood was low, unhelpful thoughts of the future crept in.

While I was in the bathroom, Alan caught my eye and we both smiled. I went to our bedroom, sat on the bed, and cried. "What's wrong?" Alan asked.

"I am frightened of losing you and then having to leave our home and all its memories after you die." There were more tears as he held me.

As I backed off our drive, our neighbour Andy caught my eye. I wound down the window. "Hazel, I don't mind going anywhere with Alan by car, bus or train, if it would help." This kind offer made me wonder whether moving away was a good idea or not.

When viewing a one-bedroom retirement apartment in Shirley, I began to realise that the work involved in downsizing to something so small, while Alan was ill, was out of the question. Downsizing and moving by myself, after Alan passed away, was a daunting thought too.

Happy music came on the kitchen radio while Alan and I were preparing food for Christmas. We downed tools and started dancing. As we whirled around the kitchen jiggling, Alan bumped into a bowl of cream on the worktop which spilt everywhere. I longed for more moments of joy like this - with or without a spillage at the end of them.

Saturday 23rd December - Alan's sister's affection
Viv and John arrived. As I showed Viv the newly decorated bedroom, I bought her up to date regarding Alan's symptoms. We hugged each other tightly before joining the men.

Sunday 24th December - The golf club without Alan - an unpleasant prospect
After Viv and John left, I drove Alan over to mum's flat to collect her. Next stop was my brother, Michael's house to pick him up before collecting his son, Connor, from across town. The five of us spent a few hours at our golf club Christmas Eve family party.

Going to the golf club felt like a double-edged sword. There was lots of support there, but it made me think what it would be like in the future when Alan would no longer be there. I wondered if I might move to another club and start again, to avoid the sadness I suspected I might feel. We ended the day with a fish pie dinner while watching a James Bond movie.

Monday 25th December - Not an ideal Christmas day
Christmas Day turned out to be a bit odd. I wanted it to be special but there was an undercurrent of tension. I suspected Alan and I were thinking the same thing - would this be our last ever Christmas?

Alan loved cooking but had struggled to prepare our meals for the last two nights. I insisted on taking charge of the Christmas meal. He wanted to help so he made the Parmesan parsnips and the stuffing, while I did everything else.

My brother and nephew giggled a lot at the dinner table, which irritated me. My stress levels rose. I wanted them to be more respectful. Mum said she felt unwell so I drove her back to her flat. Once I had taken Michael and Connor home too, Alan and I cuddled up on the settee and watched TV. It was the best part of the day.

Tuesday 26th December - Fun with our great nephews
Before setting off to visit Alan's sister, Pauline, and her husband Simon, we checked up on my mum. Thankfully she was feeling a bit better. By the time we arrived at Pauline's, Alan's mum, Joan, was there, as was his niece, Helen,

and her husband Richard and their two boys, William and Thomas. Also, Alan's nephew, Matthew, and his wife Suzanne had beaten us to Pauline's.

Everyone except Joan and Pauline went for a short walk at Creswell Craggs. The weather was a bit gloomy but it felt good to be out. Helen asked me questions about Alan's prognosis. I was careful how I answered. Misery stirred in me. After dinner we opened gifts. William and Thomas pretended to paint Alan's face like a tiger. It was beautiful watching him play with these two small boys who loved their great uncle.

We set off home taking Joan with us. Once home, in the privacy of our bedroom, Alan announced, "I am getting muscle cramps in my abdomen, weakness in my quadriceps muscles and beginning to find it difficult climbing the stairs." Stunned, I didn't know what to say. Things were moving too fast. It was only a little over one month since diagnosis! In the middle of the night, I woke and could not get back to sleep for the thoughts racing around my mind. I got up, sent some emails and returned to bed in the early hours of the morning.

Wednesday 27th December - Frustrations arranging important meetings
At 10am I got up and spent time with Alan sorting out some administration. We entered all the MND support meetings, physio sessions, holidays and dates of concerts for which we had tickets into our respective diaries.

Alan struggled to hold his pen even though I had bought him some special grips. He had beautiful handwriting, having taken lessons in calligraphy. All our wedding stationery had been handwritten by him. It was depressing thinking soon he would not be able to write at all, which would mean the end to his romantic notes to me and a lot of frustration for him.

We had a frantic couple of hours when I discovered we had not received an appointment letter for a meeting with Dr Pall, the specialist MND neurologist at the QE hospital. I spent ages talking to our GP and emailing Professor Dame Pamela Shaw regarding the referral letter for the drug trial. It turned out our GP had sent a referral letter on December 15th to a different address to the one in Professor Shaw's email. Frustratingly, Professor Shaw was now going to be away until the 8th of January.

Thursday 28th December - Red wine and fountain pen ink, not a great mixture
Mum was still not 100% well, so we only took Alan's mum, Joan to a planned afternoon tea in Stratford-upon-Avon.

Later that night Andy and Ann, from next door, joined us for drinks. During one particularly animated story Ann was telling, she accidentally knocked over a full glass of red wine. The crimson liquid flew onto our cream wallpaper, the cream carpet and over my journal. She panicked. I somehow remained calm, thinking there was no point crying over spilt wine, as I sacrificed a good glass of white wine to save the carpet! In the past I would have found such a situation annoying, but in the great scheme of things these days, it didn't matter. My main concern was for the journal which was handwritten using a fountain pen. Luckily, it survived.

Friday 29th December- The need for independence
Despite the effort and time it took him, Alan would not let me help him pack the car ready for our trip to Sunderland. Alan's desire to remain independent frustrated me sometimes. I made a mental note that we needed to discuss working more as a team and him being more open to accepting help. It was not yet clear if using failing muscles was a good idea. My instinct was that, whenever possible, Alan should rest.

Alan drove us up to Sunderland. There was not much conversation. I slept some of the time. We had a fish and chips supper with Joan and watched another James Bond movie. Before lights out, Alan announced "My right hand is getting much worse." The rate of decline was shocking.

Saturday 30th December - The 'firsts' keep coming
Alan snored a lot during the night, keeping me awake. Every time he appeared to stop breathing, I panicked. My brother Kevin called and told us the patient he had been looking after with MND, had been admitted to hospital after a fall when his legs just stopped working. I felt sorry for the wife of this unknown man.

Before breakfast, Alan and I had a conversation about his care needs if his left arm or legs stopped working. Alan did not want me to become his full-time carer. He wanted me to remain his companion and wife. We discussed the idea of a live-in carer. I didn't know what I wanted, other than for this wretched disease to go away. After breakfast, Alan and I took a gentle walk to the shops. He reminisced about the schools he had attended and the homes in which he had lived.

In the early days of our relationship, we developed a habit of counting our 'firsts'. The first time we had dinner, the first time we kissed, the first time we went to the movies, etc. I realised that, even though we had made many trips to Sunderland over the eleven years we had known each other, this was the first time we had walked to the local shops together. Also, amazingly, there were still things I was learning about him.

We left Joan's around noon, taking a pretty route to Cumbria, via Barnard Castle. Alan was in good spirits as we drove across the Pennines on the A66 with views of snow on top of the hills. My offer to drive was rejected with, "While I can still do it safely, I want to drive us."

We arrived at Viv and John's just before Pauline and Simon. Before long, Simon, John and Alan were off to the local pub. This gave Pauline, Viv and I time to talk about Alan. I found the conversation stressful, so excused myself and went into another room. When I returned, the subject had switched to Simon's health. Pauline and I were in the same boat, each worrying about poorly husbands. To lighten the mood after dinner we played *Impromptu* and all drank a lot.

Sunday 31st December - A nicer evening than I expected
Despite the rain and wind, I went for a three-mile run. After breakfast we all drove to Keswick for a gentle walk around Derwentwater, stopping for a picnic at lunch time.

Back at Viv's home everyone, except Pauline, went to the local pub for pre-dinner drinks. Surprisingly I drank a pint and a half of bitter. Unsurprisingly, I got emotional when talking to Simon about Alan.

After dinner at Viv's, we watched the pub firework display from the lounge window and those from London on TV. It was a far nicer and less emotional evening than I had anticipated, but I could not help wondering what 2018 had in store for us.

PART 3 - DISEASE PROGRESSION

2018

As the new year began, I reflected on 2017. It had started brilliantly, with wonderful celebrations of my 60th birthday but ended with a salutary lesson in how unpredictable life can be.

Before MND came we took every opportunity to enjoy life and focused on making each other feel happy and loved.

By the end of 2017, we were firefighting against an unpredictable, invisible monster.

What would the ticking time bomb of MND do to us in 2018?

Alan and I knew one thing for certain - every day we were given would be a precious blessing.

To cope with what was ahead we decided we needed to do three things:

- Live in the moment - enjoying each day, not thinking about the next day/week/year.
- Plan for the worst
- Hope for the best

We had to hang on to what little hope there was.

Without hope, we had nothing.

Tuesday 2nd January - MND symptoms start to become more obvious

On my first official day back to work, after a December on compassionate leave, I worked from home. The builders started stripping out the en suite bathroom attached to the newly decorated master guest bedroom so a walk-in shower could replace the corner bath.

One of the firm's financial advisers called saying his dad had developed MND at the age of sixty and had only lived two years.

While watching TV Alan suddenly started choking. I tried not to panic as I helped him clear his throat. Typically, Alan made light of this incident, but it seriously worried me. Had MND started to affect his swallowing muscles?

Friday 5th January - Planning Alan's early retirement

Alan left early to talk to Simon Beacham about early retirement from ABC Solutions and the payment Simon was prepared to offer Alan for his share of the business. Simon was a good man. They had been friends, as well as work colleagues, for over twenty years.

Appointments were made for Alan to see Dr Pall at the QE hospital and Professor Dame Pamela Shaw at Sheffield Hospital. As a result of immovable work commitments, I would have to find people I trusted to take Alan to these important meetings.

Workmen started removing the glass panels from the conservatory roof. One told us he knew someone with MND. It was becoming obvious MND was more prevalent than we had first understood. Over dinner Alan shared details of his meeting with Simon. An amicable arrangement had been agreed but the conversation cannot have been easy for either of them.

Saturday 6th January - Accidents happen more often

During a TV dinner in the lounge, Alan dropped a bottle of red wine from his stronger left hand. I tried to not to make a fuss as I cleaned up the mess. We didn't discuss it. We both knew what this meant.

Sunday 7th January - Land's End to John O'Groats fundraiser planning

Teresa was the first of three friends to respond saying she could take Alan to hospital on 8th January. I felt lucky to have so many lovely people in my life.

"My back muscles were stiffening when we were moving that furniture," Alan announced as we were painting woodwork in the guest bedroom. I didn't react. I felt too despondent. He added, "I need some long sleeve polo shirts. I feel the cold more these days."

It was a bright, chilly, January day. Alan fancied a walk, so we took a stroll on a local canal tow path after finding three new polo shirts in a shop in Solihull. Alan's test results arrived in the post. "There looks like some degradation of the left side and arm." Our fears were confirmed. I felt unhappy and scared.

Rob Oliver and Matt Wheeler announced on Facebook that the 1000 mile ride from Land's End to John O'Groats (branded LEJOG), would take place over ten days in April. Their aim was to raise £15,000 to support people like Alan with MND, and those suffering from Parkinson's, like the mum of the third rider, Jonathon Dicks. The ambition and determination of these men was impressive. They would be pushing themselves hard, using up their holiday allowance and being away from their families for a long time, to help others.

Alan had been a keen cyclist since his days of running marathons ended. He was humbled by what the three men were planning. I knew he would also be envious and sad that he could not cycle with them.

While I was trying to sleep, I began to feel envious of the normal lives our friends and families enjoyed. Since November our world had been thrown upside down. Sadness dominated most of my time. Every day was unpredictable and full of fear. There was no 'normal' for us anymore and things were going to get worse.

Monday 8th January - 1st visit to QE Hospital
Teresa went with Alan to meet the neurologist, Dr Pall, at the QE Hospital. My business meeting was with a man I had known for years. At the end of our time, I told him about Alan. While shaking hands he said, "I knew a man who died one year after being diagnosed with MND. I will pray for Alan." It was hard to fight back my tears.

It was odd not being with Alan on such an important day, but many friends had suggested that I try to function as normally as possible. Workdays were a useful distraction and gave me time to gather my thoughts. Teresa sent me a very comprehensive note. She was definitely a good choice for this kind of occasion. Before going home, I visited Elaine to update her about the drug trial meeting. We both agreed it would be good for her son and Alan to meet.

It was impossible to imagine how a mother felt about losing her son to MND and, how a young man of just thirty dealt with such a diagnosis. In November

Dr Thomas told Alan to focus on the happy memories he had already built. Elaine's son would have fewer memories to draw upon and a lot more future to lose.

CHANGING

What do you say,
To a man who one day,
Will have no arms to use?
To a man whose body is dying,
Bit by bit?
Every day is a day closer to the end,
A day when another small part
Slows or stops.
Invisible killer, creeping around,
Eating away at the fibres and tissues,
Claiming more for itself,
And leaving nothing behind.
Taking the person,
As well as the body.
Changing him.
Changing things.
Changing life.

Tuesday 9th January - Good advice from an MND widow

After a day in Sheffield on business I drove to Alan's sister's house in Worksop. Alan was already there. I had dinner with the three of then and then had to leave.

On my way home I called a lady named Ann. Her number had been given to me by a mutual friend, Jane, from Peterborough. Ann was a volunteer for MND Association. After explaining Alan's diagnosis, prognosis and current condition, Ann talked me through the six year journey her husband had with the disease.

Her husband had been generally mobile up till the end. They built a ramp into the house and fitted a stairlift and made the most of their time while they had it.

"What are your top tips for coping and being a good carer?" I asked.

"You need a sense of humour. Don't take angry outbursts from Alan personally - it will be his frustration coming out."

We ended by agreeing to meet if I was ever in London.

It felt weird talking to this lady. She knew where I was heading but I could not comprehend the journey. I took heart from how calmly Ann told her story. Part of me hoped that Alan's prognosis was wrong, and he would have a lot more than two years left.

Wednesday 10th January - The drug trial assessment

In Salisbury, on another business meeting, all I could think about was Simon and Alan meeting Professor Shaw in Sheffield. Later, Simon sent a text, "Eureka - Alan has done well." Alan's lung function tests were good. Phew, what a relief! Alan could live without the use of his arms, as long as we kept his mindset strong. If his breathing muscles deteriorated, things would become more critical. As I travelled home, I called various friends about the drug trial assessment.

During the evening I checked LinkedIn, for replies about MND. A lady coincidently called Hazel said that her brother, aged fifty-one, was diagnosed at the end of 2017. He was her only relative as their parents died when she was twenty-one.

Later that evening I made a couple of lists. The first was all the things Alan would still be able to do once he lost the use of both hands. (Ready for the day, if it came, when he would become depressed).

The list included:

- Talking
- Reading - with help from a page turner or audiobooks
- Walking - assuming legs still work
- Watching movies
- Watching sport - live events, or on TV
- Boccia - a specialist sport developed specifically for people with disabilities
- Listening to music - live concerts or recorded
- Train travel
- Car journeys - with family, friend, or carer as driver

The depressing thought for me was I would have to do all the domestic things such as gardening, ironing, cooking, cleaning the house, washing up, car washing or decorating myself!

The second list was all the functions Alan would need my help with once his arms/hands stopped working.

- Washing body
- Washing hair
- Brushing hair
- Dressing
- Undressing
- Teeth cleaning
- Shaving
- Scratching itches
- Blowing nose
- Eating
- Drinking
- Writing
- Toileting
- Phoning
- Texting
- Changing TV/radio channels
- Getting around (in a car/bus/train/plane, especially if baggage was involved)
- Buying things - online or in a shop (money /credit cards to be handled by me/carer)

These thoughts made me realise I would need to give up work and at some point we would need carers. Luckily we had some savings, but there would be no further income.

The biggest loss to Alan, in addition to the loss of dignity, would be that he would no longer be able to do the things he loved - play golf, ski, cycle, hug me and others. Me giving up paid work and us using up some savings, was no sacrifice compared to the losses he was going to suffer.

AUTHOR'S NOTE
Writing lists to help me organise myself had been a habit I had developed, both at work and at home. Now I found myself writing lists whenever thoughts popped into my head, so I could refer to them later when I needed them

(particularly if I might not be able to think straight as Alan became more gravely ill).

It was often very painful to consider what faced us. However, thinking about what lay ahead, planning for it and making notes about everything, was useful.

Thursday 11th January - First death

Travelling back from working in Amersham, I had a phone chat with my friend Christine. She always had good practical ideas and was keen to make things right. I loved that she was full of hope, in what felt like an utterly helpless situation.

As I opened the front door, I heard the beeping of the answer machine. "Haze, it's Kevin. My MND patient has died in hospital. It was very quick in the end." This was the first death from MND I'd heard of since Alan's diagnosis. I felt for this couple I didn't know. I wanted to write to the gentleman's wife, but what would I say to this stranger who was ahead of me on the MND path?

Friday 12th January - Not having the chance to say goodbye

Chaos at the house because it was the last day of the bathroom fitting and workmen were still putting up the solid conservatory roof. At one point Alan got tetchy with me in the morning, so I moved to another room to do some work. In the afternoon, we went shopping in Solihull. To cheer Alan up I took him to see The Darkest Hour (a film about Churchill). Our friends Alison and Adrian joined us.

At the pub afterwards, Alison talked of a lady she knew whose husband had died suddenly in his sleep. I thought how awful it would be not to have the chance to say goodbye to someone you loved.

Before bed I privately watched a video on YouTube called *The Long Goodbye*, made by a woman whose husband had MND. She sounded angry and stressed. I hoped that I would not become like her.

Saturday 13th January - A mother's hug

We spent the day finishing off wallpapering the bedroom. It looked perfect. From here on it would affectionately be known as the 'hotel room'.

I took mum shopping then she helped me prepare dinner while Alan rested. Historically, mum and I had not been close, but she had become more loving in recent years, due to her dementia and because she knew I was facing life as a widow in my sixties. She was sixty-three when my dad died.

When I delivered mum home, she gave me an unusually long hug saying, "Don't worry about Alan." It was the most tender moment we had ever shared.

Sunday 14th January – Acceptance

Alan cooked us eggs for breakfast, after I had done a short training run. He then prepared to go cycling. Sadly, he couldn't wave goodbye to me, like he always used to when he peddled away, because he needed both hands to steady himself.

At the golf club for the annual 100 Club draw, one lady member told us about a seventy-year-old who had lived with MND for two years. Another member told us about a local twenty-two-year-old girl who was diagnosed with MND six months ago. It was shocking to hear that someone so young had the disease.

Over a Sunday roast, at the local pub, we talked about the early days after Alan's diagnosis. We checked how we felt we were both coping. We concluded we had both moved out of the shock/research phase and had accepted the unfortunate hand of cards life had dealt us.

With our newfound mindset we spent the rest of lunch chatting about things we might like to do. We already had a couple of trips booked but in addition, Alan fancied going to Vienna for a weekend and hiring an Aston Martin to drive around Europe. I loved him for his spirit and romantic ideas.

I realised as we walked out of the restaurant it was 139 months since we had met. In June it would be our fourth wedding anniversary. Our first three wedding anniversaries had involved one of us surprising the other with a trip away. I chose not to think about how we might celebrate our fourth anniversary. I was beginning to think in shorter time horizons for fear of getting hopes up, only to have them dashed.

AUTHOR'S NOTE

The acceptance of our situation was critical. It freed up our thinking and gave us permission to get on with life.

Tuesday 16th January - Letting go

Not a good day. Firstly, Julie from Macmillan, phoned and introduced herself as our clinical nurse specialist. She sounded nice but the idea that we needed a Macmillan nurse at all made me feel sick. Following our notification to the DVLA a few days previously, they requested Alan give up his driving license in exchange for a three-year temporary one. It was a body blow on top of everything else he was dealing with.

"That day we ambled around that Yorkshire town was a taste of the retirement I wanted for us," Alan said as we painted the bedroom furniture. "Now it cannot happen. And I don't think we will get to Australia or New Zealand either."

"We could still go abroad, if we are prepared to risk travelling without insurance cover," I replied, to try to make him feel better,

But deep down I felt Vietnam was probably going to be our last long-haul holiday. We had to be realistic and let go of some of our more ambitious holiday plans.

Alan mentioned that his torso felt tight again. We both feared his diaphragm might be failing.

Wednesday 17th January - First MND support group meeting
We finished off painting the bedroom furniture and the electrician finished off the conservatory. At last, life would be less hectic and the house back to normal.

Late morning, we had two visitors from the Marie Curie Hospice in Solihull - Fiona, our OT, and Lesley, our physiotherapist. Lesley was a golfer and knew people at our club. Small world. Both ladies were very nice, but I found the meeting troubling especially because Alan talked more about torso stiffness.

Lesley recommended Alan do some posture improvement exercises to keep his core strong. She booked a further visit to conduct a baseline assessment and said she would make a referral to the dietician. This was standard practice, so we were prepared if Alan developed swallowing difficulties. A shocking thought.

Lesley warned, "Not to exert tired muscles too much - you need to listen to your body." I thought that's not going to be easy for Alan, who is used to pushing himself extremely hard.

The new guidance confused me. It was contrary to the initial information we were given in November, when Alan was told to carry on going to the gym. It occurred to me the neurologists wanted Alan to enjoy life while he could, whereas Lesley was trying to help Alan keep mobile for as long as possible. The last thing Lesley said was a resting splint would be organised to support Alan's weak right hand.

At lunchtime, Alan and I attended our first MND support group meeting at the Marie Curie Hospice in Solihull. The hospice was familiar to me because I'd visited a fellow golfer in his final days there. However, I sensed Alan was on edge. We were given a warm welcome and introduced to Alison, the MND regional organiser Alan had met at our home. To my relief, Lesley and Fiona were at the meeting. Alison brought everyone up to date with current news on drug trials, etc. and invited us to ask questions.

I found it tough seeing what might become of Alan in the future and worried how he must be feeling. One lady, cared for by her husband for six years, was unable to talk. Also, her legs were weak.

A gentleman called Brian had lived with MND for two years and looked well. He was not taking Riluzole tablets due to a bad reaction to them. His wife Jenny was his carer.

Another man called Bill was sitting on a motor scooter. He had lived with a slow progressing version of MND for fifteen years. Sitting next to him was his wife and carer, Lesley.

Sitting next to me was a lady diagnosed with ALS (same as Alan) in October. Her husband was not with her because he was ill. At this stage she had a weak foot.

Sitting on the other side of the circle was a volunteer, Stephanie. Her husband had died six years ago after living with Bulbar onset MND for eighteen months.

The other attendees were sisters and local fundraisers, Linda and Sue. They had lost their mum to MND seven years previously.

On the way home Alan and I agreed that the meeting was useful and not as distressing as we had imagined. I was relieved. I was hoping to attend again and to maybe collect phone numbers of wives who were carers.

AUTHOR'S NOTE
Bulbar onset motor neurone disease occurs in about 20% of those affected. The first sign is usually slurring of the speech, caused by impaired tongue movement, which may be accompanied by obvious wasting and fasciculation of the tongue.

Thursday 18th January - The power of an uplifting song
The new carpet arrived to complete the 'hotel bedroom'. Alan was singing as he cleaned the windows and put the curtains back up. His happiness made me cry.

Early evening, we went to see *The Greatest Showman* movie with Alison and Andy. "The song, 'This is me - I am glorious,' touched me" Alan said as we walked back to the car. We stopped walking and had a longer than usual hug. "I've decided I am not ashamed of myself," he said. I felt immensely proud and full of love and admiration for him. He was not going to let MND define him.

Saturday 20th January - Last ski holiday?

At 3:10am the taxi took us to Birmingham International Airport. Alan and I managed the suitcases well enough between us through to check-in. In the departure lounge the couple next to us started a conversation. "We have had a bad 2017," the lady said, "My husband was diagnosed with a serious heart condition and my sister died." I felt too emotional to share our story.

Our hotel in Saalbach was about 500 yards downhill from the hotel in which *The Ski Gang* were staying. Before dinner, Alan had to abandon writing in his travel journal because he could no longer hold a pen. It was the end of his tradition of keeping detailed records of our travels. Instead, he dictated notes on his iPhone. Over dinner I found it difficult to contain my emotions. It hurt thinking this could be our last skiing holiday.

Sunday 21st January - Short day skiing

Alan became angry as he struggled to get his right hand into his ski mitten. At one point he nearly punched the wall. His anger at himself shocked me. He was normally such a placid person. I recalled being told not to worry about such outbursts - it was Alan's frustration coming out.

It was a windy day with snow showers. Several chairlifts up the mountain were closed. In search of decent conditions, Alan and I took a bus to a lower part of the valley. On the way I smiled when Alan announced, "I feel happy," We loved ski holidays. Our entire first date had been spent talking about ski resorts.

After lunch with *The Ski Gang* in their hotel, we took a chairlift up the mountain and skied a long blue run back down. Alan became tired so we finished early and spent the afternoon chatting and drinking crazy priced beer.

Monday 22nd January - The end of a tradition

The weather was a bit better, but conditions up the mountain were tough. Phil fell first. Sarah and I both fell. Unusually Alan had two falls. Also, unusually, he needed us to help him get up. At lunchtime Alan became frustrated over something trivial. Later, he apologised to me, saying, "People offering to help me is irritating." We decided he should tell our friends he would ask for help if he needed it.

We stopped skiing early as Alan was exhausted. We found a nice café and had tea and cake. Alan had been told he could eat anything he wanted. My excuse for indulging was I needed to keep my strength up to care for him!

Après-ski drinks with *The Ski Gang* took place in Bobby's Bar. I played pool and air hockey with Sarah and shared my fears about Alan with her. She was very good at consoling me when my tears inevitably came. Over dinner, Alan became tearful when I told him, "My life was unfulfilled before I met you. I'm not looking forward to being on my own again." He shared, "I am worried about not being able to get my glove on. My legs felt weak before the falls." All I could do was to suggest "Let's take things one day at a time."

Tuesday 23rd January - A great day's skiing
At the top of the first chairlift there was freezing fog. I was worried this could cause a problem for all of us, especially Alan. As it happened, Alan safely went down the first run and the next one. He had always had excellent technique and today he had good strength. I was amazed how much skiing Alan managed. It was good to see him so happy. During the day I spotted three people using specially adapted ski chairs. I wondered who might be thinking what I was - would Alan be able to use one of these in the future?

Wednesday 24th January - Ouch!
We got up early because Angela and David were coming across from Zell at 9am. On arrival, Angela gave me a huge hug which made me cry. We had a good day skiing in the sun, but the slopes were very chopped up, making skiing difficult. We didn't see it happen but Sarah had a nasty fall.

In the après-ski bar back in the village, I slipped on the metal bar of the bar stool. I fell awkwardly, catching my right side, arm and cheek on the corner of the table as I fell onto the hard floor. Everyone in the bar gasped, then the room went silent. Very quickly the waitress helped me up. My ribs hurt a lot. An icepack was applied.

After dinner Alan and I chatted with Andy and Ruth about Alan's MND. I was pleased Alan had become more comfortable discussing his illness. The pain in my ribs was intense. It was difficult to sleep.

Thursday 25th January - Careful slow dancing
It was a lovely sunny day, but skiing was not possible for me. The staff at the pharmacy confirmed it was likely I had broken a rib and sold me a strapping to wrap around my rib cage, providing it with support. I felt like an idiot. It was

always embarrassing going home from such a holiday with a self-inflicted injury. Also, I was angry I would not be able to ski with Alan.

Later in the morning we had alfresco coffee with Julie (the non-skier in *The Ski Gang*). She gave us ideas and tips in respect of our forthcoming trip to Vietnam. Early evening, Alan and I walked up to *The Ski Gang's* hotel and listened to the Elvis and Tom Jones tribute singer. We managed a little Ceroc dancing, even though I needed to hold my sore ribs with one hand. Alan's weak right arm flopped from my waist and dangled by his side most of the time. We must have looked like a right cranky old couple!

Before the night was over Alan and I had a slow dance to "Can't help falling in love with you." He felt good in my arms. Even though I was in some discomfort, I didn't want the music to stop. I wanted this moment to go on forever.

Friday 26th January - Last day in Austria

Alan went skiing with Dave and Angela after I vowed not to worry about him. How ironic! Alan was able to go skiing, but I couldn't because of my physical incapacity!

After a leisurely breakfast I read some of *Me Before You*. It was about a young woman caring for a previously active man who had been crippled in an accident. Although it was just a novel, it provided me with some insight into caring for someone struggling to come to terms with life in a wheelchair.

Non-skiing friend, Julie and I enjoyed a pre-birthday afternoon tea at a stylish hotel. We ate delicious cakes while she explained how her family had coped when her dad had his stroke. A useful conversation. The therapist had to work carefully around my delicate ribs during my massage (another pre-birthday treat).

To my relief Alan, *The Ski Gang* and Angela and David, all turned up safely at the fateful après-ski bar. Angela and Bev gave me birthday gifts. There were hugs all round when Angela and Dave left us. "I've enjoyed this week," Alan declared while preparing for bed. I was pleased because we had another ski trip booked in March. I hoped my ribs would be better by then and his body would not be any worse.

Saturday 27th January - My sixty first birthday

We got up at 5:30am ready for the coach pick up at 6:40am. As I boarded the bus *The Ski Gang* burst into song "Happy Birthday to you... happy birthday to you..." Nice. The day ended with a fish and chips supper and a bottle of red wine - medicine for me!

Sunday 28th January - Ribs still hurting

The pain in my ribs was no better, so Alan and I went to A&E at Warwick Hospital. An X-ray showed no damage to my lungs, thank goodness, but yes, the ribs were cracked. I was told to rest and protect the injury until it healed.

Tuesday 30th January - Sunderland football team arrives in town

John and Chris Cooper came round for lunch and later, Alan's family arrived. Lifelong supporters of Sunderland football team, John, Ben and Tom took Alan to see his team take on Birmingham City at St Andrew's. Alan was not only proud of his team, but he was also proud that their supporters were incredibly loyal. His commitment to things he cared for was one of the things I loved about him.

While the men were at the game, I went to my friend Teresa's house. A Japanese style birthday dinner was cooked for me by their visitor from Japan. Teresa's husband, Phil, was also at the football match, supporting the other team!

Wednesday 31st January - A bad end to the month

My friend Jo and I had a quick informal post birthday lunch at a garden centre. We laughed as we recalled happy times when we were both single and used to go on skiing and golfing holidays together. Those days seemed like a long way off, but it was good to remember them. I felt able to share my deepest feelings with Jo, having known her for longer than I had known any of my other girlfriends.

At 3pm, Alan and I met Lesley, the physiotherapist, at the Marie Curie Hospice, for tests. "You have still got some strength left in your right shoulder, but the forearm downwards is not good," Lesley confirmed. "Your core muscles are weak... you need to be aware of your posture," she told us. "In time you will not be able to sit upright and will need a special wheelchair capable of tilting you backwards." And, finally, "It's no longer wise to do one hour work-out sessions at the gym."

None of Lesley's news was a surprise, but we were both a bit numb after the meeting. Raising his eyebrows Alan said, "It is what it is. We will have to deal with it." I felt a hole open up inside me and found it hard to be so pragmatic.

Thursday 1st February - First lung function tests

At Coventry Walsgrave Hospital we meet Dr Ali, the Respiratory Clinic Consultant who would be responsible for regularly checking the effectiveness of Alan's breathing muscles. Since diagnosis, I had been concerned about the rate at which Alan's breathing would deteriorate.

Various tests revealed Alan's baseline. He had 88% of lung function left. Dr Ali did not seem to be overly concerned. Alan asked lots of questions. I felt devastated.

Focusing on driving the car, Alan said, "I don't want to end up like Professor Stephen Hawking. I don't want a tube coming out of my throat". Without a tracheotomy it would probably be the weakening of Alan's breathing muscles that would cause the end of his life. On a subsequent meeting with our MND nurse, we were informed a tracheotomy is not offered as standard to MND patients in our area. Despite this assurance, Alan insisted on having his wishes noted on his *Do Not Resuscitate* form to avoid the risk of a tracheotomy being done automatically in an emergency.

Although I respected his wishes, I was disappointed. It didn't matter to me how many tubes went in or out of Alan's body as long as he was alive and was able to derive some joy in life. However, I didn't know how I would feel if I were in his position.

AUTHOR'S NOTE

Motor neurone disease (MND) causes muscles to gradually weaken. Over time, people with MND lose their ability to move, speak and breathe. Ventilation, using a close fitting mask (Non-invasive ventilation: NIV) or a tube in the neck (tracheotomy/invasive ventilation: TV) can help support breathing. As their condition worsens, people use ventilation for longer, until they cannot breathe without it. They can then decide whether they want to keep using ventilation. Stopping or withdrawing ventilation would result in the person with MND dying quickly.

Friday 2nd February - Time for a man bag

On a bright, fresh day in Birmingham, we met up with my ex-work colleague, Donna and her boyfriend Tim. They were genuinely interested in MND and asked lots of questions over lunch. Alan had reluctantly decided it was time to buy a man bag. Despite finding a nice one in John Lewis, Alan was unsure, so we set off home man bagless.

Monday 5th February - Right arm no longer working

As we prepared lunch, Alan admitted, "I cannot help you make the sandwiches anymore. My right arm doesn't work at all now." I hugged him hard and fought back the tears trying to burst out of me.

Tuesday 6th February - Parts of me were dying too

Working in our Amersham office it was draining having to explain the current situation to the many people who asked after Alan's progress. My boss announced he would be retiring soon. I was not concerned. I was probably going to be stopping work soon myself.

Back home Alan reported, "I was weak and uncoordinated on the treadmill at the gym, so used the cross trainer instead." I reminded him, "The physio said not to push yourself too hard," but suspected the advice was a waste of time. Alan had always pushed himself. It would be a hard habit for him to break.

I watched Alan as he prepared dinner. His right arm hung down, useless, by his side, while he used his left hand to stir the food. Tears came to my eyes, followed by an overwhelming urge to make a video for Facebook. It was almost as if the pain I felt would be more bearable if everyone could see what grieved me. Sometimes I felt parts of me were dying as pieces of him stopped working.

From the beginning of his illness Alan had been keen to raise awareness of what living with MND was like. He quickly agreed to being filmed, so I grabbed my phone before he changed his mind, and started filming.

Me: "It's the 6th of February. On this day 100 years ago, women got the vote thanks to the work of suffragettes like Emmeline Pankhurst."

Alan interjected, "Equality - so get your ruddy apron on and start cooking and do your bit."

Unphased, I continued, "So what's happening in Carter Castle right now is that Alan is cooking the dinner."

Alan: "So in 100 years we've gone backwards, men."

I chuckled and asked, "What are you doing now, Al?"

He replied, "Well, I'm making a chicken curry. It's an adaptation of a vegetable curry that we had in the freezer. I've fried up some chicken in some walnut oil and a little bit of garlic-infused oil to add to the vegetable curry. We're having it with some brown rice. It should be jolly nice I think."

Me: "So why are you stirring it with your left hand?"

Alan: "I'm stirring it with my left hand because my right hand doesn't work. Motor neurone disease has affected my right hand in such a way that it's useless just now. It's probably lost 85% of its capability, so it's just a bit of a passenger these days. So, I am doing more with my left hand. I seem to do it naturally now without thinking about it."

Me: "Hmmm… and how do you feel about that…. honestly?"

Alan: "I don't feel brilliantly about it, but that's the hand we've been dealt. I've just got to get on with it really. I'm sure there's lots of people who are a lot worse off than I am."

Me: "Do you have a message for the world?"

Alan chuckled nervously, "Ha, ha, yes. Find a cure for motor neurone disease."

Me: "Any other messages? Anything you want the world to do in your absence?"

Alan: "Hmmm. Live peacefully and happily."

Me: "Uh hum. Okay. Well, I think we'll leave it on that note. Thank you for dinner, Al. Love you."

Alan: "Love you too."

Wednesday 7th February - Sometimes it's hard to ask for help
Using his left hand, Alan painted the ceiling in the conservatory which left him exhausted. Alan didn't want to leave any major domestic tasks unfinished, but he paid a high price as physical work took so much out of him.

Alan went to bed quite early. I stayed up late listening to music that made me cry. I posted several melancholy songs on Facebook. It was as if I were trying to communicate my need for emotional support through the lyrics of songs, in the hope people would pick up on my pain. It was always hard to ask for help when I needed it. Late into the night was always the hardest time.

Eventually I went to bed around 2am, but I could not sleep. I felt terrible.

Thursday 8th February – Poems
Alan barked at me when I made a mistake doing up his watch just before we

set out to meet Julie, the Macmillan nurse, at the Marie Curie Hospice. On the journey, sensing my mood was low Alan asked, "What's up?"

"Macmillan's were heavily involved with my dad's care before he died in 2001. It disturbs me to think you need them now."

By the time we got to the hospice I was distressed and tense. Julie was great. She organised several things, including:

- A fast track application for Personal Independence Payments,
- A blue badge application,
- A referral for complementary therapy,
- A referral for grief counselling,
- A link in with local district nurses

Lesley, the physio, gave us a wrist rest for Alan's right hand.
Later that day, a poem came to me:

YOUR BODY
Your body bends and buckles, as you struggle with daily life.
You are still independent, and I'm trying to be.

This next poem was written after reading peoples' posts on Facebook.

FEAR AND ANGER
I don't want to hear,
About your happy life.
Can't cope with your days of bliss.

It's hard to watch the world go by,
People doing this and that.
Days like that for us are numbered,
Filled with challenge and strangeness.

We make memories for when you're gone,
And draw on others' kindness.

Will one sided memories bring me joy,
When you're no longer here?
Can we enjoy your remaining time,
Without the constant fear?

The fear that comes from knowing,
There is worse to face ahead.

An uncertain future,
That fills my heart with dread.

I know I am not the only one,
Who will miss you when you're gone,
But there are too many moments,
When I feel lost and terribly alone.

Those moments sometimes fleeting,
Till I look at you and see,
The most precious person in the world,
Fading away in front of me

Friday 9th February - Help needed with DIY

Sue, the wife of a neighbour Alex, popped in bringing a box of chocolates. Her kindness always made me feel emotional. My sister, Clare, and her husband David arrived after lunch to put up mirrors and pictures in the newly decorated bedroom. Such tasks were beyond Alan now.

The 'hotel bedroom' was mostly beige with statement black and gold curtains and a stylish matching throw. The final touch was a small black pillow bearing the words "All you need is love" in gold. Originally we had planned to move into this room after spending ten years in the other main bedroom. Now it was ready for us, I wondered how many nights we would be about to share it before Alan could no longer climb the stairs.

Not long after Clare and David left, Andy Gould, a golfer from our club, arrived. It was good to see how much Alan enjoyed the surprise visit. "When I get frustrated about not being able to play golf anymore," Alan told us, "I imagine myself hitting perfect shots, and scoring birdies and pars, even where I have never scored them before!" We all enjoyed a fish and chip supper before Andy headed home.

AUTHOR'S NOTE

When Alan was well, it was a tradition for us to play nine holes of golf after work on a Friday, followed by a fish and chips.

Saturday 10th February - Weakening core muscles affecting walking

Alan, mum and I travelled to Birmingham by train to see a ballet. The five-minute walk from the train to the theatre was difficult for Alan because his core muscles were so weak. Mum and I looked at each other with concern. We arrived home from the matinee, ate pizza and watched Six Nations rugby matches before Alan and I decided to sleep in the hotel bedroom.

Monday 12th February - Germ of panic

On arriving home from work, Alan looked glum and said, "I think my voice is beginning to fail." He also expressed concern at the speed at which his symptoms were developing. I too was worried but spared his feelings by not voicing my concerns.

It was less than three months since diagnosis. I had hoped the prognosis was wrong but now I feared six months might be all we would have. I tried not to be scared but a germ of panic had lodged in my gut and was beginning to grow.

Wednesday 14th February - Valentine's surprises

When I arrived in the kitchen for breakfast, I found a huge bouquet of flowers. They were from Alan and filled two vases.

We had breakfast and opened our cards. Interestingly we had both written almost the same - how much we valued having each other by our side.

In a clinic, in Chelmsley Wood, Alan's dietician, Kaye, stressed the importance of keeping Alan's weight up and talked about overcoming swallowing difficulties by using a drinks thickener. To help maintain Alan's weight, Kaye gave us a recipe for a milkshake drink which including Nesquik for flavouring, double cream, plus the thickener. Also, she told us about nutritional liquid feeds which could be taken orally if eating normal food became difficult. They could be delivered directly into the tummy via a PEG tube if swallowing failed. Alan was not keen on having a PEG tube fitted, even though without it, malnutrition would kill him before MND did.

On our way home, I surprised Alan with afternoon tea that I had pre-booked at our local garden centre. We relaxed on leather settees and enjoyed sandwiches and cakes - all in the interests of keeping Alan's weight up!

My final surprise was tickets to see *Shrek*, the musical, in Birmingham. It was a funny and uplifting show. Just the sort of light relief we needed.

AUTHOR'S NOTE

PEG - Percutaneous Endoscopic Gastrostomy - a tube is passed into a patient's stomach through the abdominal wall, most commonly to provide a means of feeding (and liquid drugs) when oral intake is not possible.

Thursday 15th February - To move or not to move?

Alan and I drove to Hampton in Arden and looked around a large bungalow which could be adapted for a wheelchair user. Back home we began to think staying at Carter Castle was probably our best option. A stairlift would make everything easier. Or so we thought.

Friday 16th February - What I know

I woke up at 3:45am and could not get back to sleep. I could hear Alan's erratic breathing. I worried about it and the prospect of him losing his voice soon. The thought of never hearing his voice, and watching him silently sitting in social situations, was distressing. I could not imagine how frustrating it would be for him. Eventually I went downstairs and composed a poem.

WHAT I KNOW

I know one day your arms won't work,
But I'm not thinking of that.

I know one day your legs will fail you,
But I'm not thinking of that.

I know one day you will lose your swallow,
But I'm not thinking of that.

I know one day your voice will leave you,
But I'm not thinking of that.

I know one day you will take your last breath,
But I'm not thinking of that.

I am thinking how much I love you,
And how I will never love like this again.

Alan came into the lounge, "What are you doing?" I read him the poem. He comforted me as I cried. We talked about his deterioration, in particular the possible loss of his speech. We talked about the lady we had met at the MND support meeting who had no physical movement, no speech, was wearing a neck support, but looked calm. Alan said, "I think she has accepted her situation." Before we went back to bed he reminded me of the serenity prayer which he found useful.

'Lord, help me to accept the things I cannot change, have the courage to change the things I can, and the wisdom to know the difference between the two.'

During the day we viewed another unsuitable bungalow. Maybe living downstairs at Carter Castle would be a better option?

We drove to Simon and Rachel Beacham's house for pre-dinner drinks. Their children were there, plus work colleagues Jo and Paul, Wendy, Chris and Christina Woolley, Norma and Dennis. At the restaurant selected to celebrate the creation of ABC Solutions by Alan and Simon in 1998, Rachel produced a 20th birthday cake made of cupcakes. Simon and Alan blew out the candles together. Alan was overwhelmed by the gifts he received. He was a modest man who had never really understood how popular he was but, on this evening, he began to realise how much people liked him.

Saturday 17th February - The big question - move or adapt?
We viewed another bungalow. The whole issue of moving house versus adapting our current home was disturbing me all day. In bed, after midnight, I posted our dilemma on Facebook. Replies were overwhelmingly in favour of staying in our own home and adapting it.

AUTHOR'S NOTE
Since Alan's diagnosis, I had joined three Facebook MND forums. They were useful for posing questions and learning practical solutions to issues caused by MND. It was always distressing seeing stories about the loss of a husband, wife, mother, father, brother, sister or friend. Even though everyone with MND suffered differently, these forums helped me feel less alone and provided a safe place for me to vent my deepest fears and feelings.

Sunday 18th February - Sheffield here we come
Unfortunately, the pretty route we had chosen to drive to Sheffield was obscured by bad weather.

As we did the long walk downhill from the car park to the hotel Alan seemed off. "You okay?" I asked. "I am tired and have a headache." He went straight to sleep as soon as he got into bed.

Monday 19th February - Big day in Sheffield
We rose at 7am. No breakfast for Alan because he was due to have blood tests. It was a difficult walk for Alan back up the hill to the car park. We would stay somewhere else next time. We arrived early at the Royal Hallamshire Hospital, so we asked the drug trial nurse to take a photograph of us in our bright blue MND tee shirts.

Dr Bell went through Alan's medical history and the details of the MIROCALS drug trial Patient Consent form. "All the fluids we will take from you will be sent to various research labs around the world," he told us. He checked that the criteria for going onto the trial were all met, including having been diagnosed within six months, being under age sixty-five and not being on Riluzole tablets. We were told: "Once all the tests are done, you can go on Riluzole and then, assuming there are no adverse reactions, you will be randomly selected by computer for the trial drug - Interleukin-2 - or sugar water." No one at the hospital would know what Alan was on. Alan would have injections, given by me, once a day for five days, every month during the two-year trial period. There would also be regular blood tests and further lumbar punctures to endure. Alan agreed to proceed.

The drug trial nurse took eighteen phials of blood from Alan's arm. Tony Hancock would have been mortified! She then did some breathing tests on him before we could go for lunch. Next Alan did some mental capacity tests which he flew through. Then came the lumbar puncture procedure.

Alan was probably more relaxed at this stage than I was. He laid on his side while the nurse tried to introduce a long, fine, needle into his lower spine. It was difficult to watch but I was fascinated. I felt slightly sick when I saw blood coming from Alan's back. Was that normal? The nurse could not succeed with the fine needle so tried a bigger one! In the end she went to get assistance.

Dr Bell completed the procedure showing us the extracted liquid. Who knew cerebral fluid looked like water! It was strange to think something so innocuous could help researchers understand what was going on in Alan's body. After a two-hour rest - which was compulsory after a lumbar puncture - Alan went for an electrocardiogram (ECG) and a chest x-ray. I drove us to Pauline and Simon's house where we had dinner and retired to bed totally exhausted.

AUTHOR'S NOTE
For younger readers, Tony Hancock was a comedian who made a classic sketch about giving blood. *youtube.com/watch?v=zcZChdM0Oil*

Tuesday 20th February - Getting news out with minimum hassle
Lying in my single bed, I could see Alan was already awake. Without a word, he got into my bed and snuggled up tight. Suddenly the emotion of everything hit me. To go on the trial Alan had delayed taking Riluzole. It felt like a big thing that he could now take one small daily tablet, even though its benefits were minimal.

Alan spent the morning relaxing while I posted our latest news on Facebook. Back at Carter Castle we updated our diary with dates for visits to Sheffield, dates for regular phone calls from the drug trial nurse and the dates for blood tests to check Alan's liver and kidney functions.

AUTHOR'S NOTE

Riluzole is an old drug used to slow down progression of respiratory deterioration by two or three months. Facebook became an increasingly useful medium for disseminating information about Alan's progress. For friends and family not on Facebook I chose to send out a blind copy 'round robin' email.

Wednesday 21st February - Riluzole started!

Alan was at home without me for the first time in ages because I had to go into Birmingham for a course. On my return home, Alan gave me a big hug and lots of kisses. He had been to the gym as planned but had not made it to the monthly MND support meeting at the Marie Curie Hospice. After two days of taking Riluzole, there were no signs of side effects.

Friday 23rd February - Get an occupational therapist involved

Fiona, the OT from the Marie Curie Hospice visited us. She advised against fitting a stairlift. She feared in our case it would not be used for long. Instead, she suggested we prepare for a few stages ahead by turning our dining room into a bedroom and building a wet room in the garage.

Fiona also suggested we needed to build a ramp off the wet room to provide the means for wheelchair access in and out of the house. Her experience was invaluable. She gave us hope when she said she knew people with only the use of a thumb or small head movements who could still use a computer. Fiona mentioned Alan might need a 'tilt in space' wheelchair and a shower chair because of weak core muscles. It was unsettling and depressing thinking about what the future might bring and hard to take in everything Fiona was saying.

Alan busied himself getting the house tidy and clean ready for friends visiting later. I started to worry about what it would be like in the future, looking after the house myself, caring for Alan and being responsible for my mum too. One friend, Alison, was good with Alan. Like some of our other male friends, Adrian, went very quiet during conversations about Alan's health.

AUTHOR'S NOTE

Up until meeting Fiona, I was ignorant of the role of an OT. Fiona had a keen interest in helping people with MND and would remain involved with us till end of Alan's life.

Saturday 24th February - The "one"

Alan and I went to the engagement party of my nephew, Andrew, and his fiancée, Lauren. My sister Clare and I both cried when talking about how my married life to Alan was due to be cut short. Back in 2006, Clare was the first person in my family I talked to about meeting Alan. At that time, she excitedly said, "He's the one."

"How do you know?" I asked.

"Your face lit up when you talked about him."

During Alan's illness I confided in her many times that I was afraid that losing him would break my spirit.

Monday 26th February - Anxieties about coping

Looking online at wheelchairs agitated me, so I called our friend Andy Boyes, who worked for a wheelchair company. He offered to call Alan to talk about wheelchair customisation. It occurred to me I was struggling emotionally and psychologically. I began to worry how I would cope on our ski holiday in March if Alan's legs gave way on the slopes. It was difficult not being able to share my deepest fears with Alan, but I didn't want to distress him. Also, I didn't want to become a burden to friends. I felt isolated, confused, worried, heartbroken and scared all at once.

MARCH 2018

Thursday 1st March - Walking getting very difficult

At mum's flat I met her OT to talk about mum's care needs. Coincidentally the OT's uncle had died from MND, so she was very supportive of my request for extra help for mum. Back at home Alan said, "It was hard work walking to the post office today."

Every time Alan said something about his deterioration, it felt like I had been hit in the stomach with a hammer. As a competent individual normally, I was not used to feeling so helpless and went to bed feeling disconsolate.

Saturday 3rd March - Off skiing, or are we?

We arrived at Birmingham airport at 4:15am only to face a three hour wait at check-in. Snow had fallen heavily overnight. Our 6am flight had been delayed to at least 4pm because our inbound flight had been redirected to Manchester. "What do you most like to eat Al?" I asked to kill some time. His list included steak and kidney pie, roast pork, and sausages. He added, "I enjoy nibbling on your neck too." Unfortunately, his joke made us both burst into tears.

There was a long wait for our skis at Geneva airport and a long walk up a hill to the coach. Alan struggled, so I asked the tour company rep for help with our baggage. Alan and I slept on the journey to Morzine.

Our hotel was halfway up a mountain, so the bubble car had to be opened specially to transport the dozen or so of us staying up there. Other holidaymakers saw me struggling with the bags and offered help. I thought how embarrassing this must be for Alan who had always been the first to assist others in need.

At 1:30am we finally got to our room, totally exhausted. This ski holiday had been booked before we knew Alan was ill. He had insisted that he wanted to go, rather than cancel it. It had started badly and, I feared, worse was to come.

Sunday 4th March - First day on the slopes

We slept until 8:20am resulting in us being late for breakfast. The views from the dining room were stunning. If this was to be our last ski holiday it was not a bad choice.

As we walked to the ski locker Alan became angry and lashed out with, "I am a fumbling bastard," and "I am beginning to think coming skiing was a bad idea." Despite his outburst, we put on our ski boots and carried our skis out onto the slopes. Within seconds he said, "I don't think I can do this. Maybe I should ask for a refund on my pass." He was scared.

"Try to do at least one run Al," I urged. "If you feel unable to go on, we will stop."

We chose an easy looking blue run. Alan jetted off and surprisingly went a long way before he stopped. We managed three more easy blue runs before having lunch high up the mountain. Shortly after lunch we went back to our hotel and both fell asleep while watching TV.

I was really pleased Alan had managed some skiing. It was clear he was not going to manage the whole week. At least, he would have felt the wind on his face and his skis sliding across the snow a few more times, before he retired from the hobby he loved so much. It was also obvious to me now, part of my role would be that of motivator and provider of moral support.

We both ended up sobbing after talking about favourite past ski holidays over dinner. "If we had known this was going to be our last ski holiday Al, where would you have chosen?"

He had two suggestions: "Where we had our first ski holiday together, Val Gardena in Italy, and the Three Valleys in France because of its vastness."

When our rep, Leanne, came to see us, she confirmed it was possible to exchange a ski pass for a walker's pass if necessary. She held my hand when I started crying, until I was calm again. After dinner, Alan and I talked about the worst and best hotels we had stayed in on any holiday. "The worst one," Alan said, "was the one on Sunset Strip in Hollywood." The best he said was, "Four Seasons, Mauritius, where we had our honeymoon." Then he started to cry.

Monday 5th March - Alan's skiing days come to an end
Alan and I made it onto the slopes around 10am. It was a beautiful day - deep blue sky, tons of white snow everywhere, very little breeze and snow kissed pine trees galore. We tackled two of the blue runs we had done on Sunday. Alan rested at a bar at the bottom of the valley while I took the nearby chairlift to the top of the red run beside it. As I travelled down the wide-open piste I thought, if this is to be Alan's last run, it is a beautiful one.

Alan struggled to stand up from his deck chair when I returned, but he did manage to do the red run. At the end of it I made a video.

Me: "How do you feel today Alan?"

Alan: "I'm still apprehensive about my skiing so I am just going to take it steady. I'm very weak in the legs. My right arm is useless. I'm putting turns in on blue runs now which is unheard of."

80

Me: "What's making you feel apprehensive?"

Alan: "I am worried about falling over and not being able to get up again. Also, I am concerned I may not be able to react quickly enough if someone cuts across in front of me."

Grinning, I said, "Don't worry, if you fall over, I'll pick you up."

Chuckling, Alan replied, "That's very good of you."

Realising it would be impossible for me to haul him up if he fell, I added, "Or maybe I'll just scream for help."

We both laughed.

We took the chairlift back up the mountain and had a lazy lunch outside a restaurant in the warm sunshine. Alan turned to me. "I am finding it too tough now. I'm going to quit on it." His tone told me he didn't mean just for the day, he meant forever. My heart sank.

As we disembarked from the final chairlift back to our hotel, a French man and his son crashed into us. We all went down hard on the ice. I landed on my shoulder (which still hurt a week later). I pulled myself up thinking, tomorrow I will still be able to ski, but my dear Alan will not.

The idea of skiing solo for the rest of the week - and on future ski holidays - was incredibly dismal. Like a lot of things in life, skiing holidays are always better when shared with someone, so you can talk about them days, months and years after.

Before bed we spent an hour in the bar where people were singing karaoke. Alan started to cry at the Christina Perri song, *A Thousand Years.*

Tuesday 6th March - End of life care
Snow was falling so Alan and I had a lazy morning at the hotel. Around 11am, we took a lift down to the village where it was raining and walked around. We came upon a ski and bike shop called 'Alan'. Alan smiled from ear to ear as I took his photograph standing under the shop's sign.

We stopped at a hotel for a hot chocolate when Alan found walking hard. It was a nice place, so we agreed to stay for lunch. We were the first people in the restaurant. Three hours later, after pizza, salad and a nice bottle of white wine, we were the last out! Over lunch we talked calmly about Alan's end of life care. "I want to remain at home rather than die in a hospital or hospice," he confirmed.

We took a welcome afternoon nap back at the hotel. Live jazz was being played in the bar after dinner. We were both calm and relaxed, which was a bit bizarre after such a significant discussion over lunch.

Wednesday 7th March - Practical matters

During the night I was awake between 2am and 4am thinking about Alan and trying to work out how I could resign from my job. Over breakfast we discussed how we might adapt our home. We would need a TV aerial in the dining room if it were to become Alan's bedroom. Fiona's idea of making a wet room in the garage, with a ramp out of the house via the garage, looked viable.

After breakfast Alan gave his ski pass to the rep and insisted I go skiing. We had an emotional goodbye as I set off onto the slopes without him. It felt strange covering slopes Alan and I had been on, so I didn't stay out long. To stop myself overthinking things I made some videos. Alan enjoyed seeing my amateur documentary, which was a relief as I had worried about causing him hurt.

After dinner, our rep confirmed that she had secured a part refund of Alan's ski pass and had exchanged it for a walker's pass. So that was it. Alan was officially never going to ski again.

Thursday 8th March - Brave adventures without Alan

Another night passed with me thinking about Alan coming to the end of his skiing life. Rather than staying local, I skied down to the village, travelled across town and took the lift up to Avoriaz. I was well outside my comfort zone, but it felt better than skiing on Alan's last runs. The conditions in Avoriaz were excellent. The sky was bright blue and the slopes well-groomed. Alan would have loved it. I made several videos for him. During a snack stop, I created a poignant photograph of my crossed skis sticking out of the snow with the mountains in the distance. It became part of a posting on Facebook where I told everyone Alan had hung up his skis.

On a long chairlift, I tearfully told a nice English couple why I was skiing alone. It was often easier sharing our story with strangers, because I could be more honest about how I felt. Alan and I ate a late lunch at the hut across the piste from our hotel, sharing a bottle of rosé. Due to lack of sleep, the altitude, stress or maybe too much wine, I developed a headache. I took some painkillers and had a nap before dinner.

Friday 9th March - The birth of Alan's 'Perfect World'

It was a grey morning. I skied locally during the morning, at one point taking a wrong turn and ending up in Les Gets. Unfortunately, Alan's pass did not allow him to travel up to the mountain to Avoriaz. Plan B was eating at an Italian restaurant in Morzine village with great views of the mountains. We shared a large pizza, a plate of chips, a bottle of white wine and a chocolate dessert. "Life's good," Alan said, "It's the disease that's the problem."

While in the town, we made enquiries about the specialist disability equipment at the ESF office. It cost €100 for two hours to hire a ski instructor to steer a specially adapted chair. Alan thought it was a lot of money. I felt it was well worth it. We discovered people with disabilities qualified for a 70% discount on their ski pass! It didn't occur to me Alan would be far too ill to enjoy the mountains next ski season.

"How do you fill your time while I am skiing?" I asked Alan over dinner.

"I imagine myself in a world where I am without disability - a perfect world where I cycle on open roads with no potholes, play great golf shots on lush fairways and ski on beautiful pistes. Also, I have been thinking about all the people I know and wondering how many will come to my funeral." We both ended up crying.

I found it difficult to sleep after our intense conversation. I suddenly felt a strong inclination to stop work as soon as possible. Time with Alan was beginning to be more precious. I fell asleep imagining myself discussing my resignation with my boss.

AUTHOR'S NOTE

A lot of my time was spent thinking of ways to give Alan hope. Without hope we had nothing. Keeping Alan's morale up, while his body shut down around him, was very important. Alan's mental strength amazed me. The perfect world daydreams he started in Morzine would sustain his mental health right up till the day he died.

Saturday 10th March - Airport special assistance needed

We had to get up at 5am for the coach at 6:20am. There was an emotional farewell with our rep, Leanne. We took the télécabine down the mountain for the final time. At Geneva airport, special assistance staff did an excellent job of looking after Alan. I was pleased we had the foresight to book them once we realised Alan would struggle at the airport. "I feel like a VIP," Alan declared when we found ourselves being deposited in the Pilots' lounge before boarding our plane.

Getting on the plane with various injured skiers was less glamorous. A special vehicle hoisted us up to a door at the back of the aircraft cockpit. It was not a glamorous process, but it was very effective. At Birmingham airport we had special assistance again. I made a mental note when the chatty lady assisting us said, "Alicante and the Caribbean are the most popular destinations for wheelchair users."

Later, I drove mum to my sister Clare's house, where I presented Clare with her fiftieth birthday gift. Clare cried when we talked about Alan. Her husband, Dave, offered ideas for finding a buyer for Alan's MGB. Mum was very chatty. She had been having carers all week and it was working out well. Once mum was deposited in her flat, Alan and I watched recordings of Six Nations rugby matches and ate a takeaway curry. We slept in the 'hotel room'.

AUTHOR'S NOTE
Special assistance at both airports was first class. I had personally used it following a skiing accident in the past, so I knew exactly what to expect, including fast tracking through security and passport control.

Sunday 11th March - Mother's Day
We set off early for Sunderland. On the three-hour journey we chatted about me resigning and taking early retirement in June. On arrival, we took Alan's mum out to lunch at one of her favourite hotels.

AUTHOR'S NOTE
We had to manage Alan's mum's understanding of Alan's condition very carefully so as not to alarm her. Joan was ninety-six. We worried she might think she could outlive her only son.

Thursday 15th March - Telling my team
In Plymouth I told my team I might be leaving the company soon. I felt it was important to manage their expectations. They were not surprised and were incredibly supportive.

Friday 16th March - Blue Badge
At the Genting Arena, we used the disability blue badge for the first time and parked in the wheelchair users' car park. The struggle up the steps to our seats was worth it. Alan smiled a lot during the Joe Bonamassa show. Next time, I would suggest we use a wheelchair and sit in the special seating area.

Wednesday 21st March - A scary glimpse at the future

Alan and I went to the MND support group meeting at the Marie Curie Hospice. It was shocking seeing Brian now wearing a mask attached to a non-invasive ventilator. We met Melvin, who was also struggling with his breathing but who was not on the ventilator mask full time. Melvin's wife, Wendy, told me that Mel had also developed some dementia as a result of MND.

Alan was agitated and frustrated when we reached home. While washing up, he smashed a sieve against the sink. I didn't know what to say. It was impossible to imagine what he was feeling. I tried to imagine what it was like for him looking at the men earlier, seeing what may be ahead for him. I wondered if I should go to these meetings without him in the future.

AUTHOR'S NOTE

Brian died five months after Alan. Mel was diagnosed in 2013 and had been on a ventilator from early on. He died in March 2021.

Thursday 22nd March - Preparing for voice loss

An OT, supplied by the NHS, visited us. Her mother had died from MND about two years ago. Later we met, Katie, an NHS speech and language therapist. She explained Alan could have a synthesised version of his voice made using voice banking. All he had to do was record 1600 pre-set statements which would capture elements of his speech! The final meeting of the day was with our financial adviser, Patrick.

AUTHOR'S NOTE

Voice banking was useful because it meant that when Alan would need to use a machine to speak for him, it would sound like him, rather than a robot. Professor Stephen Hawking, who had MND, was instrumental in developing such technology.

It was essential to capture Alan's voice early before it became too weak. Alan was successful banking his voice, but the big mistake we made was not practicing with the technology while Alan could still speak. By the time his voice stopped working he was too weak to learn how to use it effectively. Since starting to write this book, advances in voice banking have been made, so the process is now much less arduous.

Friday 23rd March - House adaptations

We had a busy morning. Firstly, the builder, Martin, came round to check if part of our garage could be converted into a wet room. His firm had built a wet room for his mother when she was diagnosed with MND. Then a man from the council arrived to fit a grab rail on the staircase wall.

I had a long telephone chat about my leaving options with the HR manager at my firm. She was incredibly sympathetic because she had nursed her father with MND. In the evening we went to a Blues Brothers show at the golf club. A lot of people caught up with Alan, some had only just heard his news.

Tuesday 27th March - Forming Alan's Army
At work in the Amersham office, various people said, "I don't know how you cope."

I explained, "Work feels like a safe haven... keeping busy here gives me a little break from worrying about Alan."

Viv and John had arrived by the time I made it home. Alan announced, "I want John to have my Levi's and Simon Beacham to have my bike." Alan and Simon had done many cycle rides together, including The Wessex 100 mile ride. It was hard hearing Alan talk about who was to have his possessions, but he was being practical and sorting things out while he could.

While I was at work Alan had seen his GP. Blood tests were okay, and the GP would help us sort out a non-invasive ventilator if we needed him to. Having heard horror stories from other families affected by MND, I realised we were lucky to have a supportive GP.

Before going to bed I set up a JustGiving page in respect of the September 10k run, with an initial target of £5,000. Viv confirmed that she wanted to join in. I felt excited about pulling together a group to run with me. 'Alan's Army' was beginning to form.

Wednesday 28th March - Not going to Dignitas
Viv and I went for a run before breakfast. Our physio, Leslie, visited to check up on Alan's progress. Alan could no longer stand up straight. I took photographs to help him see how his posture had changed. Lesley demonstrated what Alan needed to do to keep himself upright and also gave him exercises to help work his core muscles. I could see that he was beginning to treat these physio sessions like trips to the gym. He had found new ways to drive himself hard.

Later in the day we went to see the movie Three Billboards Outside Ebbing, Missouri. The scene where a key character committed suicide because he had cancer made me feel sick inside. I was worried it might give Alan the idea of going to Switzerland to end his life. We knew one person at the MND support group who had said he had already booked his place at Dignitas.

When we discussed the film, I was relieved Alan showed no interest in the idea of voluntarily shortening his life.

Friday 30th March - Choking episodes
We drove to the house of our friends, John and Bev. John offered to lend us a lightweight wheelchair that folded up neatly into the boot of the car. I wondered how Alan would feel about the idea of being pushed around in it.

En route to Wokingham, for a stay with Angela and David, we bought a packet of midget gems. It was my job to feed them to him as he drove. The packet was almost empty when he started choking. Terrifyingly, initially, he would not stop the car. He only pulled over when I shouted at him. He insisted the choke was random. Eating breakfast cereal recently had caused him to choke, so I suspected his swallowing muscles were weakening and that he was in denial.

Later in the day I carefully raised my concerns. "Al, it will not be helpful if you start to deny what's happening, or if you hide symptoms from me," I explained, "It's distressing seeing you choke."

I also suggested he let me drive more often. He agreed to be more open and to share the driving more equally in future.

Saturday 31st March - Remembering the Ice Bucket Challenge
I met Angela and David in April 2006, just before meeting Alan in the June. Like us they were golfers and skiers. We had enjoyed many ski holidays with them so had plenty of memories to talk about together. Ironically, I was with them when I did the ice bucket challenge.

AUTHOR'S NOTE
The ice bucket challenge originated in America raising funds for ALS (also known as Lou Gehrig's disease there, and as motor neurone disease in the UK). The campaign raised over $220 million. Part of that money raised in the UK funded our specialist MND nurse.

Sunday 1st April - Easter Sunday

During breakfast Angela and David gave us a handmade basket filled with various chocolate Easter eggs. On the drive home, Alan and I talked about the idea of him coming off the drug trial and increasing the dose of his Riluzole tablets. He chose to stay on the trial.

We briefly popped in to see my mum. Her behaviour had changed recently. She often accused people of hiding her handbag. I didn't understand much about vascular dementia and had no time to educate myself. We chose not to tell her much about Alan's condition in case she inadvertently told Alan's mum too much. I felt it was beginning to become impossible to try to look after mum and Alan allowing for their two differing sequences of decline.

While closing the garage door, I accidentally caught Alan's shoulder. I felt angry at myself for causing him injury. Before going to bed I checked the JustGiving fundraising page. We had already reached 25% of the target!

Tuesday 3rd April – Complementary therapy

Alan and I went to the Marie Curie Hospice for a meeting with Alyson, the social worker. It was unsettling listening to her talk about care package options. While at the hospice, we both had a massage from the complementary therapist. It was blissful!

Over dinner at Carol and Graham's we chatted about our forthcoming holiday to Vietnam and the three-week tour of Wales they were planning. A quick check on JustGiving before bed showed donations totalling £2,240 - 44% of target!

AUTHOR'S NOTE

Because of the degree of Alan's care needs we were eligible for care in the home funded by the state, provided by a company who would bid for the contract. We had been saving for retirement, so were lucky we had sufficient money to cover other costs and our lifestyle.
nhs.uk/conditions/social-care-and-support-guide/care-services-equipment-and-care-homes/care-and-support-you-can-get-for-free

Complementary and alternative medicine is treatment that falls outside mainstream healthcare. Generally, treatments can range from acupuncture and homeopathy, to aromatherapy and colonic irrigation. When a non-mainstream practice is used together with conventional medicine, it's considered 'complementary'. When a non-mainstream practice is used instead of conventional medicine, it's considered 'alternative'. At the Marie Curie Hospice, both Alan and I were offered complementary treatments.

Wednesday 4th April - MND tee shirts
The MND merchandise arrived. I hoped Alan's Army of 10k runners would be about ten people, so I'd ordered a dozen tops. Next time I trotted around the village, with my face the colour of a beetroot, instead of thinking why on earth am I doing this, I would proudly advertise my support for MND via my new orange, blue and white running vest!

Thursday 5th April - The kindness of a stranger
Whilst chatting to the man who did our oven cleaning, I discovered that his partner's ex-husband had died from MND. One day when the man was being fed by his carer wife, he removed his ventilator mask and refused further care.

On my training run I cried a lot thinking about the oven cleaner's sad story. I stopped to take a short drink break. A young, skinny, door-to-door seller came towards me in a dazed state - was he spaced out on drugs, or drunk?

"What's the vest all about and why are you running in the rain," he asked.

I blurted out, "My husband is dying from this disease that will paralyse him."

He offered to donate. Respectfully I declined,

"You need the money more than we do." I replied.

Moved by his kindness and feeling guilty about my wrong first impression of him, I hugged him, saying, "You look after yourself."

Our neighbour, Steve, popped around for a chat. He was a regular runner and instantly decided to join Alan's Army when I told him about the 10k race in September.

Friday 6th April - Breathing issues
We set out for Stoke Royal Hospital at 9:30am. On arrival, Alan had a battery of breathing tests and an assessment to see if it was safe for him to make the long-haul flight to Vietnam. Worryingly, the test designed to check his ability to sniff had to be done twice because the first time the results were extraordinarily low. The respiratory consultant reported that his results were borderline, and it would be a good idea to use a non-invasive ventilator at night to aid sleep. To our relief he confirmed Alan would be okay to fly!

Nurses demonstrated how the ventilation machine worked. Alan looked uncomfortable using the mask. "It will make your life better," the nurse stressed. I was not sure Alan would see it that way. From Stoke we drove north to Cumbria.

AUTHOR'S NOTE
MND does not affect the lungs themselves, but over time the breathing muscles around the lungs deteriorate. Oxygen is not needed (we were told it could be harmful) but a non-invasive ventilator (NIV) pumps filtered air into the lungs at regular intervals and at a pressure that is set dependent on how weak the breathing muscles are.

An early indicator that breathing muscles are failing is when the person with MND wakes up frequently in the night. CO_2 builds up in the lungs and triggers the brain to wake the individual. We were told at the outset to check if Alan was getting headaches or becoming very tired due to lack of sleep.

Breathing masks attached by tube to the NIV came in various designs: some for over the nose only, others go over both nose and mouth. The choice of mask depends on whether the person is a nose or mouth breather. The benefit of a nose only mask is it enables the person to stay on the machine while eating. At the time, these masks were intrusive and drew attention to the person's condition. New designs have since been developed.

Using an NIV at night helped Alan to sleep, but it kept me awake due to the machine's noise (subsequent designs are smaller and less noisy). In any event I found I could not sleep easily for fear that Alan might stop breathing at any moment. Using an NIV at night was one thing, but using it in the day, when everyone can see the unattractive mask, was a different matter.

Saturday 7th April - Carter family party
In Penrith I did my first Park Run. My beetroot face ran the course with Alan's sister Viv, Ben and Tom (Viv's sons) Pauline (Alan's other sister) Matt (Pauline's son) and Matt's wife Suzanne. We played party games with Helen's two boys (Pauline's grandchildren) back at the house before having a family dinner at the local pub. The last time we were all together was November at Richard's fortieth birthday, just before Alan's diagnosis. Unbeknown to us at the time, the Yorkshire trip would be the last time Alan would walk with his whole family.

AUTHOR'S NOTE
The problem with MND is things change suddenly. You don't always know

when you are doing something for the last time. In the early days of our relationship, we used to count the first time we did something. Nowadays we made note of the last time we did something. These 'last times' took different forms. The last time Alan would walk, or breathe unaided, or sign his own name were major things. The last time he would be able to scratch an itch, comb his hair himself, clean his teeth, clean his glasses, wipe his own nose were all small things, but were equally frustrating for Alan.

Sunday 8th April - Birthday celebrations
All the family gathered round for a breakfast Buck's Fizz, followed by cake and more drinks before most of the family had to leave Viv's birthday celebrations. What sort of surprises would I be able to spring on Alan for his sixty fourth birthday on June 21st? I hoped all his family would be able to attend any party because there was no guarantee he would make it to his sixty fifth birthday.

Monday 9th April - Feedback from sister-in-law
Alan, Viv, and I visited their auntie Freda who lived with their cousin Christine and her husband Dennis. We had tea and cake in the garden before the weather grew too cold. Back at Viv's house, Alan and his two brothers-in-law went to the pub for pre-dinner drinks. Alone with Viv, she told me I was doing a good job and that she loved me. It meant a lot to have her support.

Tuesday 10th April - Keeping more relatives informed
We left Viv's house straight after breakfast and drove to Chester. I dropped Alan off at a hotel and continued to my firm's Chester office. Back at the hotel another one of Alan's cousins, Kathleen and her husband Michael, had lunch with us while we brought them up to date about Alan's condition.

Wednesday 11th April - Legs getting weaker
"I am worried about my legs… they are getting weaker … it's hard getting up the stairs," Alan mentioned as I left the house. We needed to talk about creating a bedroom downstairs. On my journey to work I phoned Stephanie whose husband had died from MND. In her role as a volunteer visitor for people with MND, she was able to provide useful information about installing wet rooms.

In a letter from my cousin Pam in Barnstaple, there was a donation in respect of the 10k run. She also said the proceeds from the annual charity Christmas Fayre at the garden centre she and her husband owned, would be donated to the MND Association this year. I immediately called her to thank her and promised I would visit when possible.

Thursday 12th April - More to Life friends

After work meetings in London and before catching the train home, I met up with Jill Duffin and other ladies I knew who had been supported by *More to Life* - a charity for people who were involuntarily childless. Judy and Lesley had been friends since 2005 but I only met Sally and Melanie years later. We had dinner at Carluccio's in St Pancras. It was tough bringing them up to date and answering their questions about Alan's progress, but the love and support I received was incredible.

Friday 13th April - First time using the wheelchair

The day started with Alan saying, "I am worried I have changed in your eyes."

"Oh Al, you are no different on the inside and that's what I really love about you," I assured him.

He looked forlorn.

"I feel bad because I cannot do my fair share of chores around the house, and I miss being able to move around with ease like I used to."

All I could do was let him talk. The right words would not come to me.

It did not feel strange pushing Alan in the loaned wheelchair around Solihull because of the type of voluntary work I had done in the past. I hoped that Alan was not too self-conscious and would appreciate still being out and about rather than being stuck inside, ruminating about his legs not working.

Saturday 14th April - Trip to Brighton

We set off to visit Jill and Steve Duffin at their house in Surrey. Lesley and Roger joined us. Jill cooked a fish pie and a Spanish cake with orange sauce for us all. We chatted about holidays, shows, movies and I took plenty of photographs. Alan and I drove to Burgess Hill and checked into an Airbnb property. At a nearby pub, we bought dinner for Alan's business partner, Simon, his wife Rachel and their daughter Maddie because Simon was running a marathon the next day, raising funds for the MND Association.

Sunday 15th April - Getting used to the wheelchair

We took the train to Brighton. Because Alan could not walk far, he had allowed me to bring the wheelchair, so I pushed him down the hill to the front of the marathon course. Finding the fourteen-mile marker post where we had agreed to rendezvous with Rachel and Maddie took ages. When Simon passed us wearing his MND running vest we all cheered wildly, then nudged our way into a front row position at the eighteen-mile marker post.

Once Simon had passed us we pushed Alan in the direction of the finish line. The pavement was too crowded to get through, so we abandoned the idea of seeing Simon cross the line and went to the MND Association tent in the charities village instead. The volunteers in the tent made us very welcome and before long Simon arrived, brandishing his medal. Despite his weak legs, Alan was determined to stand up from his wheelchair to hug Simon. Rachel and I burst into tears.

Inside the tent, we met a chap called Dave and his wife, Helen. Dave had an impressive high-tech wheelchair. Dave's son had proposed to his girlfriend on the finish line so there was a lovely atmosphere. It was good to know Alan and I were not the only two romantics. Simon was given a leg massage and some refreshments then insisted on pushing Alan in the wheelchair up the long hill to the train station in the cold, damp early evening air.

Just before Alan and I boarded the train, Alan's camera slipped out of the man bag he had recently purchased and fell under the carriage. He became angry when he realised it could not be retrieved. There was a tense moment on the train too. Alan wanted to stand because the carriage was so busy.

"You cannot do that Alan," I implored, insisting he stay in the wheelchair.

"You are making a scene," he accused.

I felt hurt. I was just trying to keep him safe. I also felt angry. In my view he was being too polite and thoughtful to others when he probably had greater needs than everyone else.

Once all the emotions died down, I delicately asked, "How do you feel about me posting my pictures of you in the chair on Facebook?" He agreed and even got excited when I suggested heading the post "The Wandering Wheelchair." It was a sign he was getting comfortable with the idea that he would not be walking much in the future. We drove to Heathrow and checked into our hotel. We needed a good sleep ready for a special holiday we had booked before Alan's diagnosis.

Monday 16th April - Vietnam holiday time
Alan slipped when taking a shower and ended up in a heap in the bath. It took me ages to get him out. He was wet and heavy, and his legs were weak. It was very stressful for us both because time was short. We left our car containing the wheelchair at the hotel and took a taxi to the airport. Special assistance personnel took us through to departures without any hassle.

We suspected this would be our last long-haul holiday, so had treated ourselves to premium economy seats. We hoped the extra comfort and the lower cabin pressure of The Dreamliner aircraft would cause less jetlag after eleven hours in the air. Alan slept for most of the flight. I couldn't settle so watched four films in a row.

Wednesday 18th April - Where there's a will…

Min, our local tour guide in Ho Chi Minh City, collected us from the Reverie Hotel at 9am. I explained Alan's challenges and the need to use the wheelchair. Despite Vietnam not appearing very wheelchair friendly, Min gave me confidence we would be well cared for. With the hotel's wheelchair safely stowed in the boot, and Alan carefully transferred into the taxi bus, we set off.

The streets were crazy. Hundreds of families on motor scooters, everywhere. Clearly some sort of etiquette was at play, as there was no evidence of accidents.

Min told us, "Both parties are deemed to be at fault if there is a crash, so everyone is super careful." What a good idea.

The tour included a moving visit to the War Museum and a trip to the Post Office where Min and I had to carry Alan in his chair up the entrance steps.

At a Buddhist temple, we each paid to send a prayer via the suspended spiral incense sticks. I didn't know what Alan wrote on his burning paper, but there was only one prayer I wanted answered. Outside the temple a local 'doctor' spotted Alan and offered to heal him. I was amazed that Alan was up for it. I winced several times as the doctor helped Alan from his chair, laid him on a blanket and moved Alan's neck and legs into unusual positions. It hurt me to think it was all in vain, but I said nothing, for fear of dampening Alan's enthusiasm. Maybe Alan had prayed for a cure too.

Our final stop was the Reunification Palace where unfortunately the lift down to the underground bunker was too small for Alan's chair. He waited for me as I went down and took videos for him. In the afternoon, I took Alan out in the wheelchair in search of a shop that sold cameras. Having failed in our mission, we took a lift up to the viewing gallery close to the top of the tallest tower in Ho Chi Minh City. Over a relaxing cocktail we took in views across the whole city.

Our plan for dinner was to go to the Romeo and Juliet restaurant on the first floor of our hotel. The problem was it was not accessible to wheelchair users, so we went to the restaurant on the 6th floor instead. Not wishing to be defeated, after dinner we tried various routes to get into the Romeo and Juliet. Eventually we discovered we could do it via the underground car park and past the huge cold storage area. I felt embarrassed for Alan. It was degrading having to come into the restaurant via the back door. He was not deterred, however, so we booked a table for dinner the following night. On this holiday, our catchphrase became, "Where there's a will, there's a way."

Thursday 19th April - Was there something he was not telling me?
We were collected at 7am for a trip to the Cu Chi tunnels. The place where the Vietnamese fought off the Americans. Alan had extensively studied both World War I and World War II books for many years and was particularly keen to visit this part of South Vietnam, even though it meant a tricky manoeuvre to get him and his chair, into the speedboat.

We sat next to a couple of German nurses on the boat and a lady from Australia and her daughter. These people proved very valuable during the two-hour trek around the tunnels. At one point a tyre came off the wheelchair and several people were needed to hold Alan while the chair was turned upside down and fixed.

There were a couple of elements of this tour that Alan could not enjoy. One was the opportunity to shoot an AK47 rifle because the wall over which you had to fire was too high. The other was going inside a forty-metre-long tunnel to experience the pitch black and cramped conditions. He insisted I did both. Alan looked awkward for a lot of the day. As he sat staring at a tank, I took his picture. Afterwards he said, "I now know what it feels like looking down the barrel of a gun."

In the afternoon I went for a run in the hotel gym, while Alan was parked up in the shade on the decking around the pool. I ran 3k in fifty minutes on the treadmill - nowhere near the 10k I would be doing in September.

Back in our bedroom I was in a rush to get ready for a massage and accidentally spilt a bottle of water over Alan. Uncharacteristically, he barked at me. I felt guilty for being selfish but, we had agreed I should take some time out to be pampered.

The massage was ninety minutes long and was followed by an overdue haircut. The whole time I was away from him I worried about Alan. Was there something he was not telling me? We were getting ready for dinner when Alan finally opened up. "I feel weak and am worried that I haven't opened my bowels for a long time." We agreed to monitor things and buy appropriate medicines as necessary.

We had a lovely romantic dinner in Romeo and Juliet's restaurant while listening to a female jazz singer. Alan's mood seemed lighter which in turn helped me to relax. After helping Alan get undressed, I packed our bags before retiring to bed. Sleep did not come as most of the night I worried about Alan's newest symptom. What was going on with his digestive system?

Friday 20th April - Anglo-French relations
We checked out of the hotel and were collected by Min at 8:30am. We rested on the four-hour journey to the Mekong River. At the shoreline Alan and his chair were lifted into a small speed boat. It was a short trip to the bassac boat that would be our home for the next twenty-four hours. Our guides on the boat were, Ann and French-speaking Tuyet, who told us her name translated into Snow White.

The only other guests on the twelve-cabin boat were an architect and his wife from France. Alan's French was good, he was able to engage with our fellow travellers. The boat glided gently down the river. The French couple and I went on shore to meet some local farmers. Their conditions were basic, but their smiles were wide as they proudly presented us with local delicacies.

At dinner, the French couple bought us a bottle of wine. In the moonlight, as we drifted silently down the river, Tuyet sang a beautiful French song which made me cry. She joined me as I dredged up basic French songs from my school days. My spirits lifted` and with my head softened by the wine, I slept well.

Saturday 21st April - Back on dry land
I woke up with a startle when the boats engines fired up at 6am. In the morning glow I did yoga stretches on the deck. Tuyet's attempts at some of the movements left us both rolling around in laughter. I felt young and carefree.

The French couple, our two guides, Alan and I toured the floating markets in a sampan boat. I took several photographs to show Alan of another trip on shore so he would not feel too left out. We said our goodbyes to our companions, who had helped us create some very special memories.

Our driver took us to a hotel at Can Tho. Unfortunately, we had to change rooms as the one we were allocated did not have the wet room we had pre-ordered. We ate an excellent tiger prawn lunch in the town. Snoozing around the pool, happy hour cocktails and a delicious dinner rounded off our day.

Sunday 22ⁿᵈ April - A paradise island and ticking time bomb

It took four hours to reach the airport, for the final leg of our Vietnam adventure. Sitting in the special assistance part of the airport, I watched the muscles in Alan's legs twitch uncontrollably and wondered how irritating it must be for him.

We had a smooth, short flight to the Vietnamese island of Pho Quoc. The Salinda Resort courtesy transfer bus drove us to the hotel that would be our home for the next eight nights. On arrival, we were given an exotic cocktail to celebrate Earth Day. The hotel was modern and easy to navigate. Paths down to the beach were wheelchair friendly and surrounded by lush tropical gardens.

Alan wasn't hungry so we had room service. "My left arm feels much weaker," he declared. As he slept, I lay listening to Alan's shallow breathing thinking how much longer do we have? I felt like I was waiting for a ticking time bomb to explode. The holiday had been beautiful but it had presented many challenges. We were doing another 'last'. I felt sure there would be no more foreign holidays after memories were made of this one. It was the end of an era.

Monday 23ʳᵈ April - Preparation for difficult feelings

In the gym I did my first ever 7K run. My beetroot face had a huge smile on it when I told Alan. The hotel's Guest Services Manager helped find a better wheelchair because the one initially supplied by the hotel was too small. Apparently, for many years, an Englishman whose wife had MND, visited the hotel. The man used to wheel his wife to the beach so she could watch the sunset. I felt both comforted and upset by this story. Comforted because the hotel would be accustomed to seeing a person with disabilities around the place. Upset because I felt for this unknown man whose wife was on the same journey as Alan.

When we arrived at the beach, Alan could not stand up from his chair, his legs would not hold his weight. Walking was out of the question. My heart sank as I watched the young beach staff, either side of Alan, manoeuvre him across the sand to a beach bed. Eventually, we enjoyed chilling on the beach, even when a short heavy shower arrived.

A much more suitable wheelchair arrived, enabling me to take Alan to dinner in comfort. During the meal Alan barked to the waiter, "I want to see the chef - his lasagne is too sloppy." I was shocked. Alan seldom complained about anything or raised his voice. On deeper investigation he confessed, "I feel angry. No one prepared me for how I was going to feel psychologically, and no one is checking up on my progress."

It was true. Most of the information we received from medical professionals and the MND Association focused on the *physical* changes people with MND could expect. Alan needed help to deal with the emotional impact of his diagnosis and deterioration. I made a note to source some counselling when we got home.

Tuesday 24th April - Beach bathing
Alan had a fitful night's sleep. During our morning cuddle, I could see his breathing was more laboured. On the beach I saw a lady reading the same book I was also reading. I introduced myself to Daniella from Germany. "I am frustrated at the speed the disease is taking things from me," Alan announced during the daily rain shower. His mood matched the grey clouds.

Wednesday 25th April - Shoreline sadness
On a taxi tour of the island, we saw a fishing village, pagodas, the Coconut Prison and a pearl farm. The afternoon was spent on the beach. I ventured into the ocean for the first time. Walking along the shoreline alone was heart breaking. Without Alan by my side, too many unhappy thoughts entered my mind.

Thursday 26th April - Wet room specification
At the gym I did 3k ride on a bike and 3k run on the jogging machine, plus 1k warm down. It was beginning to feel that running 10k in September might be achievable. After breakfast, Alan and I created the specification for the wet room. As a qualified quantity surveyor, used to designing office spaces, our little project was easy for Alan to tackle. I was given the fun job of thinking about the colour scheme.

The afternoon sun warmed our skin on the beach. Talking with Daniella I found it impossible to keep my emotions in check. Although she was much younger than me, she was incredibly mature and supportive. She made me promise that I would visit her in Hamburg after Alan passed away.

Friday 27th April - Branching out
It was extremely hot on the beach. Plenty of beers were needed to keep us cool. My courage up, I suggested we venture outside the world of our hotel. I struggled to steer the heavy wheelchair down the hill to the roadside until one of the hotel porters came to my rescue. We came across a barbershop. It was awkward getting Alan onto the bed but eventually, his face covered in white

lather, a young Vietnamese lady started work with her cut throat razor. Alan looked terrified!

All smooth and shiny, Alan decided we should eat at the restaurant opposite the barber's. The restaurant owner spotted us trying to cross the busy road and helped us. He earned himself a large tip, which guaranteed we would get help returning to our side of the road. We drank cocktails in the hotel lounge bar. I cried at some of the songs the services manager sang from our favourite movies.

Saturday 28th April - Chats in the rain
Daniella left for home, and I went for another long, lonely walk along the seashore watched by Alan. Evening cocktails were taken undercover because it was raining. The Guest Services Manager told us about Plum Village in France where people go to meditate. She showed us pictures of the lady with MND who visited each year with her husband.

We had a chat with the head waiter in the Indian restaurant who told us about places in Kerala where people go for internal and external detoxing. It was heart-warming and overwhelming that these two strangers wanted to help us cope with the emotional stress of our situation. It was upsetting realising it was unlikely we would ever return to this heavenly place.

Sunday 29th April - Last day in paradise
A lifetime best run of 7.15k in thirty minutes was achieved in the gym before I joined Alan for breakfast, sporting my best ever beetroot face.

"I had a cry when I struggled to dress myself," Alan whispered.

My joy dampened, and guilt hit me - I should have been there to help him.

"What have you been thinking about lately?" I asked.

"My funeral arrangements," he said without hesitation.

My heart sank.

"I want a church service, and the song *Time of my Life* played, from the film *Dirty Dancing*."

Then, his new favourite saying came again. "Life's good. It's the disease that's the problem." I took a deep breath and stayed calm while inside a pain gnawed in the pit of my stomach. A strong desire to howl like a wild animal rose within me.

It was our last day in Phu Quoc - a tiny tropical paradise island off the coast of Southwest Vietnam. The last beautiful island Alan would see.

Monday 30th April - Leaving Vietnam

We woke up at 6:30am. Torrential rain fell outside. The island looked like I felt - sad. Hanoi, in north Vietnam, was hot and humid and bursting with hundreds of family laden motor scooters darting around. I wanted to stop the clock and flee back to the peace and calm of Phu Quoc.

Our schedule included a half day escorted tour. At the Confucius University something went wrong with the wheelchair when we tackled a difficult pavement. Within seconds, three local people appeared from nowhere. One magically produced a spanner and quickly fixed the damaged chair. I decided I loved the Vietnamese. Alan and I didn't talk much on the flight back to London.

MAY 2018

Tuesday 1st May - Surprising the cyclists

Driving back from Heathrow, via a tracking device, we could see the three cyclists would be passing through Staffordshire on their way to John O'Groats. We decided to spring a surprise. However, Alan's BMW inconveniently got a puncture. We lost three hours getting it sorted out and eventually arrived on the outskirts of Newcastle under Lyme just ahead of the cyclists. The look on their faces when we flagged them down was priceless. Alan had a beaming smile and was full of appreciation for their efforts. They were delighted to see us.

Wednesday 2nd May - No need to struggle without NIV

At mum's mental health clinic we were told the vascular dementia with Lewy bodies was getting worse. Drugs were prescribed to reduce hallucinations. "I am sorry for adding to your burdens," mum said mournfully. "Don't worry mum, I am coping at the moment." Little did I know how different things would be in just a few months.

While changing my sweater something caught on the fabric. I felt sick when I discovered a stone was missing from my engagement ring!

Later, Alan struggled to get out of his chair when the phone rang. Joan, Alan's mum, lived in Sunderland and didn't see much of Alan so rang regularly. Naturally she spent a lot of time worrying about her only son, especially now. It was hard listening to his emotional conversation with her.

Later in the day Alan became extremely tired. He decided to try the non-invasive ventilator for thirty minutes to help regain some strength. The ventilator nurse had stressed, "You can use it anytime." Trying to live without it would not make him a hero.

Thursday 3rd May - Planning Scotland trip and special chair

The MND Association local fundraiser dropped off a large banner for when the three cyclists ended their epic journey in John O'Groats. We also had MND balloons, some Scottish hats, champagne and beer for their welcoming party. It was exciting planning a road trip through Scotland, tracking the boys and encouraging them on the final stages of their fantastic fundraising journey. Alan insisted on booking our B&B's so he could ensure each venue was wheelchair friendly and in the right location to meet up with the cyclists. He enjoyed having something to do.

The riser recliner chair arrived - on loan from the MND Association. It was unattractive, but I was grateful for something to help Alan stand from a sitting position and reduce the risk of him falling.

Friday 4th May - Scotland here we come
We set off for Cumbria - our staging post. Just like previous trips to Viv's, Alan and John went to the pub, giving Viv and I to time to have an emotional heart to heart, while quaffing a glass of wine, or two.

Saturday 5th May - First day in Scotland
Before leaving Cumbria we called at the house of Alan's second cousin, Lindsey. To give time for Alan to chat with Lindsey in private I asked if her husband would show me the barn they were converting. It was a long drive to Fort William, but the guest house Alan had chosen was perfect. Over dinner with the three cyclists and Pete, we listened to stories of challenging steep hills in Cornwall and Devon. They suggested they might raise over £9,000!

AUTHOR'S NOTE
Pete, the father of Matt, drove the motorhome in support of the cyclists. The four of them slept in the motorhome at camp sites along their route.

Sunday 6th May - Stocking up on Scottish whisky
Before breakfast I managed a 4.25 mile run which included a steep hill up to a war memorial. Momentarily I felt downcast. Prior to MND, Alan would have run with me and would have enjoyed seeing this tribute to the commandos who had fought for our country. I took some photographs for Alan.

On the way to The Morangie Hotel (not far from the Glenmorangie distillery) we took photographs of the cyclists at a rest stop. It was a beautiful day with the sun shimmering on the Lochs. We bought some bottles at the distillery - it would have been rude not to!

Monday 7th May - The end of the line
The drive to John O'Groats was long and hilly. The conditions were difficult for the cyclists, especially for Rob who was the least experienced of them. He had to push his bike up several long hills - partly because he was exhausted and partly because he said his bottom was too sore. His grit and determination were admirable. We fed the cyclists sweets, biscuits and cakes at rest stops.

Our car and the motorhome arrived in John O'Groats about thirty minutes ahead of the cyclists. Pete helped me get Alan into his wheelchair and wrap him in two thick blankets to keep out the biting wind.

The three of us located ourselves under the famous fingerpost. I put up the banners and balloons and placed the beers and Scottish hats close by. It was incredibly emotional when the cyclists arrived. Alan was in tears. I was in tears. The cyclists were elated and drained. After hugs and a quick beer in the chilly Scottish wind we parked up at a local campsite.

Alan could not lift his own weight up the motorhome steps. Pete and the exhausted cyclist physically lifted Alan up and placed him inside the warm vehicle. While we all thawed out I asked the cyclists, what the trip had meant to them. Rob spoke first. "Without your motivation over the last three days I would not have made it."

Matt said, "What we have endured is nothing compared to what Alan is having to deal with."

We cracked open the champagne and toasted the LEJOG team.

AUTHOR'S NOTE
The cyclists raised a magnificent £12,000. Two thirds were donated to MND Association. The other third to Parkinson's Association, as Jonathon had a relative living with that disease. When we met Rob, months later, his sore bottom was still troubling him. I didn't ask for proof!

Tuesday 8th May - Driving south through Scotland
On the beautiful drive south through the Cairngorms, we played a Faith Hill CD in the car. The lyrics of one song were poignant. "I will take a part of you with me. Wherever I am, there you will be." Before crossing into England, we had lunch with Lindsey's sister, Jill. Jill's nine-month-old daughter sat happily on Alan's knee. Alan looked happy. At times like this, I regretted we had not met earlier in life - he would have made an excellent father.

Wednesday 9th May - Brief stop in York
In York we met Eric, another of Alan's cousins. Eric had designed his house upside down. The 'through the floor' lift in the hall enabled Alan to get to the upstairs living area without the use of stairs.

Friday 11th May - Hard talk
On the way to the Marie Curie Hospice, as gently as I could, I shared some of my recent feelings with Alan. Firstly, "I am a little frustrated you don't use the non-invasive ventilator during the day when you are clearly struggling to breathe." Then, I told him, "Sometimes you are too stubborn - you try to do more for yourself than you are capable of. I would probably be the same in your shoes, but it's heart-breaking watching you."

He understood but confessed, "I am sorry. I hadn't realised how hard it is on you watching me. Truth is, I don't want you to have to help me."

"I don't mind helping you Al, it gets things done quicker and is less frustrating for both of us."

Our bereavement counsellor, Jane, listened to us for a long time, "You are both suffering from anticipatory grief." I'd never heard the phrase, but it explained a lot. She went on, "You are both living with the thought that your future life has died. Not only is Alan's life being cut short, but your lives have changed irrevocably and all your plans have been smashed."

She was spot on.

Alan told Jane about his elderly mum being deaf and how hard it had been to explain to her what was going on. Jane recommended that Alan write a letter to his mum so she had something tangible to help her understand what MND was and how Alan was feeling. Jane suggested Alan consider who he personally wanted to say goodbye to - before it was too late. Finally, she said Alan needed to think about where he wanted to spend the end of his life if he had a choice - at home, in a hospice, or in hospital.

It was a difficult and painful meeting, but we were grateful that some tough topics, neither of us had raised, were brought out into the open. Back home we invited our neighbours around for drinks. We explained we might need to call upon them for help from time to time. They were all keen to assist in any way possible. It was comforting knowing we had good support close by, just in case.

Saturday 12th May - Sleeping together despite the noise
Christina and Vikki, from Alan's office, popped in bringing lemon cake. Privately, Christina asked me, "Would it be okay to send a Father's Day card to Alan?" She had always regarded him as a father figure. I knew such a card would mean a tremendous amount to Alan.

My sister Clare and her husband David came round together with my nephew Darren, his wife Suzanne and their twins. Alan and my mum took care of the twins in the house while everybody else helped me clear out our garage to make room for the future wet room. The Eurovision song contest came on TV. Alan and I did what we always did. We ranked each song individually to see if we could spot the winners. I batted away the thought this could be the last time we did this. We managed to sleep together despite the noise from the non-invasive ventilator. It felt good to hold Alan.

Sunday 13th May - Becoming Alan's carer

While getting Alan up out of bed, washing him and dressing him, Alan complained I was being too rough. I was shocked and hurt. It was hard getting both myself and Alan ready every day. Somehow I needed to manage things differently in the future. I drove us to Lewis. Our hotel bedroom was supposed to be an accessible one, but there was no walk-in shower. I went to bed dreading how I was going to get Alan ready in the morning.

AUTHOR'S NOTE

Alan liked to have a shower, his hair washed, teeth cleaned and a shave every morning so good bathroom facilities were important to us. Finding suitable hotel rooms was not easy. Places advertised that rooms were accessible, but often they were too narrow to get the wheelchair around the bed to the bathroom or the bathroom did not have a level access shower or a shower chair. Be cautious - there is no set standard.

Monday 14th May - Brain scans

Alan and I had volunteered to assist a medical researcher at Brighton Medical Centre who wanted to compare healthy brains, supposedly mine, and MND affected brains. Due to the time it had taken me to get us both ready, we were running late. In my haste I accidentally hit the kerb while parking the car. Alan became angry which escalated my frustration levels.

In reception while waiting to meet the research doctor, I spoke with a lady whose husband had lymphoma. After explaining MND and my forthcoming 10k race she gave me a donation of £20 and said she would pray for us. I regretted not asking this kind stranger her name. Andrew was a kind doctor, appreciative of us driving so far to help the clinic. Alan and I each spent forty-five minutes in an MRI scanner. It was the most rest I had had in ages.

Tuesday 15th May - Busy day

I was due to have some complementary therapy at the hospice but had to cancel because my car would not start. So frustrating. Luckily Tom and Ben were staying with us and sorted out the vehicle. Later in the day an old ex-boss, John, and his wife Sarah, arrived for afternoon tea. Tom and Ben helped me clear up the dining room after our visitors left. Some neighbours popped in adding to an already busy day.

Wednesday 16th May - A near death incident

In the middle of the night, I woke with an overwhelming need to talk to someone. On my iPad I could see my friend Fiona in Australia was online, so I messaged her. She called me immediately. I brought her up to date about Alan.

She talked about her son who had been born with no eyes or hearing and was undergoing ground-breaking treatment. Her story reminded me there is always someone worse off. Fiona and I agreed our loved ones were living on borrowed time and we had to be brave.

During the morning the hospital bed arrived complete with an inflatable mattress. We could now create a bedroom in the dining room. A shower chair also arrived for the wet room. Slowly, our lovely home was turning into a hospital. Early evening, I caught a train into Birmingham for a meal with my friends Teresa, Christine and Jenny. It was the first time I had been out in months. I was due to catch the 10pm train home but felt uneasy leaving Alan alone for so long, so I caught an earlier one.

In the lounge I found Alan lying on the floor with blood on the carpet near his head! His eyes were open, but his face was flushed. For a split-second, time stood still. Then I blurted out, "Oh my goodness Alan, what happened?"

"I was trying to walk but fell backwards and hit my head on the coffee table."

For the first time in my life, I dialled 999.

To stem the bleeding I was told to put a rolled up towel under Alan's head. The ambulance arrived quickly. Because Alan was mostly paralysed the paramedics used an inflatable cushion to raise him up and get him onto a stretcher. Alan was driven to Warwick Hospital, followed by me in my car. Luckily there was no concussion, so by 4am we were allowed to go home. The part of Alan's head that was shaved revealed a neat row of stitches.

For hours I felt sick and shaken up. I was angry with Alan for putting himself at risk and angry at myself for assuming he would be okay if I went out. I decided he was never to be left alone again. Before long I had created a list of all the people who had said they would 'help anytime' and a list of responsible people I felt I could trust to handle Alan's care if I needed to go out.

AUTHOR'S NOTE
We were told it was important that the mattress was kept fully inflated to prevent Alan getting pressure sores, due to his immobility.

Thursday 17th May - Not coping very well
While I was at work in Birmingham Teresa and her husband Phil stayed with Alan. At the office I negotiated the terms of my exit from my job. It was time for me to be with Alan all the time.

During supper Alan said, "The fall was a significant wake-up call." I was pleased that he had come to his senses and would now accept more help. Alan received a heartfelt letter from his sister Pauline. It made him cry.

Simon, Alan's good friend and business partner, came to visit. As I was saying goodbye to Simon in the hallway he asked, "How are you doing?"

Initially I said, "I'm fine" but followed it quickly with, "I'm not fine really. Things are getting tough. I am not coping very well."

It was the first time I had admitted out loud that, perhaps, everything was getting too much for me. I had got used to getting Alan up, washed and dressed every morning and getting him ready for bed every evening, as well as managing the house and finances. But the constant worry and the total responsibility for his every need, was taking its toll. I was dealing with my own feelings of loss and dreading a future without Alan and looking after mum too. Nothing felt normal anymore. Our lives were upside down. It was hard work physically and mentally, and on top of that, I felt heartbroken most of the time.

Friday 18th May - The Midnight Sapphires
Alan's niece Helen arrived for lunch with her youngest son. We ate outside on the decking in the sunshine. The afternoon was frantic with lots of phone calls coming in, including one from my sister, Rowena. I was a bit short with her, so texted later to apologise.

I drove Alan to Wilmcote where Simon's wife, Rachel, was performing in a band called The Midnight Sapphires and fundraising in aid of MND Association. In the hall, Alan looked self-conscious. It was Alan's first evening out in the wheelchair. I was unable to be by his side all the time because, I was helping with the sale of raffle tickets. He spent a lot of time talking to a friend in a side room. During the interval, Alan made a heartfelt appeal for patrons to buy raffle tickets. People cried.

We were introduced to a gentleman who had recently lost his young wife to cancer and a lady who had lost both her sister and a friend to MND. One kind gentleman donated £200. Originally, we had said we would leave the event at the earliest opportunity. But there was so much love and support for us we stayed almost to the end! Before we left I made a short speech thanking everyone for their generosity and appealing for runners to join Alan's Army. The husbands of two ladies who worked in Alan's office signed up immediately.

Saturday 19th May - Stages of death

My sister Rowena and I had a long chat. Her husband was a stroke victim. She was worried how I was going to cope as Alan degenerated further. Mum watched the wedding of Prince Harry to Meghan with us.

Our friend and ex-lodger, Jaki, arrived and told me, "I spent time looking at the stages of death, so I was prepared for my father's passing."

I began to worry when she mentioned, "A person's heart can stop beating if their lungs don't work properly." After she left, I Googled 'stages of death'.

AUTHOR'S NOTE

It was not my intention to be morbid, but I searched the internet a lot to help me prepare for what was ahead. This was my first experience of caring for a dying person. Learning what happens to a person as their body dies was emotionally painful, but helpful from a practical point of view.

Sunday 20th May - Mastering the pee bottle

Alan and I had a long chat about his feelings. His left arm was not working now, his legs were very weak and he was concerned about his lungs. There was never much I could say when we had these chats. We just took stock every so often, so Alan had a chance to get things off his chest.

The timetable for the building of the wet room looked good, but it was going to cost a lot. Luckily the local MND Association group approved a small grant which helped a little. At a chemist I bought a pee bottle for Alan to use while he was sitting in the wheelchair. It turned out to be a challenge trying to keep the bottle in place while his pee spurted out. I didn't always get it right!

Alan sat in the sun by the front door while I re-organised parts of the garage and cleaned the cars. There were many jobs Alan used to do which now fell on my shoulders. How do younger women manage to care for a spouse, look after kids and go to work? Later, I couldn't get off to sleep so did more research on the stages of death. When I became consumed with grief, I poured my heart out in an email to my friend Fiona in Australia.

AUTHOR'S NOTE

MND Association offers some financial support to help with: cost of living (household bills and food shopping), funding of equipment, home or wheelchair adaptations and services that people with MND have been assessed as needing. Many grants are not means tested and several can be applied for by a carer, or a health or social care professional on behalf of the person with MND.

For up to date information go to -
mndassociation.org/support-and-information/health-and-social-care-
services-for-mnd/benefits-and-financial-support

Monday 21st May - Some 'me' time

The morning was frantic as I sorted out the paperwork ready for the Continuing Health Care (CHC) assessment. My brother Kevin arrived to help with chores around the house. It was great having his assistance. He even cut Alan's toenails - a job I had been putting off.

Alan and I had a brainstorming meeting with Pam Leek who was due to be Lady Captain at Shirley Golf Club from November. Pam had chosen the MND Association as the charity she would support.

Our next meeting was to sort out our wills and our Lasting Powers of Attorney (LPA).

At 3pm our neighbour Alex arrived so that I could play my first round of golf since September. I needed some down time. After warming up, my playing partner, Richard, and I decided to take on another couple in a friendly fourball. To inspire me I used a golf ball with Alan's initials on it. My clubs had been stolen from my car several months earlier, so I used Alan's. Surprisingly I played well, and we won on the fifteenth hole. Then I broke down and cried. "It's good to have you back," Richard said as he hugged me.

AUTHOR'S NOTE

Arranging our wills and the LPAs ticked off an item on Alan's *Peace of Mind* list. The LPA would provide those chosen to be executors with the necessary authority to act on financial and property matters in the event one of us lost mental capacity.

Tuesday 22nd May - Carbon dioxide building up

While Alan was busy having a massage at the Marie Curie Hospice I caught up with Lesley, our physio, and mentioned, "Alan's been having vivid dreams and talking a lot in his sleep." Lesley pointed out it could be a build-up of CO_2 in his brain, and suggested, "He needs to use his non-invasive ventilator every night." As I cried I realised the hospice was the place where I felt safe letting go of my emotions.

One of the other physios gave me a raised toilet stand for use back at the house. She would be a key contact for us in disability aids and gadgets to support Alan's changing needs. Not long after we arrived home a lady from social services arrived to talk about Alan's care package. Alan agreed to go on the non-invasive ventilator while I sorted out the kitchen and found linen for the hospital bed in the dining room. Armed with a packed supper, we set off for Sheffield at 7pm. I was feeling frazzled.

On this trip to Sheffield, we stayed in a recommended hotel close to the Royal Hallamshire Hospital. The room was not 100% suitable but the staff were extremely helpful when we pointed out what we needed. Alan shouted out in his sleep, "I've got to get out of the water to avoid the shark." The dreaded CO_2 was building up.

Wednesday 23rd May - End of hope

Like every morning, I got Alan out of bed and showered and dressed him. I brought the car to the front of the hotel, put him in the passenger seat, and bundled the wheelchair into the boot.

We arrived in good time for the randomisation appointment. The drug trial nurse took thirteen phials of blood from Alan before he could have breakfast. While the nurse made notes of the long list of things Alan could no longer do for himself, Alan started sobbing.

Shockingly Dr Bell told us, "Now that you are using a non-invasive ventilator you are ineligible to go forward on the trial."

I pointed out "That was not clear in the original eligibility paperwork," and pleaded, "Alan only started using the NIV a few days ago."

Dr Bell tried to comfort us. "The many blood samples and lumbar puncture fluids you have given have already gone to various research clinics, helping researchers understand the disease better."

It was of little comfort.

The journey back home was sombre. I tried to lighten the mood, "There will be other trials Al." He didn't respond. He didn't reply either when I joked, "At least we won't have to put up with inadequate Sheffield hotel rooms anymore." Being excluded from the trial after everything Alan had gone through - like delaying going on Riluzole drug - was a body blow. We were both disappointed. Alan had found a purpose in being part of a trial. I feared his mental health would deteriorate without this little ray of hope to keep him going.

It was six months and two days since diagnosis.

AUTHOR'S NOTE

Randomisation is the stage in a drug trial when a computer in a remote location, decides which patient (identified by a number, not a name) receives the trial drug. In this double-blind trial, staff at Sheffield didn't know who was on the trial drug and who was on a placebo.

Thursday 24th May - Without you

Pauline, Alan's sister, arrived to care for Alan while I attended a conference. While driving south I came up with my first poem in ages.

WITHOUT YOU
Life will go on without you.
I will play golf where we used to play,
Climb the same Lake District hills,
Eat at some of our local restaurants,
Listen to our favourite songs,
Without you.

But I don't want to.
I don't want to go back to places we have been,
Without you.
Go to places we dreamed of visiting,
Without you.
See new things,
Without you.
Be with our friends,
Without you.

Life will go on,
But without you.
It will never be the same,
Without you.

Saturday 26th May - MGB for sale

Pauline left after breakfast. Despite being haunted by memories of Alan and I on the golf course together I played well in the competition. It was sad realising I would never see him on the fairways again. On my way home I called Bev. She was with Alan and confirmed he was fine.

My final task was a post on Facebook saying Alan was selling his beloved red MGB called Morris. To make letting go of Morris a little more palatable I suggested, "Maybe half of the sale proceeds could be donated to the MND Association." Alan liked the idea.

As always, I helped Alan get ready for bed. For the first time he slept on his own in the single hospital bed in our dining room. I cursed MND for separating us in this way.

Sunday 27th May - Struggling to use the stairs
When I went downstairs to Alan's new bedroom I found him wide-awake. We briefly discussed his ideas for our fourth wedding anniversary. Alan really wanted a shower, so he struggled up the stairs, bent over like an old man. I shaved his face and gave him a shower. It was equally hard for Alan to get back down the stairs. When I looked at Facebook there were fifty-eight shares of my post about Morris being on the market!

Monday 28th May - Bank Holiday
Wendy phoned sounding distressed. She had received an end of life medicines pack because it was deemed Mel was in the final stage of life. This news, about a person we had recently met with MND, dismayed us. In the past Wendy had tried to assure me by saying Mel had been on a breathing machine for four years and that Alan's condition could plateau. I feared Alan may not survive another twelve months.

My sister, Rowena and her husband Steve, visited in the afternoon. Alan listened intently as Steve talked about the functionality he had lost due to his stroke. Alan said nothing about his lost functionality.

Tuesday 29th May - Comfort eating and bottom wiping
Having spent most of the night worrying if Alan was okay downstairs, I got up feeling tired and lacking motivation to do any office work. Having a full-time job, looking after Alan's increasingly complex needs and being responsible for mum was now too demanding. I decided I would now resign on 1st June.

Alan was sleeping when I popped into his bedroom. When he awoke, he decided he would relax in the lounge in his pyjamas while I went for a run. I fitted the ventilator mask over his face and left him resting on the settee watching TV. My knees ached and complained when I lifted Alan and tried to wash him in our cramped cloakroom. Alan went on the ventilator again and rested in front of the TV when I took my car for its MOT.

Before going home, I bought and ate three chocolate bars and a cake. I had developed an unhealthy comfort eating habit. During the afternoon I had telephone conversations with our social worker contact at the Marie Curie

Hospice, Fiona, our OT, and Kaye, our dietician. Everyone was lovely but I felt low.

On Facebook I noticed that some of Alan's Army were worrying about their low running speed or fretting about running the distance. I sent a motivational email to all the runners, reminding them why we were undertaking the challenge and assuring them it would all be okay on the day if they put in the training.

"I am getting more nervous about going out," Alan remarked.

He was now unable to do most things for himself so we created a list of people who would be prepared to help with personal care and, with whom, he would be comfortable in that situation, when I could not be with him.

Wiping Alan's bottom later in the day, I smiled as I thought, after eleven years, eleven months of knowing each other, we are still having 'firsts'! At the same time, I dreaded to think how Alan felt about me, and or anyone else, having to perform this task for him. When I went to bed, I mulled over a statement Alan had made in the day. "Our future has been stolen." Another poem came to me.

MY LOVELY MAN
The tank is almost empty,
No more fuel to burn.
Everything is too hard to do,
Every task a struggle,
For my lovely man.

Each day he grows weaker,
For my lovely man.
Each day another function leaves him,
To depend on someone else.

How much longer must he suffer?
How long will he hang on?
He talks of a future stolen,
Dreams dead and gone.

He's not ready to leave me,
And I don't want him to go.
But each day there is less of him,
Is he still the man I used to know?

Every day I look at him,
His eyes dull and strained,
His face so thin and haggard.
And then he smiles, or sings a song,
And I know he's still there,
Underneath the broken body,
And the muscles that twitch and fade,
There he is, my lovely man.

AUTHOR'S NOTE

It was no longer safe for Alan to use the stairs to the bathroom, but he had been used to a daily morning shower. Because we didn't have a wet room yet, I gave Alan a wash, shave and cleaned his teeth, in our small downstairs loo, while he perched on a high stool to steady himself. We learned the hard way that we needed to anticipate future needs as best as possible and be one step ahead of the unpredictable MND progression.

Wednesday 30th May - Worrying about choking and feeling groggy

The morning was hectic preparing for various visitors. In the cloakroom handbasin I washed Alan's hair before giving him his shave. He looked well, but his face was flushed. He had declined to take his Riluzole tablets for the last two nights. I wondered if withdrawing from them was causing side-effects.

Fiona, the OT, and Lesley, the physiotherapist, arrived at 2pm. Fiona went away with a long list of items she said she would source for us. Kaye, the dietician, arrived unexpectedly with fortified milkshake drinks for Alan to try. "They are easier to swallow than food and will provide much needed nourishment," she said. Friends, Andy and Jo, arrived around 5pm for nibbles and drinks. They were cheerful and comfortable around Alan, and a pleasure to have in the house.

It was a busy but sad day. On Facebook, I shared some of my feelings. Alan's cousin in America, Renee, responded to my Facebook post saying she thought Alan should consider a feeding tube. He was totally against the idea when I raised it. I dreaded the idea of witnessing him wasting away from malnutrition. He had been choking on food more often lately, but he dismissed the idea that his swallowing was failing, which frightened me. Most mornings Alan woke up very groggy, which also worried me. It was impossible to sleep due to circling thoughts about Alan's health. When I started to think about all the things I loved about Alan, another poem came to me.

SUCH A GREAT MAN

You know you are married to a great man,
When he thanks you for looking after him,
At the end of every day.
When he apologises for needing your help,
To keep him clean.

When he never complains,
About the disease that's wrecked his life.

When he raises a smile,
Every time you take his picture.

When he puts you first,
Even when his needs are greater.

When he would rather exhaust himself,
Than put upon you.

You know you are blessed,
When you are married to
Such a great man.

Thursday 31st May - At an advanced stage

At the Marie Curie Hospice, our first meeting was with Katie, our speech and language therapist. She said she would order a special headset so that Alan could sit at a computer, repeating 1600 sentences to bank his voice. I feared he was already too weak to undertake such a huge task.

Next, we saw Caroline, the MND nurse. We discussed what stage Alan was at but she would not give us a one to ten rating of his condition. She did confirm, "Alan is at an advanced stage." When I suggested that meant he was probably eight out of ten she didn't disagree. It was just over six months since diagnosis. I felt stunned.

We then saw Julie, from Macmillan. Alan needed some drugs to help with saliva production because his glands didn't appear to be working - a home visit from the GP would be arranged. Alan announced, "I am coming off Riluzole." He asked questions about tube feeding. A cheerful man at the earlier MND support meeting had shown Alan the tube in his stomach saying, "It's there, just in case." Simon Beacham, Rachel and Maddie came around at 5:30pm. By the time they left three hours later, Alan was completely shattered.

AUTHOR'S NOTE

Every person we met with MND had a different set of symptoms and had lived with the illness for different lengths of time. It was therefore sometimes difficult to relate to the experiences others had of the disease. Instead, we gained insight for each of them in different ways.

Friday 1st June - Sorting out CO2 levels

At our house Marie, the ventilation nurse from Stoke Hospital, took various readings. His CO2 level was 7.9. Too high, as suspected. (It was 5.5 in April). To help it to get back down to level six, she adjusted the setting on NIV. Marie carefully explained everything about having a feeding tube fitted and its benefits. It was a massive relief when Alan confirmed he would proceed. He didn't want to die from malnutrition.

Before she left, Marie checked and corrected the way I fitted the mask onto Alan's face. Poor Alan, I hadn't been doing it quite right. Within seconds Alan fell asleep. Marie explained "It will take weeks to get the CO2 levels back down but using the NIV every night will make a difference."

Friends, Alison and Adrian, arrived just after 7pm. They brought a bottle of champagne. We celebrated my resignation.

AUTHOR'S NOTE

The operation to fit a feeding tube is called Percutaneous Endoscopic Gastrostomy (PEG). Such operations for people in our area were undertaken at Stoke Hospital. The patient must be awake so the camera and tubes necessary to fit the PEG could be introduced down their throat. It was possible to do the operation while the person is on their breathing machine.

Saturday 2nd June - Professional carers

At 7am a carer called Hayley arrived from a care agency allotted to us. She was a great help with Alan. Unfortunately, she was the manager in the office, so would not be our regular carer. These carers were funded by the local authority. The idea of having carers in the house put me on edge. I was concerned about their experience of MND, their punctuality, hygiene standards, etc. Letting go of doing Alan's care did not come easy. I was worried on many levels. Could I trust others?

Friends, Moraig and Mark, arrived in the afternoon, bringing home-made gifts before Alan and I joined *The Ski Gang* for dinner at Robert's house.

Sunday 3rd June - Feeling useless

At 8am, a carer called Ann arrived. She said she had been caring for many years and tried hard to make me feel confident in her. She was very talkative, which made me more nervous than ever. I wanted her to concentrate on what she was doing. Anita, the owner of the care company, appeared genuinely moved by our story as she undertook a full risk assessment.

Just before lunch Christina, from Alan's office, and her husband Chris arrived. It was supposed to be a surprise visit, but eagle eyed Alan saw their car pulling up to the front of the house. Nothing wrong with his powers of observation! I left them to chat while mum and I did some shopping. Back at our house, mum, Alan and I enjoyed a visit from my brother, Kevin and his wife Sue and their two sons Martyn and Alex. After Kevin and his family left, I did some gardening and washed the MGB.

"I feel useless and frustrated because I cannot help you," Alan remarked.

I didn't know what to say, so we both felt useless sometimes.

Monday 4th June - Choking getting worse

A carer called Chelsea arrived. Alan's personal care was still being managed in the cloakroom. When I did it, I usually stripped to my undies to save me getting wet through - much to Alan's delight. The poor carers had to endure being squeezed into a small space wearing their full uniform and a plastic apron. It must have felt to them like being in some kind of kinky sauna.

Alan was now struggling to walk any distance. With help from me or a care worker, he could stand and be transferred from his recliner chair to his wheelchair and back again. In the confined space of our downstairs loo, moving him around was far more challenging.

While eating his usual Weetabix breakfast, Alan choked badly. I had to pull him forward and beat his back. He was not amused when I suggested, "Maybe you should break your habit and have a less risky cereal or poached eggs on a weekday." I laughed when he vehemently denied being a creature of habit.

With Alan's permission, for the first time, I included a photograph of him wearing his ventilator mask on a Facebook post. A man came to fit a key safe box outside the house. From now on the carers could let themselves in. Yippee, one less job for me!

Tuesday 5th June - Tough decisions

In a long, tearful telephone conversation about my fears with my friend Angela, she told me, "Dave and I are impressed by your Facebook blogs, which help us understand what you are going through. Maybe you should write a book. It will inspire people to live well and encourage them not to put things off or take things for granted."

Hmmm? I thought.

My sister Clare chatted excitedly about her forthcoming cruise when she visited. I was pleased for her, but I also felt a bit depressed because it was unlikely Alan and I would ever experience such a holiday together.

Alan had a tough conversation with our Marie Curie consultant regarding his preferred location at end-of-life. He settled on hospice as his first preference, followed by a care home, followed by home, followed by hospital. The decision was captured in his *Do Not Resuscitate* form (DNR) and *Respect* form. I was pleased he had not chosen to die at Carter Castle because living in the house afterwards would be heart breaking. The thought of witnessing him dying anywhere was scary. I had no experience and did not know how I would cope. I feared I would be like some demented woman when they came to take his body away. The Marie Curie Hospice was a wonderful place. It was a good decision.

Co-incidentally, that morning, a Radio 4 programme included Professor Higginson talking about assisted dying. He suggested there should be more palliative care available so the need for assisted dying was reduced.

"I would not choose assisted dying if it were available," Alan declared. "I don't want to die, not at this stage."

Simon Beacham popped in for a short visit. "I cannot stop thinking about Alan's situation," Simon confided. The two men had been mates as well as work colleagues for a long time. I felt for Simon.

When Alan wanted to pass a bowel movement, I manoeuvred him onto the loo, but nothing came. He got distraught later when he pooed his pants. My hugs and reassurances didn't help him get over the embarrassment. Our evening carer did not arrive until 8.30pm and, unexpectedly, it was a chap called Matt, because there had been a bereavement in Chelsea's family. That evening, Alan and I discussed the quality of our carers. We both agreed Hayley was the best.

Wednesday 6th June - Planning Alan's sixty fourth birthday
Another new carer, Sadie, arrived. She was less warm and friendly than the others but good at her job. Martin and Phil came from the building firm. It took a long time to identify where the foul water would exit the wet room. Alan knew their firm through his business.

Alan's sister, Pauline, called me asking if a six-month subscription to Sky Sports and cinema package would be okay for Alan's sixty fourth birthday present. It was a perfect idea. Out of Alan's earshot, we hatched a plan for a surprise party at Shirley Golf Club. Our friends, Iris and Ron, arrived at 7pm, bringing treats - vodka and red wine. They knew us well! Catching up with work emails kept me up until 2am.

Thursday 7th June - Electric wheelchair arrives

Jenelle, another new carer, showed me how to help Alan stand up with me acting as his 'spine'. As I held him upright I could feel the warmth of his body against mine. I hadn't hugged him so intimately for a long time. Unfortunately, Jenelle was going to live in Yorkshire in August. Such a shame. She was a good care worker.

The local district nurse, Roz, delivered supplies of barrier cream and Tena pads. Alan was not amused. A shiny, new Sunrise Midi electric wheelchair arrived, complete with a joystick that Alan would be able to operate with his left hand. The NHS OT and wheelchair technician set it up, trained us how to operate it safely and stressed indoor use only! It was clear some of our doors and walls would be at risk of damage, until we mastered the bulky machine.

Wendy and her husband Mel arrived, a surprise I had arranged for Alan. Wendy owned portable ramps, so Mel was able to come into the house via the internal garage door. Having two big wheelchairs in the kitchen was fun. Wendy was wonderful caring for Mel. I was not sure I would ever be as good a carer as her.

We looked at photographs of Mel's wet room and Wendy explained the routines of turning, cleaning, and flushing the PEG feeding tube going into Mel's stomach. I felt a bit squeamish at the idea of having to do the procedure for Alan, but I was not going to let the carers do such an important technical job. Rob (one of the three cyclists) and his wife, Yvonne, arrived. This was another arranged surprise for Alan. I popped out shopping and left them to chat.

Early evening the neighbour of Alan's mum called saying Joan was due to go to hospital for a check-up. Alan got stressed when he called Joan - she was more interested in his situation and wouldn't give him straight answers about hers. Later we found out from Alan's sister Pauline that Joan had experienced some unusual bleeding which needed to be checked out. Without going into detail, it was not an easy conversation for a man to have about his mum.

Friday 8th June - Negative feelings

Carer, Sadie came back and appeared in a lighter mood. I took Alan to the dentist in Redditch, where we discovered his gums were getting diseased. I received training on how to clean his teeth effectively with an electric brush. I would need to train our carers.

Alan fell trying to step over the threshold of our front door. I had to summon the gardener working on next door's lawn because I could not lift Alan on my own. It turned out Alan had been rushing because he wanted to go to the loo. When we got there, we discovered, it was too late. Luckily Alan had started wearing the Tena pads.

Back in his recliner chair, with tears in his eyes, Alan declared, "I am beginning to feel sorry for myself. It's not fair that two good people have to go through this. It's not the life I want for you or me."

Trying to hold back my own tears, I had to remind him, "We said at the outset we would not feel sorry for ourselves, and not get angry. Today is a bad day - that's all - tomorrow will be better."

At 5.30pm the HR Manager from my company texted me to see if I was okay. I had completely forgotten to call her at 4pm. After a brief chat she said, "The company do not want to lose you. I have drafted a letter and a proposed self-employed contract for you to consider." She had first-hand experience of MND so was sympathetic to my situation. She finished with, "You are highly rated, Hazel. We will do what we can to make life easy for you while you work through your notice."

Over dinner Alan mentioned he experienced discomfort during bowel movements. I asked for more information. "The pain is eight out of ten and has been going on for some time." I berated him and eventually he conceded it had been silly not to mention it sooner.

AUTHOR'S NOTE

Alan and I had adopted a numerical ranking system for quantifying everything. For example, when discussing pain, zero was low - ten was unbearable. There were many times we were able to explain to others how bad a particular situation was using this method. Things like, how satisfied were we with treatment or how hard was it dealing with a particular problem, could all be ranked out of ten.

Saturday 9th June - Support from golf club friends

Carer Chelsea was back on duty. We liked her and felt sorry she had lost her grandma. Our skiing friend Robert arrived at 10am for his turn as carer. In the same way that I did with all those who sat with Alan, I demonstrated the ventilator and stressed the need for care when giving Alan drinks and using the pee bottle. Robert would brief the next helper from *The Ski Gang*, Malcolm.

By the time I arrived at the golf club for the Lady Captain's Golf Day, I was a bit stressed. One of the ladies I played with had lost her husband, also called Alan, six years ago. "It still hurts when I think of him." I felt for her. Six years of grieving was not a pleasant thought.

I recalled telling my sister Clare that Alan's death could break me. Of course, I knew it would not, but emotional pain is a powerful force. It was impossible to predict how I would react when my Alan passed away.

Neighbours, Sue and Alex were with Alan on my return, having stepped in when Malcolm had to leave. "I enjoyed listening to Malcolm playing songs on his guitar," Alan declared "I wore my breathing mask for a lot of the day." Good man!

Sunday 10th June - Mum needs care too
Another new carer - Ligita from Lithuania - turned up on the doorstep, and loudly announced, "I am here to look after Alan," before marching into the house. She turned out to be a very capable and engaging woman, despite her direct style.

Mum rang complaining of a severe headache, so I popped in to see her. Shockingly I discovered she had mistakenly taken the wrong pills. It was time to start getting some help for her.

Alan complained of discomfort in his bowels. I noticed his tongue was very coated and his thinking was slow. I made a note in my blue notebook to discuss these symptoms with appropriate medical professionals as soon as possible.

AUTHOR'S NOTE
From the outset of Alan's condition, in addition to my journal, I kept a separate blue notebook of every meeting or significant telephone call, with every medical person or care provider. It turned out to be an invaluable tool because whenever I met a district nurse, or OT or physio, etc. I could refer to various meetings and provide them with a full history of everything that had been happening to Alan.

Monday 11th June - Wet room build started

The dietician, Kaye, arrived to discuss the PEG operation and PEG feeding. I could tell Alan was nervous about the procedure, but it was more urgent now that choking episodes were frequent. The builders arrived to kick off the wet room build. Yippee!!!

Late morning my brother, Kevin, arrived to help me with some domestic chores. At noon the ventilation nurse, Marie, from Stoke Hospital, arrived. She made some tweaks to the ventilator settings after checking Alan's readings and introduced us to a new device - the cough assist machine. As Alan was now depending on the ventilator so much, she left us with a spare one, in case the main one broke down.

Alan enjoyed a visit from golf club friends, Andy and Dawn Gould. It was a tiring day. I was ready for bed once I had undressed Alan, cleaned his teeth, got him into his pyjamas and transferred him to his bed. I would be glad when the wet room was built - abluting Alan in the cramped downstairs loo was no longer fun.

AUTHOR'S NOTE

The cough assist machine was to be used three times a day. We had to take Alan off the ventilator, fit the cough assist machine mask over his face, and turn on the machine. The machine forced air into his lungs for three breaths, and sucked air out on the fourth cycle. It helped draw up mucus from Alan's lungs, because he was now unable to cough for himself. The tricky bit was getting him back on the non-invasive ventilator quickly afterwards.

Wednesday 13th June - Last day in the office

After helping Alan with the cough assist machine, I had to take mum to the doctor's for a twenty four hour blood pressure test to be set up. In the Amersham office, it was emotional saying farewell to my work mates for the last time. Back at the house, Christina and Wendy, from Alan's office, were still with him and he was cheerful and relaxed.

Thursday 14th June – A happy anniversary

The most special day in our calendar. The twelfth anniversary of our blind date, and the fourth anniversary of our wedding day. I surprised Alan with a string of red heart shaped lights and fresh flowers on the kitchen table.

After breakfast, he read my latest heartfelt Facebook post, stating, "It's not bloody fair."

We had an emotional meeting with three people from the Marie Curie Hospice and a social worker to discuss Alan's continuing healthcare requirements. Not the way we usually spent our anniversaries, I thought to myself.

Flowers and a huge balloon turned up for me - organised on behalf of Alan by Christina. Even though he was now very poorly, Alan still found ways to make me feel special. I opened cards from friends and family and the bottle of champagne my mum had bought us. The highlight of the day was Alan being able to drive his electric wheelchair out of the garage via a newly built ramp and into the bright sunlight at the front of our house. He looked like the happiest man alive. My heart ached with love for him.

Friday 15th June - Preparing the MGB for sale
Simon Beacham arrived first thing and helped me get the MGB started, ready for a viewing.

Alan's nephew, Tom, arrived - passing through on his way to Cumbria. Unusually, Alan was not quite himself during Tom's visit. After Tom left, I had to ask, "What's up?"

Alan spoke of his (negative) feelings. I suggested, "You are letting the disease limit your life and there is no need to. Do you think it will help if you change your mindset?"

Alan agreed to try to think more positively and to my relief, said, "I am not ready to give in." Phew.

Saturday 16th June - Buyer for the MGB and Captains' Dinner
Frustratingly, our carer, Matt, arrived late, throwing our morning plans out. Soon after Matt left, Harry, a business contact of mine from Bristol, and his wife, arrived to look at the MGB. On their return from a test drive, Alan showed Harry the owner's manuals and the neat file of paperwork associated with the car.

Harry said he would buy Morris for the asking price. There was no haggling because he knew Alan planned to donate half the sale price to MND Association. It was an emotional morning. Alan had owned Morris for thirty-nine years and had enjoyed over 80,000 miles in him. I was dreading the day Morris left us.

Mum had lunch at our house. For weeks she had been saying she wanted a dog but, I knew that would be a disaster. Instead, I gave her an animated toy dog I had found for her. I don't know why, but she named him Ben.

I got Alan ready for the annual Captain's Dinner at the golf club. He looked handsome in his pink shirt and shiny Dune shoes. If it weren't for the fact that he was going to arrive in a wheelchair, no one would know the extent of his condition. I packed up the car with the ventilator and cough assist machine and, after getting Alan into the vehicle, folded up the manual wheelchair and put it in the boot. At the club we were warmly greeted by Gary, Club Captain and Jackie, the Lady Captain.

We had been allocated seats on a table close to the exit. That was useful because, at one point during dinner, we needed to go to the private room where I had left our medical equipment.

At one point, I overheard a man make an unkind comment about Alan while I was applying the cough assist machine. Somehow I stopped myself screaming, or worse, at the ignorant man!

During his speech, the Captain said, "It's nice to see all the ladies looking so glamorous, but the most beautiful person in the room is Alan Carter." There was a spontaneous round of applause and everyone stood up to honour Alan. Alan did well to hold back his emotions. I was not so successful. Later, Alan became short of breath and needed the ventilator. He was not yet ready to be seen in public using the machine and wearing the mask, so we retired to a private room for fifteen minutes.

Sunday 17th June - Lunch with friends
Matt, the carer, arrived and before long Alan was proudly telling him about the previous evening's speech. We all agreed it was good if people spoke out more, publicly, about their positive feelings towards others. An email arrived from Harry confirming he had transferred the agreed sum to Alan's bank account for Morris. So that was it, the end of another era.

I drove us to Redditch for lunch at the house of Bev and John. We had to get Alan, in John's loaned wheelchair, into the house via some wooden ramps John had cleverly made. Bev told us she had not cooked a meal for guests at home in the four years since the traumatic loss of her mum. We felt like honoured guests. Bev had made soft food, easier for Alan to chew and swallow and had purchased a spoon with a special grip, easier for Alan to hold. So thoughtful.

Back at home, we watched the gripping final day's play of the US Open. Once Alan was in bed I emailed friends and family about the forthcoming surprise sixty fourth birthday party at the golf club.

Monday 18th June - Visitors from America

The morning was busy with housework. The wet room build was in full swing, so I was chief tea maker and supplier of biscuits. Also, I had a conference call with my boss who asked, "Is there any way you could delay your early retirement?" He didn't get the answer he wanted.

After lunch, I drove to the local train station to collect Alan's cousins from America. Joni and Jim were staying with us for one night at the end of their European tour. I nodded off during a World Cup football game. Joni had to wake me so I could get Alan ready for bed.

Tuesday 19th June - Request granted

Our American visitors were delivered back to the station before Julie, our Macmillan nurse, arrived with a Marie Curie doctor to discuss medicines which would help get Alan's bowels moving. Despite having to leave Alan alone, I grabbed an hour's 'me time' at a local salon and had a much needed massage on my tight neck and shoulders.

During the ritual of getting Alan ready for bed, he stated, "I prefer it if you wake me up in the morning, rather than the carers." It was his way of making a request, one I could not deny, even though it meant I would get less sleep.

AUTHOR'S NOTE

'Me time' was an increasingly rare treat. From the beginning of Alan's illness, nearly every medical professional, family member and friend told me I should look after myself, but it was extremely difficult because of the overwhelming sense of duty I felt for Alan's care and well-being and the many plates that needed spinning.

Wednesday 20th June - WAV needed

Amy, fundraiser from MND Association for the Midlands region, arrived. I gave her two cheques and we discussed the items I needed to support the 10k runners in September. She offered to lend us a large banner for photo shoots.

At the monthly MND Group meeting we met Marie, an Irish lady who looked after her husband, Parmar. They had been married for forty years. Marie was dreading losing Parmar. Alan allowed me to show Wendy and Mel how his cough assist machine worked. The meeting chairperson said she found that sometimes people living with MND made some decisions too early. They decided they didn't want a PEG fitted, or to use a ventilator machine, only to change their minds as their condition progressed. She implored, "Please try to keep an open mind and only make such decisions when you need to."

Almost as soon as we were home Alan wanted to do research into wheelchair accessible vehicles (WAV) to enable us to go on journeys using the electric wheelchair. Alan qualified for Personal Independence Payments (PIP) because he had a terminal condition, so he was eligible to obtain a vehicle under the Motability scheme. We learned we would need to pay a deposit and enter a three, or five, year lease. A pro rata refund of the deposit would be payable in the event of death before the end of the lease. Unless he plateaued, I wasn't sure Alan would last twelve months, let alone thirty six or sixty. Despite his short life expectancy, getting a WAV was, without doubt, going to be life changing.

Thursday 21st June - Alan's birthday
As soon as I entered his bedroom I sang "Happy birthday" to Alan. I switched on the fairy lights in the kitchen and arranged his cards and presents on the kitchen table. After breakfast, I helped Alan open his cards and gifts in the lounge. There were two cards from me because I didn't know if Alan would be alive for another birthday. He cried on seeing them both.

During the day I tackled some overdue gardening. I lost myself in removing weeds, putting in new plants and trimming back shrubs. When I returned to the house Alan was angry with me because he had needed me for something. We agreed I should check on him more regularly in future. I was cross with myself for causing him distress on what might be his last birthday.

There were several occasions I needed to use the cough assist machine to help Alan clear mucus. It was getting more difficult to clear built up secretions. Just as I was about to pop out to the shops, my friend Christine from Pershore turned up unexpectedly. She stayed with Alan while I popped out to buy a birthday cake. Alan had said he didn't want any fuss for his birthday and that's what he got. He didn't say anything about me not creating a surprise party the weekend following his birthday!

Friday 22nd June - Surprise party planning
Today was supposed to be the last day of building on the wet room. Alan had predicted it would take at least three weeks to complete. Six men were now working on the foul water drainage challenge. I gave Teresa and Phil a heads up on everything they needed to do for Alan before setting off for a business meeting in Chester.

The long journey gave me time to call Alan's sister and niece and collude with them about the surprise party. It was useful having them as my partners in crime! On my way back from Chester I delivered balloons and other party pieces to my golf club friend Dawn - another useful partner in crime.

Saturday 23rd June - Party time!

There was a high risk something could go wrong with the party plan. All I could do was hope for the best. Bit like living with MND. Stuffing a scribbled welcome speech in my handbag, I worked to my hidden agenda of getting to the club just after all of Alan's family arrived for lunch. He was still very alert and would guess something was going on if he spotted a single member of his family or one of their cars!

At the club I wheeled Alan around to the back of the building, parked him up and peeked into the dining room. To my horror only Pauline, Simon and Alan's mum were there. Apparently, Helen and her family, and Matt and Suzanne were held up on the M40! We were not expecting Alan's sister Viv, and Alan's nephew Ben and his partner Claire, because they were on holiday, or Alan's nephew Tom because he was on a training course.

I busied myself taking photos of Alan by the 9th green, for next year's Captain's charity posters, until I received the 'all ready' text from Pauline. Alan's reaction as we entered the dining room was priceless. Helen's two boys jumped out, from their secret hiding place under the table, to surprise their great uncle. I had expected tears but, instead, there was laughter and happiness. Alan was delighted.

During lunch I sneaked into the lounge to check on progress. Dawn had done a great job dressing up the room and a large crowd was gathering. After we had eaten, I wheeled Alan out of the dining room. As we turned the corner into the lounge, he noticed the room was unusually full of people - and he knew all of them! For a brief moment he didn't realise they were there for him. His face was a picture when the penny dropped.

In my welcome speech, I introduced our guests to our golf club members: Alan's family, my family, Lesley and Fiona from the Marie Curie Hospice, Jo and Andy, Val and Richard and Pat, ski buddies Bev, John, Robert and Nina, friends from *More to Life,* Teresa and Phil, Sue, Chris and John, cyclists Rob and Matt and their driver Pete, and Simon Beacham's wife, Rachel and her daughter Maddie.

Gary, Club Captain, made a brief speech. Alan made a short speech. My brother made an emotional speech, and kissed Alan. Then Alan made a second speech thanking me "for everything." Everyone sang "Happy birthday" when the birthday cake arrived. The party he didn't want, was perfect!

Monday 25th June - The loo incident
Another hectic morning. The builders were in the wet room; Kevin was helping with housework; the man from the wheelchair accessible vehicles showroom arrived with a Volkswagen to demonstrate, and Julie from Macmillan nurses arrived, all before lunchtime! Julie and I took the VW for a test drive and realised immediately it would be a massive asset.

We placed an order for one straight away.

Julie then discussed Alan's *Respect* form with us. This purple framed document outlined Alan's do not resuscitate decisions and his preferred end of life location. It would travel with Alan wherever he went, so that hospitals, hospices, etc., would understand his wishes even if he could not speak. Alan could no longer write, so Julie filled in the form and signed it in her official capacity once he approved its contents. It felt like a sad thing to have to do, but necessary.

In the afternoon Alan wanted to use the loo. I struggled to support him as I transferred him from his wheelchair to the toilet, and he ended up in a heap on the toilet floor. Luckily two strong builders were available to help me pick him up. It was a very distressing incident for everyone. Alan was now too disabled for me to handle on my own. In desperation, I called the manager of the care company to see if we could get any more support.

That evening, a carer called Holly helped me with Alan's bedtime routine. She was good. Another corner had been turned in our journey. It was seven months since diagnosis, and we had moved to a new level of care need.

Tuesday 26th June - Frank discussions
There was a lot of noise outside the house as the digger continued to make a trench for the foul water pipe from the wet room.

Four people arrived from Accessible Communications and Technology (ACT) to discuss how Alan would communicate when his voice failed. They talked about voice banking, Eyegaze screens, etc. I felt sick. Communication was a cornerstone of my relationship with Alan. Being able to chat with friends was one of the things that had kept Alan going. After the ACT people left Alan and I were fractious with each other. We were both ill prepared for this stage and scared of its implications.

I went to the Marie Curie Hospice for a complementary therapy session. I was in tears most of time during the massage. The therapist hit the nail on the head when she said, "You have probably been holding everything in for a long time and you are trying to be strong for everyone else."

Alan and I had yet another deep conversation. I revealed, "I feel helpless and like I am firefighting all the time." Alan felt bad too, "For piling so much onto your already busy days." We both agreed life was not as good as we hoped we could make it, but it would be better when the WAV arrived and when the wet room was finished. If only we had been better organised!

A carer arrived early evening, but we turned her away because we wanted time to ourselves. As it happened, that night it was difficult for me to get Alan into bed. I vowed never to turn away a night-time carer again.

Wednesday 27th June - Ready to retire
While I was in Surrey, and various people sat with Alan, I met up with my friend Jill. I talked calmly about some of my plans for my future as a widow but, deep down, I knew I would be devastated for a long time after Alan died.

The journey home was horrible due to an accident on the M25. I hurriedly contacted people who could keep an eye on Alan, fearing he might choke to death if he was left on his own. Sitting in the traffic queue, I thought about the early days of our courtship. I suddenly felt more excited than normal to be driving home to Alan. I couldn't wait for my retirement. All I wanted to do was be with Alan and make his life as happy, comfortable and calm as possible.

Thursday 28th June - Considering self-employment
My day started with an emotional phone call with two of my staff in Plymouth, effectively saying our goodbyes. Alan spoke with them too. We promised to make a trip to Plymouth sometime. A promise we were not able to keep. Late afternoon I spoke with the HR Manager. I raised issues over the offered self-employed contract. "I will arrange for you to talk to the main board director you would be working for," she offered. I felt no enthusiasm for such a conversation.

I spoke with a district nurse about using special sheaths (Conveens) to reduce the need for a pee bottle. A box of incontinence pads, and mesh knickers to hold them in place, had turned up but they were too small. Grrrr!

No evening carer turned up, so the carer agency manager herself did the shift.

Friday 29th June - Last day at work

It was my last official day at work. There was a final conversation with my boss and one with the main board director who wanted to meet me in August. He was vague about what he might want me to do. I couldn't decide if I trusted him, so decided not to progress further. It was a sad end to a forty-six-year career in one industry.

The bio-toilet was fitted in the wet room which Alan christened with a poo. The wash and blow dry of his bottom brought a smile to his face. Alan's friend from work, Dennis, arrived at 1pm. My sister, Clare, and her husband, David, arrived soon after. The men stayed with Alan while I took Clare out for her final fiftieth birthday treats. She smiled a lot at the beauty salon and, over afternoon tea, told me she and Rowena were worried they might not be able to hold themselves together at Alan's funeral.

Matt, the carer, had difficulty getting Alan into bed on his own. It was becoming apparent we now needed two carers and needed to start using the hoist that had recently arrived. However, to make a change to the care plan we needed a meeting to re-assess Alan's care needs. The volume of meetings was beginning to feel overwhelming and intrusive.

Saturday 30th June - Fun in the wet room

After six weeks of strip washes in the cloakroom, Alan had his first shower in the newly completed wet room! He grinned ear to ear as the warm water sprayed over him. It might have been fun for him, but it was frantic for carer, Ann, and me. We got nearly as soaked as Alan did!

Before dressing Alan, Ann put on one of the Conveens. Alans's pee would be directed via a tube into a bag. The bag was strapped to his calf. Later in the day I discovered Alan, and his chair, were soaking wet. Too late I learned it was a good idea to check if there were any bends in the pee tube! Urine had bubbled up the tube and out of the sheath and found anything but the bag to land in. Neither Alan nor I were impressed and neither keen to continue using the contraptions.

Our neighbours, Alex and Sue, invited us for early evening drinks in their garden. While Alan enjoyed some beers, my mood was lifted by the large measures of Pimm's that Sue poured me. I hoped there was no law against being drunk in charge of a wheelchair!

PART 4 - DISEASE TAKES HOLD

JULY 2018

Sunday 1st July - Goodbye to a car, and a dream

My neighbour Steve and I did a training run near Stratford-upon-Avon, with Simon Beacham, his wife Rachel, and their daughter Maddie. A Scottish gentleman gave us £10 when he heard why we were all running wearing MND vests. He knew someone with MND and knew about international rugby player, Doddie Weir. My face was its usual bright red by the end of the 3.5k distance and, as I drove home, I realised my knees were not happy.

"You might not want to watch him being driven away," I suggested as Harry came to collect the MGB, but Alan stayed by the door. We both cried as we waved goodbye to our ambition of driving Morris around Europe in our retirement.

Tuesday 3rd July - Come on England

Alan spent the morning carefully reciting and recording 200 of the 1600 phrases for the voice banking synthesiser after the speech and language therapist got him started using a bit of kit called Model Talker. He was very motivated, despite the difficulties he had using the mouse with his weak left hand.

The GP called, He had signed the *Respect* form and approved a prescription for oral Morphine. The idea of Alan going into arrest and no one trying to resuscitate him scared me. How would I resist throwing myself at him and trying to beat him back into life?

Wednesday 4th July - Independence Day

To celebrate the fourteenth anniversary of the day I bought the house that became Carter Castle in 2008 when Alan moved in, I did a 5k run thinking about writing a book about life with MND.

One of our wet room builders finished off the snagging and told us how his dad was struggling caring for their mum. Martin agreed to join Alan's Army and said his wife would too.

Alan's bedroom (formerly the dining room), our kitchen, the wet room and Alan's dressing area (formerly the garden room between the kitchen and the wet room), were all like hospital rooms now.

Feeding Alan his dinner was a challenge. The shredded Peking Duck in pancakes was delicious, but not practical!

Thursday 5th July - Anything but convenient

Handing us the external condom catheters called Conveens, Eric, a district nurse, said, "I will be back later to prepare you, Alan."

This we deduced meant shaving Alan where it mattered!

The packaging stated, "These alternative and discreet solutions have proven to improve quality of life compared to absorbent products." Alan's face told me he was not so sure about that. I wasn't so sure about them either. The wheelchair technician fitted a better headrest to support Alan's weak neck. Unfortunately, it made getting Alan in and out of the chair difficult, so we reverted to the previous one.

Alan's ventilation nurse, Marie, ran her tests. Alan's CO2 levels were down to five point five and his HCO3 (bicarbonate) levels were also going down. Marie left us with a nose-only mask as an alternative to the full-face mask. It would allow Alan to eat while on the NIV. Alan's voice was stronger when using the ventilator due to the air pressure on his vocal cords. Finally, Marie gave us a nebuliser, in case Alan's secretions became too sticky.

More hospital equipment to find a home for and another bit of nursing for me to learn!

Some of our carers were nervous about the ventilator. I personally taught them how to put on and take off the masks, without hurting Alan's face, and how to respond if the ventilator started to alarm. Right up to the end of Alan's time living at home, some carers struggled with these skills, which meant I had to be on hand most of the time.

Friday 6th July - I miss those days

The day started with a long meeting reviewing Alan's care needs, his continuing health care (CHC) package and our current care plan, with the social worker from the Marie Curie Hospice, and manager of the care company.

New arrangements were agreed commencing the following Monday. Carers would arrive at 7:15am for an hour, 1pm for thirty minutes, 5:30pm for thirty minutes and 9:30pm for thirty minutes. That meant a lot more people coming and going, less private time for Alan and me, and less stress on me - in theory at least.

It was difficult to sleep. My mind was racing, and I was too hot. In my head I thought through a packing list for our forthcoming trip to Wales. I felt even less like sleeping when I realised how much equipment we would need to take, and the difficulties of fitting it around Alan, in the wheelchair adapted vehicle!

The thought of how much our lives had changed since the beginning of the year spawned a short poem.

I MISS THOSE DAYS
I remember the smile on your face,
When we first we met.
How it felt to hold your hand,
To walk with you.
Now your body fails you,
We will never dance again.
Never hold each other,
Wrapped in each other's warmth.
I miss those days.
I miss you.

Saturday 7th July - Trophies up for grabs

Since I joined my club in 1992 I had hardly ever missed playing in the annual thirty-six-hole Club Championship competition. So that I could participate without worrying about Alan, I arranged for four lots of people to be with him during the times no carers were at the house. My playing partner, Stacey, had a promising start but neither of us won the prestigious prize. It was a bit optimistic of me to enter such a major competition with little or no playing practice in recent months, but it felt important to uphold some traditions and stay connected to the golf club.

My friend Dawn won one of the trophies, so we celebrated with a quick drink, and I picked the brains of Gina, a retired nurse. The moral support from golf club friends became more vital as the months rolled on. England defeated Sweden in the World Cup quarter finals. For Alan's sake, I hoped they would go on to win the trophy.

Sunday 8th July - Pulled in all directions

The newly plastered conservatory wall needed painting and I had limited time. Neighbour Steve offered the help of his son for the price of some pocket money. I gained a useful spare pair of hands and the time to do the job was halved.

After taking mum shopping, I brought her back to our house. There was an angry message on the house phone "Haze, it's me, mum. I have been waiting ages. DON'T BOTHER COMING ROUND." She must have called when I was on my way to her. Her state of mind worried me. I felt pulled in all directions and helpless on all fronts. Another poem formed in my head.

DAYS, WEEKS, MONTHS

Days go by, and I don't see,
The way you used to be.
I only see the man you are,
With a disease leaving its scar.

Weeks go by, and I don't hear,
Your complaints, I just feel your fear.
We soldier on brave and strong.
To give in now would be all wrong.

Months go by, and I don't know,
How much further this will go.
What will happen as time goes by?
What will it be like,
When you come to die?

Tuesday 10th July - Turning corners

Alan and I were sitting at the front of the house chatting when Vikki and Christina, from his office, came to visit. They became excited when I talked about my ideas for a book.

Something red, possibly blood, appeared in Alan's secretions when I used the cough assist machine. I didn't mention it to him but made a note to speak to a nurse about it. Alan's legs were too weak to safely transfer him manually, so we started using the hoist to get him in and out of beds and chairs. Another corner turned.

While tucking Alan into his bed, I joked, "So now your left arm and hand don't work you need me to be your secretary, as well as your skivvy, quartermaster, carer and matron." I then gave him an extra big kiss.

Wednesday 11th July - Have WAV, will travel

The carers were leaving as I descended the stairs. I had overslept. To try and get ahead of schedule, I started packing for our forthcoming trip to Wales.

District nurse, Eric, arrived with a trainee and more condom catheters to try. Eric shaved Alan before checking which size of Conveen would be best. During the day I checked if the condom was working and breathed a sigh of relief when discovering Alan was dry. The bag strapped to his leg looked like a mini, yellow hot water bottle. It was tricky getting the Conveens fitted correctly. Should we risk using them in Wales?

The wheelchair adapted vehicle (WAV) arrived, a dark blue metallic VW Caddy with just 190 miles on the clock. Alan needed my help with the WAV paperwork and paying the deposit. Tax, insurance, servicing, tyres, windscreen repairs and MOT would all be funded via the monthly payment (which was taken directly from his personal independence payments). All we had to do was put fuel in the vehicle and hand it back at the end of five years, or earlier, if Alan did not survive that long.

After lunch I took the WAV for a short test drive. It was bigger than my own car, so I was glad we had paid extra for reversing sensors. It was exciting thinking about the freedom the vehicle gave us. England played Croatia in the World Cup semi-final. It went into extra time, but, unfortunately, we lost.

AUTHOR'S NOTE

There would be a pro rata refund of the WAV deposit if death occurred within the lease term.

Thursday 12th July - Getting ready for Wales

My hairdresser arrived and cut my hair and tidied up Alan's. We would both look smart for our first holiday in the WAV. While Alan struggled to use his iPad with his left hand, he mentioned "My left ankle is stiffer than my right one." When I was giving Alan his lunch I noticed his breathing was very shallow. The ventilator showed a reading of 78% instead of the usual 100%. He would need to use the ventilator as much as possible over the next few days.

Alan's sister Viv, and her husband John, arrived early evening. They observed the carers undertaking Alan's bedtime routine so they would be able help me with his care in Wales.

Friday 13th July - Wales here we come!

By some miracle I managed to squeeze everything into the WAV. Around 11am we set off. Viv and John had sat nav in their car, so we followed them. On the

M5, just before the M50 turn off, we stopped as Alan wanted a cough assist machine session. The machine needed to be plugged into a power source as it had no battery pack. Embarrassingly, we had to do the procedure near the entrance of a service station.

We stopped for a pre-planned picnic lunch and a comfort break at Tredegar House, where we rendezvoused with Alan's nephews Ben and Tom, and Clare, Ben's girlfriend. There was a further cough assist stop at the services on the way to Swansea. Here we also used a disability toilet facility. Thank goodness we had purchased a Radar key in advance!

The long, slow, traffic ridden journey was made easier by listening to an exciting semi-final from Wimbledon on the radio. The tiebreak in the third set one was won by twenty points to eighteen! We finally arrived at Apple Cottage around 7:30pm. Before bedtime we watched the thrilling tennis match on TV.

In the absence of a hoist, at bedtime the three of us had to use one of the red slip sheets to manoeuvre Alan into bed. Alan's legs were too weak to support him, so John had to take most of the strain. Exhausted, I dropped straight off to sleep once in bed.

AUTHOR'S NOTE
Cough assist machines now have battery packs. Radar keys work on public disability toilet doors. *disabilityrightsuk.org/radar-keys*

Saturday 14th July - A perfect day
After sorting out Alan and clearing away the breakfast things, we packed Alan and his equipment into the WAV. With John driving, we set off for St. David's in glorious sunshine. Using the joystick near his left hand, Alan steered himself, in his electric wheelchair, across the stone slabs to the cathedral. He looked less self-conscious and was clearly embracing the freedom the new chair gave him. A nice man welcomed us at the cathedral door. Later we had to go back to him for permission to use a power socket near the front entrance when Alan needed the cough assist machine.

An orchestra and choir were setting up to perform Hayden's *The Creation* later in the day. I would have liked to have listened to rehearsals, but Alan was not bothered about going back inside after our picnic. The nice man at the door told us where we could find the special wheelchairs I had heard about on Radio Four.

The beach wheelchairs at Whitesands had huge, inflated rubber tyres and were a bargain to hire - just £5 for the day! I was pleased Alan was up for giving one a try despite all the manhandling it took to get him into one. Strolling across the huge empty expanse of white sand, wind in our hair, watching the surfers playing on the waves, felt like heaven. Alan smiled a lot. I filmed him a lot.

Back at the cottage, it was a challenge for John and I to manoeuvre Alan, in his heavy electric wheelchair, around the side of the cottage into the back garden for the BBQ, but worth it. Eating alfresco and drinking cold beers in the softening, evening sunshine was a lovely way to end a perfect day.

Sunday 15th July - Moving a giant slippery fish

We drove to Fishguard after breakfast and took Alan along the Marine Walk until we found a suitable place for a picnic. The day was cooler, but there was a sweet scent in the air. The sky was blue and clear. Back in St. David's we enjoyed delicious, organic ice cream made locally. After a coastal drive back to the cottage we watched the men's final from Wimbledon.

It was too cold to eat in the garden again, but John still bravely cooked our evening meal on the BBQ outside, earning him extra beers! The three of us struggled to get Alan into bed. This time using the red slip sheet felt like trying to move a giant slippery fish on a marble table!

Monday 16th July - Challenges

Heavy rain meant packing away everything into the WAV was not fun. We had only been on the road a short while when Alan needed the cough assist machine. At a restaurant we could not get the wheelchair inside the building because one of the double doors was locked and no one knew where the keys were! At the back of the building, there were two steps to scale and a threshold to negotiate. I muttered under my breath that the establishment was not accessible and returned to the front door where we managed with an extension cable.

After all that Alan also needed to pee, so I moved the car to the far corner of the car park and found the pee bottle. My blood pressure was off the scale. We caught up with Viv and John at a service station just before the M4. The cough assist machine was needed again - this time in full view of the public. We also used the disability toilet when a couple with a baby vacated it. Eventually we were on our way to our next destination.

Worryingly Alan wanted a third cough assist machine session but there was nowhere to stop so he had to wait until we reached our hotel in Cardiff. The so-called accessible hotel room was so cluttered there was no room to get

Alan into it in his electric wheelchair. I had to ask for a table and chairs to be removed.

We took Alan into town where we met Ben, Claire, and Tom for an Italian dinner. The restaurant had lovely views but was noisy. Alan looked unsettled. He needed to have his breathing machine mask on after eating. I was feeling very tired, so we decided to head back to the hotel for drinks. It was an exhausting, challenging day. I hoped Alan had enjoyed some of it and that the noise from his breathing machine would not disturb my sleep too much.

Tuesday 17th July - You've got a friend
We reached the National Trust property, Dyffryn House, just outside Cardiff by 9.30am. Ben and Tom were delayed so Viv, John and I escorted Alan around the house. We were touring the wheelchair friendly gardens when the boys arrived.

Back at the hotel, Alan watched the Tour de France while I got changed for our second night out in a row! Viv and John came with us in the WAV to Cardiff centre. We had a quick pizza and beer before meeting Ben's girlfriend, Claire, who worked at the Motorpoint arena. She escorted us through the building to the VIP box.

Bonnie Raitt performed her act before James Taylor came on with an excellent band of musicians. It was good to hear *Fire and Rain* and *Sweet Baby James*, but the words of *You've got a Friend* set off my emotions. Lucky for me the lights were so low, no one saw my tears.

Wednesday 18th July - Back home
We had a straightforward journey home from Cardiff. Viv and John stayed at our house while I took mum for a check-up with her anticoagulant consultant. He was pleased with her progress and signed her off. Phew! One less thing for me to deal with in the future.

Thursday 19th July - Too much fluid
We had a visit from Alan's GP about the swelling in his arms and ankles. She was concerned that the hot weather was causing fluid retention and arranged a prescription for some surgical stockings and a referral to a lymphedema specialist.

Friday 20th July - Poorly family members
Before driving mum to her appointment at the mental health clinic, I managed a six-mile run. Looking at his notes, the consultant advised us that mum would always have hallucinations because he could not give her the usual dementia

drugs, due to her heart condition. Fortunately, he could prescribe anti-anxiety drugs.

During the afternoon I had to take Alan to the local fire station. Carers had tried to remove his signet ring, but it was stuck fast and beginning to cut into the flesh of his swelling finger.   The firemen and women made light of our situation, while skilfully sawing at the back of the ring. They gave me the ring in three pieces. I gave them a donation for their charity box.

It was sad saying goodbye to Jenelle, one of our best carers, after she got Alan ready for bed. She was off to new pastures 'up North' with a small gift we gave her for her new home.

Saturday 21st July - Single bed space

For a change we had a quiet day at home. Alan looked handsome in his new grey tee shirt, so I squeezed myself onto his single bed and hugged him while watching TV. With tears in his eyes, Alan protested, "This isn't fair." I knew he didn't mean how little room there was for me on the bed.

"I would be happy if things could stay just the way they are," I replied, adding, "All I want is for you to be happy."

He reminded me, "We don't know how long we have got left."

I couldn't reply to that.

In the middle of the night Alan called out, so I went downstairs. Looking anxious he said, "Air is leaking from this ventilator mask." It looked fine to me, and the alarm on the machine was not going off. I wondered if he needed some of mum's anxiety tablets or, did he just want me to get back into bed with him, as I returned upstairs.

Sunday 22nd July - Good night, "I love you"

We had a lazy day indoors, despite the lovely sunshine outdoors. We watched the German Grand Prix, the Tour de France, and the exciting conclusion of last day of The Open. While Alan was in a good mood, I asked, "How do you feel about doing the September 10k in your wheelchair, with the rest of Alan's Army?" He declined. I didn't push the matter. He probably felt awful about the idea having run several marathons in his life before MND.

Aware of Alan's fear of leaks from his ventilator mask, I checked the readings on his NIV machine. It showed his ability to take a good breath had gone down. I offered him an additional dose of oral morphine to calm his anxiety, which he accepted.

When the carers arrived at lunchtime we had a chat about using the hoist instead of manually handling Alan. They agreed but insisted I have a go in it first, so I could feel what Alan would experience. That was fun, not!

Preparing Alan's medicines, I asked, "How are you feeling about the forthcoming PEG operation Al?"

"I am not keen, but I need to go through with it," he answered.

"You will go with *The Ski Gang* to Wengen in January, won't you." Alan insisted.

After a moment of thought, I replied, "Only if you are well, and Viv comes to oversee your care that week."

At lights out Alan said his usual, "Thank you for looking after me," but unusually added, "I love you," before his usual, "Don't let the buggies bite."

The added "I love you" made me realise a little something had shifted in his mind. I couldn't sleep - my mind mulling over how Alan would be affected by the PEG operation. It was getting harder for both of us to stay positive.

Monday 23rd July - Nurses uniform needed

Alan was stern with me while he was trying to sign some legal documents for our financial adviser. "What's wrong Al?"

My heart broke when he said, "I can't make my left-hand work anymore."

Following his revelation, we ended up having a long chat about what was on our respective minds. To try to motivate him, I talked about the various things he was still able to do even though his arms and legs weren't working any more. I shared how I felt the pressure of an ever-increasing list of tasks and told him, "I worry about what's on your mind, when you don't talk to me." He admitted being scared about the operation. We agreed that it was essential to keep communicating with each other. Finally, we concluded that when a man says he is fine - it generally means he is, but when a woman says she is fine, generally she is not.

One of my friends called when I was out at the Post Office. I told her I felt guilty, taking time away from Alan, to do enjoyable things. She said she thought Alan would want me to have time to recharge, laugh and be happy, because he loved me. My brother, Kevin, arrived with his grandson Tyler. They helped me with housework and watering the garden plants.

Our OT, Fiona, arrived at the same time as the people from ACT. We had a long session working out solutions to communication challenges. The PEG nurse, Jane, arrived to show me the fundamentals of keeping the PEG stoma site clean and how to flush the tube. It was all a bit scary. While practising the techniques I joked, "Perhaps I should wear a nurse's uniform when I do this for real in the future." Jane said, "I will arrange training for the carers to relieve the pressure on you." I wasn't sure I would trust anyone to undertake such a tricky task.

Drinking a beer in the back garden while I was weeding, to my delight Alan said, "I want to go out more on nice warm days like these."

Wednesday 25th July - PEG operation day
As instructed, I called Stoke Hospital at 11am but no bed was available. I tried again at 2pm and still no bed. I packed in anticipation. Late afternoon we received a call advising no bed was going to be free that day. We treated ourselves to a huge portion of raspberry ripple ice cream and settled down to watch a film - a far nicer experience than surgery. Tommy's Honour was a true story about a golfer who died from a broken heart aged twenty-four after his wife died in childbirth. Not the best film for cheering ourselves up!

"My left leg is really bad," Alan said, "and I feel strange and lonely at the end of each evening when you close the door and go to bed without me." He ended with, "I feel like a useless lump." Keen to cheer him up I hugged him and said, "I would rather have you as you are than not have you at all." There were tears when I shared a poem with him that I had written a couple of days before.

DOWNSTAIRS ALONE
I don't want to leave you,
Sleeping in your bed,
Downstairs, all alone.
I can't sleep upstairs,
All on my own.
I want to hold you,
And never let you go.
Feel you,
Never let you know,
How the pain cuts deep,
Tugging at my soul.
How the tears fall,
Staining as they go.

Thursday 26th July - Alarming calls

For some reason the electric wheelchair would not work properly. The problem appeared to be with the battery. I called the service centre and, after much pleading, secured an appointment for the next day. It was good to get an early night for a change. I fell into a deep sleep.

At 11:30pm Alan woke me up by activating the newly acquired alarm button, via a slight turn of his head. I cleared his airways using the cough assist machine and returned to bed. Around 3am, Alan activated the alarm again. Looking apologetic he said, "Sorry, I hit the alarm by mistake." So much for an early night!

Friday 27th July - Worrying test results

At Stoke Hospital Dr Mustafa did a routine check-up of Alan's respiration. Alan's CO2, oxygen and bicarb levels were okay. His peak flow test however was not good - the readings were low. His sniff test was also low, proving what I feared - Alan's diaphragm and breathing muscles were being affected a lot by MND.

Dr Mustafa recommended using Oramorph in the day, to relax Alan's breathing, rather than depending on the non-invasive ventilator (NIV) so much. Depressingly, the doctor said, "Your breathing has deteriorated faster than the average person with MND." Sitting behind me in his wheelchair in the WAV, I could see Alan in the rear-view mirror as we travelled home in silence. He looked as low as I felt.

From the beginning of Alan's diagnosis I had feared his respiratory muscles failing. Thoughts and questions whirred around my mind as I drove. It was now clear. He would not live the typical two to five years that people with his form of MND usually did. He was probably not one of those rare exceptions who lived more than five years. In fact, the prognosis of six to twenty-four months, given to us just eight months earlier, was looking more realistic.

Could we still get lucky? Could Alan's former peak physical fitness help him defeat this disease? Could I help him stay strong mentally as he headed towards total paralysis?

Saturday 28th July - With this ring....

Alan managed without the ventilator for most of this grey, wet day. In the evening I drove him to Redditch for the sixtieth birthday party of our friend, and ski gang member, Bev. At the pub, so he could drink without the need for anyone's help, I rigged up the newly acquired Hydrant bottle. It was filled with beer and the tube he could suck on was placed over his shoulder. People were fascinated by it. Alan loved it. Outside, I had a particularly emotional conversation with Julie.

Alan and I had to leave early because we were due at a surprise fiftieth wedding anniversary party for our friends Val and Richard, organised by their daughter. We arrived just after the main course had been served and sat with past and current members of Shirley Golf Club. During the speeches Richard made an emotional mention of Alan. His daughter told us later that it was a rare thing for her dad to be so emotional. When we came to leave, our golfing friends could not hide their feelings. Iris cried. Pat said she had no idea things were so bad. Val told us she loved us.

That night, while the carers were getting Alan ready for bed, Holly brought me Alan's wedding ring, saying, "Alan asked me to give you this. He doesn't want it to have to be cut off in the same way as his signet ring was." My heart sank. It felt odd to be holding something so symbolic in my hand - especially as it was handed to me by a relative stranger out of the blue. Alan probably wanted to avoid the heartbreak of asking me to take it off him. Later, there was a huge response to my Facebook post, showing a photograph of the ring in my hand.

AUTHOR'S NOTE
The Hydrant is a hydration bottle with a drinking tube which can be hung, hooked or clipped almost anywhere. It gave Alan some independence due to its hands-free design.
hydrateforhealth.co.uk/our-products/the-hydrant

Sunday 29th July - Freedom of the mind
The wet weather continued, which didn't bother Alan. With a glint in his eye he said, "Being snug indoors with you is all I want to do. When you're not around I imagine myself cycling the mountains with the Tour de France racers." His body might not be free to roam, but his mind certainly was.

While I was out shopping with mum she spoke of seeing my dad. He had died in 2001 so I decided it must be her dementia. I didn't want to make her feel stupid, so I merrily chatted about dad as if he were still alive, which had the effect of making me feel stupid! It was bizarre that mum's mind was degenerating, but her body was okay, at the same time as Alan's body was degenerating but his mind was sharp as a pin.

Alan and I did a FaceTime call with his sister Viv, after which I cooked one of his favourite meals - a roast chicken dinner. Before lights out Alan and I had a nice hug which felt good. More than usual, I wished I could sleep with him in his downstairs single bed.

Monday 30th July - Wash and blow dry anyone?

The adviser helping us sort out Lasting Powers of Attorney arrived. Alan could not sign his name so put a mark in place of a signature. I wondered if our neighbours, who were our witnesses, had a lump in their throats, like I did.

We discovered a technical problem with the bio bidet toilet. The plumbing-in had gone okay but the latest commode chair was too narrow to fit over it. Alan would no longer experience the joys of a wash and blow-dry to his undercarriage.

Tuesday 31st July - Disturbed sleep

Gina, an ex-nurse from our golf club, looked after Alan while I played in a match, which I lost. Just after midnight Alan hit the alarm button. "I am in pain," he said. I gave him paracetamol. Then he wanted a pee but when I brought him the bottle he was unable to go. Slightly worrying.

Further on in the night, Alan buzzed me again. The unit at the bottom of his bed, which pumped up his mattress, was vibrating against the foot board. At 2am, the buzzer went off again. This time the tube from the NIV had slipped and was dragging his face mask to one side. He tried to pee again without success. More worry.

I struggled to get to sleep after all the interruptions. Also, I could not block out the sound of Alan's breathing and the NIV machine coming through the intercom. I needed ear plugs but, if I wore them, I might not hear the alarm calls. It was hard not to feel sorry for myself.

AUGUST 2018

Wednesday 1st August - Alan's Army meeting

Most of the day was spent preparing for a meeting of 'Alans's Army' at our house. With five weeks till the 10k race, I felt it was time to get some serious training done.

I treated the runners to a buffet meal and one of my signature strawberry and orange trifles.

Jaki, who was a regular runner, gave us hints on how train without gaining injuries. She also gave me some exercises to strengthen my weak knees.

Thursday 2nd August - Shower chair and hoisting issues

For some reason I woke up with a hangover. I had only drunk one glass of red wine the night before. It was 14% proof Malbec though. Despite my throbbing head I ran for over four miles around the village.

Alan's work contact, Kevin, visited. I had not met him prior to Alan's MND diagnosis, but he was very likeable and kind. Kevin talked about how becoming a vegan had helped his health. Alan liked my roast chicken dinners too much to become a vegan.

A new shower chair arrived but, unfortunately, it too did not fit over the bio bidet toilet. At 9pm, three carers arrived for the bedtime shift. Afterwards, I asked Alan how it went. Rolling his eyes, he said, "It was a circus. They struggled using the hoist." Oh dear. I hoped he would not refuse to be hoisted in future.

Friday 3rd August - Garage space at a premium

Carers, Terese and Olivia struggled with the new shower chair. It was much bigger than the previous one, making it harder for the carers. Also, it retained a lot of water.

My sister, Clare, and her husband David arrived after lunch to help me put things back in the garage. However, space was limited now the wet room was in place. I had not factored this in, so a lot of reorganising would be necessary.

Saturday 4th August - The problems with NIV masks

At 2am, I needed to go to the bathroom. Twenty minutes later Alan's alarm went off. He needed his mask to be adjusted. Not long after I returned to bed I heard Alan calling me via the intercom. "You forgot to turn the alarm buzzer back on. I've been trying to call you. I am getting a pain in my right hip," he barked. "I think it's because I am not fully straight in the bed." He looked perfectly okay to me. To help him feel more comfortable I raised his knees a little higher and crossed my fingers. Please let that work.

During the afternoon, Alan and I took a trip to see my other sister, Rowena, her husband Steve and their son, Darren. The three of them helped me get Alan round to their back garden. In the bright sunshine Rowena and I found ways to stop Alan's skin burning as he was wearing shorts and didn't have a hat.

Back at our house, the local carpet shop representative arrived. We needed a quote for changing the hall and cloakroom floors from carpet to a hard surface to make it easier to wheel the shower chair between the kitchen and Alan's bedroom. Unusually, Alan took no interest in the project. Was he getting fed up with MND causing us to change our lovely home into a hospital? I knew I was.

AUTHOR'S NOTE

The tightness of the NIV face masks was critical, but it was difficult to position them comfortably. The muscles in Alan's face relaxed when he was sleeping on his back - his usual position these days. This meant that a mask that fitted well when he was being put to bed, often became loose as his face relaxed, allowing air to escape later in the night. As such, he needed to wake me up several times in the night to make mask adjustments.

Sunday 5ᵗʰ August - Loss and making people cook their own lunch

In Alan's room, just before the carers arrived, Alan admitted, "I haven't slept well. I kept feeling cold." I chastised him for not waking me up. Looking up at me from his bed, he said, "I didn't want you to have two bad nights in a row." He was selfless to his core.

Our friends Jill and Steve from Surrey, with Lesley and Roger from London, arrived armed with food and wine. While the men were outside sorting out the barbecue, I told the girls, "Alan told me the other day, he is grieving the loss of his left-hand functionality, grieving the loss of his independence and is also worried that his voice is weakening."

Lunch was eaten outside in the sunshine. Alan and I had to endure jokes about us inviting people for a meal and making them cook their own food. Cheekily I invited Steve and Roger to do some odd jobs. I was taking advantage of offers to help, at last. Jill and Steve stayed the night. Alan looked happy when I tucked him into bed. Different company had made a nice change.

Monday 6ᵗʰ August - Behind schedule

After Jill and Steve left, I drove Alan to Stratford-upon-Avon so I could familiarise myself with the route of the forthcoming race. Seeing it made me realise I needed to do a lot more training or I would be walking, not running, the 10k in just over a month's time.

Tuesday 7th August - Voice banked

Once the carers were done, our day started with our daily dose of *Frasier* on TV. During the morning, Alan finished saying the last of the 1600 sentences into the model talker software so his voice could be banked. To celebrate we went out in the WAV. We made it as far as the local municipal tip to drop off some rubbish. Where had all the romance in our lives gone?

En route home we checked out a new retirement development in our village. It was an easy decision not to move into one. Bungalows with one bedroom cost half the price of our house! An unexpected new symptom popped up - excessive dried mucus in Alan's nose. I made a note in my blue book, ready for our next discussion with one of the medical team.

Wednesday 8th August - Funds raised and fears about choking

Judith, an ex-work colleague of mine from the 1990s, arrived with flowers and good news. Her company had selected MND Association as its charity for the month of July. Although she and her colleagues had never met Alan, they had raised £550!

Inconveniently, the man who was supposed to fit a threshold ramp between Alan's bedroom (previously our dining room) and the conservatory, did not arrive. When I took mum shopping she started talking about her funeral arrangements. Her awareness that Alan had a terminal illness prompted her to share her wishes with me.

It was difficult to get to sleep. I was terrified of Alan developing pneumonia due to food going down the wrong way, or him choking to death before he had the operation to fit the feeding tube.

Thursday 9th August - Wheelchair adaptations and physiotherapy

Looking at some old pictures of Alan standing up and walking around saddened me. It seemed like a long time since he was fit and able bodied.

The wheelchair technician came and fitted bolts to the chair's handlebars so that I could hang the non-invasive ventilator machine on the back of his chair. This would give us the opportunity to travel further distances. Yippee! I pointed out Alan could no longer use his left hand. Unfortunately, no further adaptations were available. Sadly, from now on Alan would need another person to steer the vehicle for him.

Alan's physiotherapist, Lesley, arrived and showed carers Terese and Olivia some arm exercises to save Alan's shoulders from seizing up and becoming painful. I made a video so that I could show other carers when they came to do their shifts.

AUTHOR'S NOTE
Many carers do not have much experience of the specialist equipment and procedures needed when caring for a person with MND. It's important to explain everything carefully and train carers in the correct practice.

Friday 10th August - More visitors
The rainy, cold day started with our usual dose of *Frasier*, followed by a lazy morning. Phil, from the golf club, visited during the afternoon. Jo and Andy came early evening for nibbles, wine and beer. Eating our usual fish and chip supper, I pondered how much longer Alan would be able to enjoy this Friday night treat?

Saturday 11th August - Both feeling robbed
Alan pressed his alarm at 2:30am. He had a pain in his left foot. I couldn't see anything obvious. Could he be developing a bedsore?

My old boss Martin and his wife, Fliss, looked after Alan while I was out, followed by Malcolm from *The Ski Gang*.

Later, after relaying Malcolm's recent experience of dating, Alan gently asked me, "Have you thought about your future?"

"I cannot imagine living with someone else," I replied.

Alan then made a fair point, "You might feel differently if you move out of Carter Castle."

But I wanted to grow old with him. Sadly, MND had robbed me of that. An alternative was hard to imagine.

While watching TV Alan announced, "My lower tummy is painful."

We both agreed it was probably something to do with his bowel again.

"How are you in yourself?" I asked.

"It's the simplest things I feel robbed of, like not being able to scratch an itch."

I held him for a long time and told him how much I loved him.

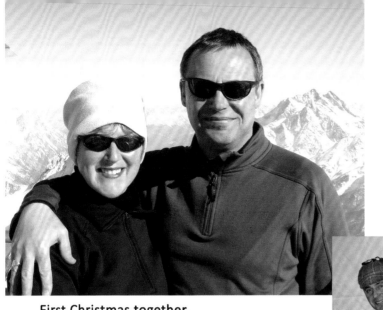

First Christmas together,
in the Italian Alps - Dec 2006

Shirley Golf Club fancy dress
party - Aug 2012

Wedding speeches- June 2014

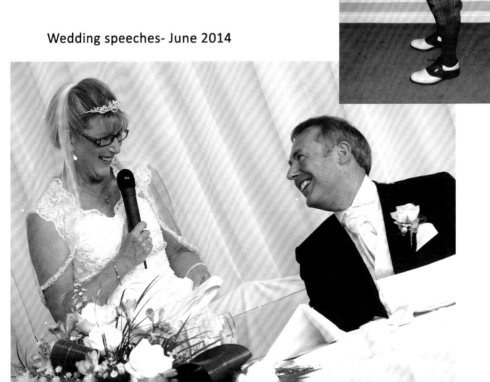

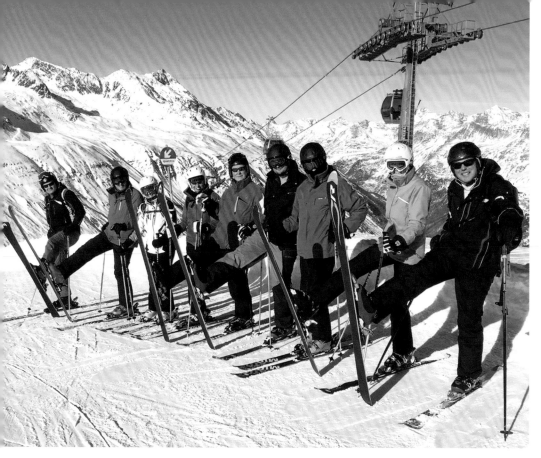

The Ski Gang in Obergurgl for Hazel's 60th - Jan 2017

ABC Christmas dinner - Dec 2017

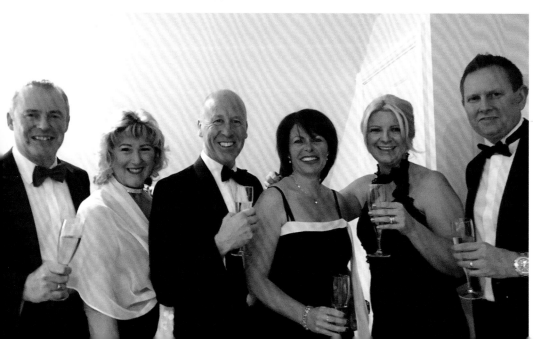

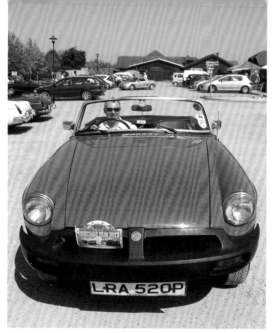

Morris the MG out for a summer
spin - July 2013

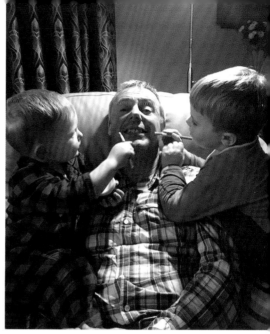

Great nephews painting
Uncle Alan's face - Dec 2017

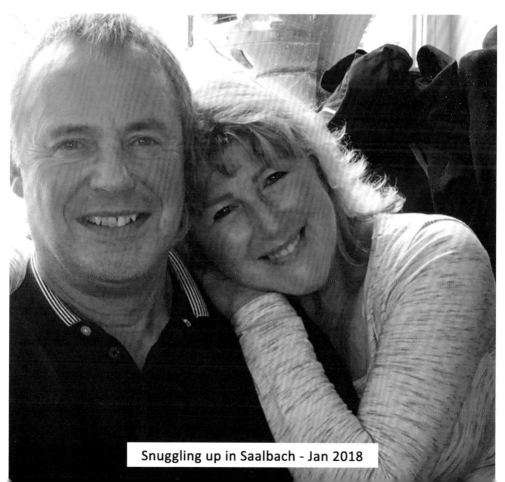

Snuggling up in Saalbach - Jan 2018

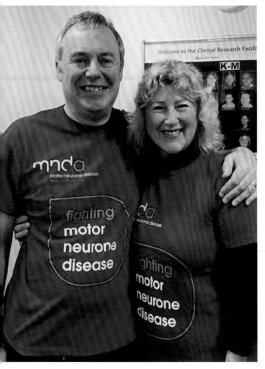

Ready for drugs trial assessment at Sheffield Hospital - March 2018

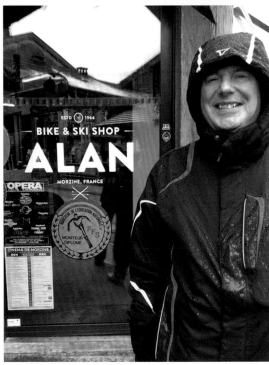

Alan's shop in Morzine, he can no longer ski or cycle - March 2018

Shaving, Vietnamese style
- April 2018

Easter with Angela and David
- April 2018

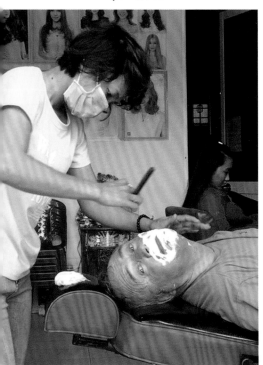

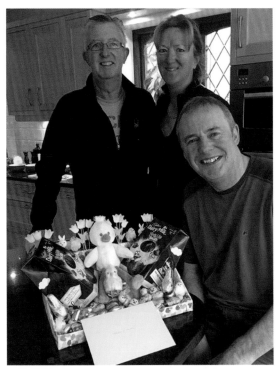

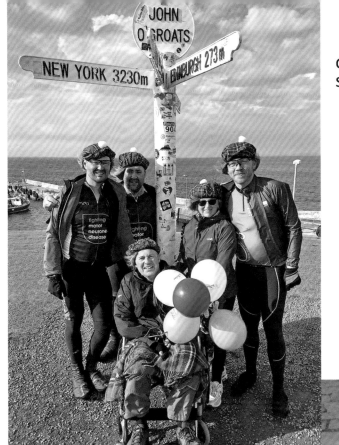

Celebrations at John O'Groats, Scotland - April 2018

64th birthday surprise at Shirley Golf Club - June 2018

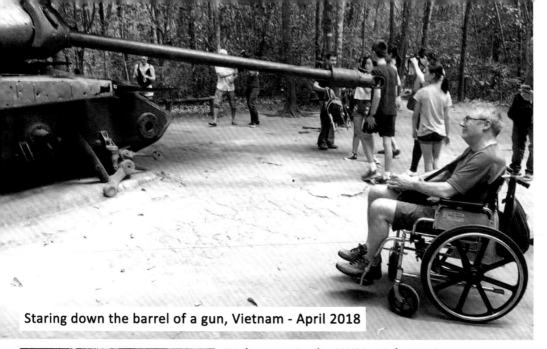

Staring down the barrel of a gun, Vietnam - April 2018

Wales tour in the WAV - July 2018

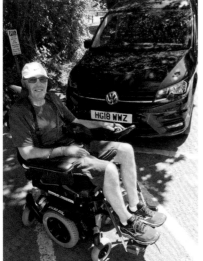

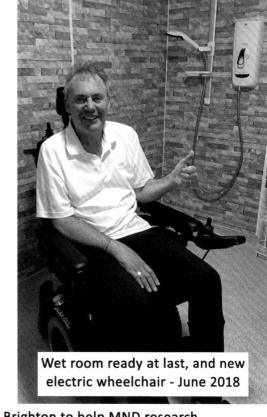

Wet room ready at last, and new electric wheelchair - June 2018

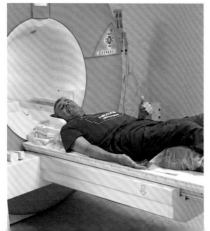

MRI in Brighton to help MND research - May 2018

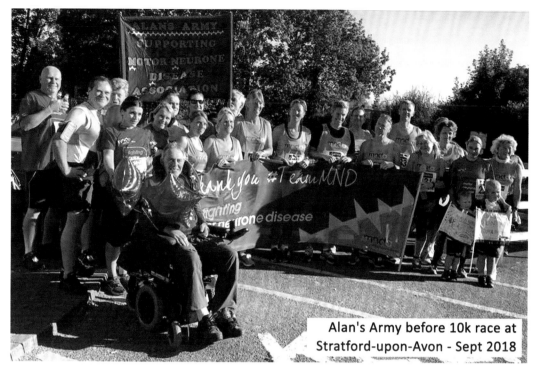

Alan's Army before 10k race at
Stratford-upon-Avon - Sept 2018

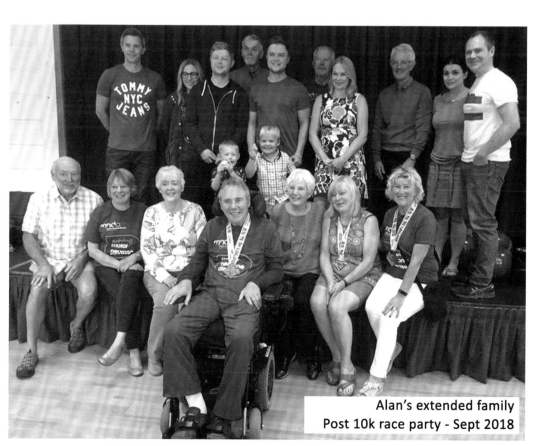

Alan's extended family
Post 10k race party - Sept 2018

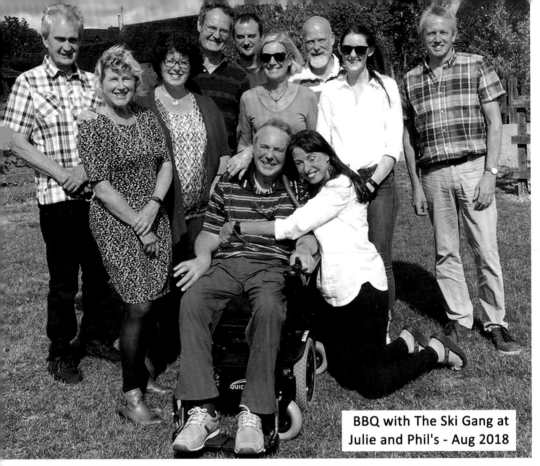

BBQ with The Ski Gang at Julie and Phil's - Aug 2018

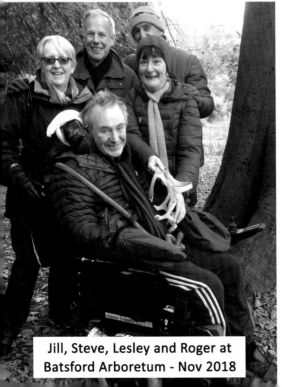

Jill, Steve, Lesley and Roger at Batsford Arboretum - Nov 2018

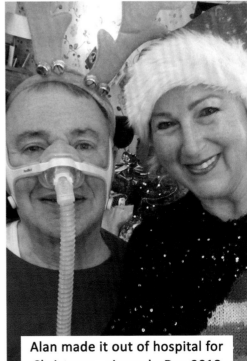

Alan made it out of hospital for Christmas - yippee! - Dec 2018

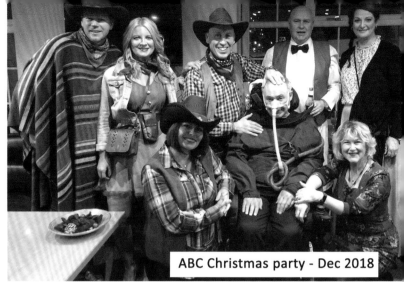

New Year's Eve in Coventry Hospital - Dec 2018

ABC Christmas party - Dec 2018

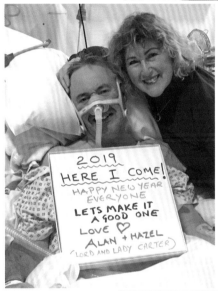

2019 HERE I COME!
HAPPY NEW YEAR EVERYONE
LETS MAKE IT A GOOD ONE
LOVE ♡
ALAN + HAZEL
(LORD AND LADY CARTER)

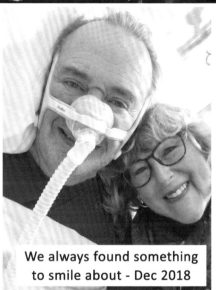

We always found something to smile about - Dec 2018

Helen and Tom at the Marie Curie Hospice, Solihull - May 2019

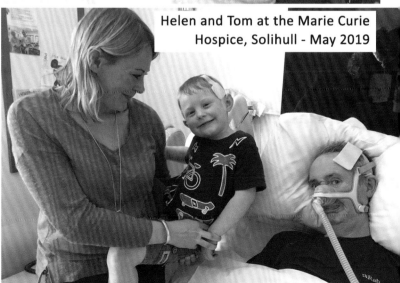

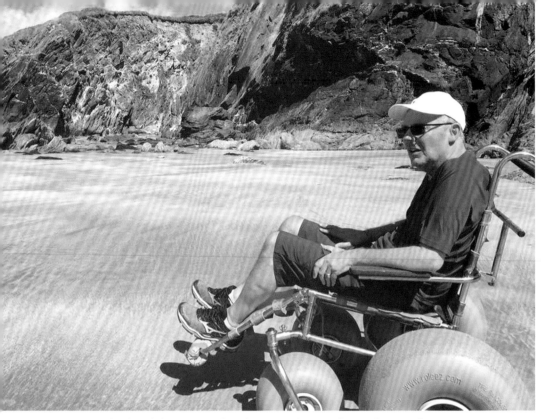

Special wheelchair rental, Whitesands Beach, Wales - July 2018

It's not Christmas without some
tinsel, Coventry Hospital - Dec 2018

Kevin, Sue and Tyler at the Marie
Curie Hospice, Solihull - May 2019

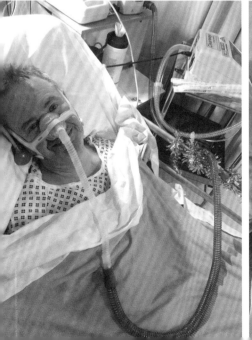

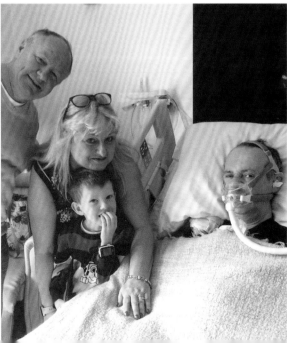

Sunday 12th August - No meeting with James

Alan alerted me at 5:30am. I re-fitted his NIV mask. "The pain in my bottom is worse and I need a pee." I put the pee bottle in place, but in my tiredness, let it slip. Pee went everywhere, leaving me with a sore ear from the telling off Alan gave me and a lot of cleaning up to do.

After my short early morning run, Alan reported, "The pain in my abdomen is much worse. I don't think I should go out." I cancelled our trip to Doncaster to meet a couple affected by MND. By mid-afternoon I had developed a headache, was shivering and felt excessively tired. I feared I was getting a cold. Alan had to be kept safe from germs as his breathing was already compromised. How could I care for him if I was infectious?

Monday 13th August - Bad bowels and bad choking

As soon as the GP surgery was open I called and booked a home visit. The doctor diagnosed that Alan had a compacted bowel. He needed to take Senokot. A specialist cream and a pessary could be prescribed if things did not improve. The threshold ramp between the bedroom and the conservatory was finally fitted. For the first time in ages Alan was able to sit in the conservatory and get a decent view of the garden.

Our neighbour, Sue, popped in. I trained her in how the ventilator worked and the tricky art of putting on and taking off masks. She was due to sit with Alan on Tuesday. Alan was now using the NIV most of the day so, everyone sitting with him would have to be trained in future. While drinking through his Hydrate bottle straw, Alan had a serious choking episode. It really worried me. Earlier in the week he had choked on a pea. We had another discussion about the delicate topic of taking liquid food via the PEG, rather than eating by mouth.

Tuesday 14th August - Letting out the 'pain'

Tom, from the club, looked after Alan, followed by neighbours Alex and Sue, so I could play in a competition. It was hard to concentrate on my golf. By the time I got to the fifteenth hole I was constantly thinking about the days I used to play with Alan. It occurred to me I may have to join a different club one day, to avoid painful memories. Walking up the final fairway I became emotional. The 14th of every month up until Alan was diagnosed with MND had always been so enjoyable, but now…….

Before taking my last putt on the 18th hole, I felt a strong emotional pain inside me. It made me want to cry out. My playing partner, Lady Captain Pam, noticed my angst and approached me about it in the changing room. Then the floodgates opened. Several ladies comforted me. I heard someone say, "You need to let out the emotion."

Wednesday 15th August - 'Barbara' arrives

Alan's speech and language therapist delivered a communication aid she called a Barbara book. The book contained a number of pre-printed requests, such as I need a drink, which I could point to. All Alan had to do was blink once for yes, twice for no, so that I could establish what he wanted. We could add to the list of the requests and it also had a page with the alphabet on it. We were advised to practise using it so we would be experts by the time Alan's speech left him. I felt sick thinking about it. Alan did not appear very interested.

We attended the monthly MND meeting at the Marie Curie Hospice. This time we met Paul. He used to run a transport business in South Africa, until he developed MND and returned to the UK. He was still very independent despite having some limited arm and leg movements and slurred speech. He had been diagnosed a couple of years before Alan. Seeing him made me realise how much more aggressive Alan's condition was.

Back at the house my friend Jenny, from Sutton Coldfield, visited bringing fresh eggs from her own hens. They would make a nice breakfast at the weekend! Simon Pointon, Simon Beacham and Norma from Alan's office came to visit. Simon Pointon encouraged me to continue to write my Facebook posts.

Thursday 16th August - Climbing up Clent Hills

Alan alerted me at 4am. He was cold. I added more layers to his bedding. After the usual morning carers' routine, we drove to Stourbridge and collected Viv and John from the place where they had deposited their motorhome for servicing. Before returning home we stopped at the Clent Hills. Remarkably, Alan managed to steer the electric wheelchair himself over the rugged terrain during our short walk. I could tell he was frustrated about the failing ability of his left arm because he snapped at me a couple of times. I had to work hard not to take it personally, even though his words cut through me.

Mum's care company called to say that mum had fallen and hurt her ribs, so Viv and I visited her to check she was okay.

Friday 17th August - Hoist training

Fiona, OT and Julie, Macmillan nurse, visited. For the first time, respite care was mentioned, so that I could get some rest. How could I rest while Alan slept at a hospice while I stayed at home worrying if anyone would go to him when his mask slipped? The whole idea grieved me.

Alan's sister Pauline and her husband Simon arrived, followed shortly by their daughter Helen, and her two boys. We all had lunch in the back garden. Simon and John fixed the broken door handle to our cloakroom while I collected mum, who joined us for afternoon tea. The wheelchair team came with ideas for alternative steering controls to the wheelchair. None were suitable.

Alan had bowel pains again, so I increased his regular doses of Senna and Laxido. It was difficult getting the balance of these treatments right. Too much would end up with more movements than any of us would want to clean up! We steered Alan over the ramp into the conservatory and all ate my homemade chilli together. Maybe it would help short out Alan's stubborn bowels! Tom, Viv's youngest son, arrived. The bedtime carers showed Viv and I how to operate the hoist and transfer Alan using the slings while Pauline made comprehensive notes.

Saturday 18th August - Poignant songs
The Coventry 5k park run left me redder faced than Viv, Pauline and Tom. Later, Viv, John, Pauline, Simon, Alan and I went to the KT Tunstall, Pretenders and Simple Minds concert at The Butts, Coventry. It was a blessing to discover the stadium was wheelchair friendly. Before long, pints of beer were being enjoyed and we were singing along to poignant songs like *Stand by you, Won't let nobody hurt you* and *Don't you forget about me.*

Viv and I handled Alan's care at bedtime, as we had deliberately cancelled the carers. Pauline's step by step notes on the hoisting technique were invaluable as Viv and I tried to make sense of the various coloured straps which looked like a bowl of giant tangled tagliatelle.

Sunday 19th August - Stressful situations
The BBQ at Phil and Julie's house with *The Ski Gang*, and Alan's family, went well. Everyone, except me, was drinking alcohol. I felt in an odd mood following some difficult conversations earlier in the day about plans for the 10k race.

During the evening back at the house I felt pained when someone suggested I sit down for a while. I had lost the ability to rest. I was constantly in a state of high alert and felt the overwhelming burden of everything that needed to be done. I didn't realise it at the time, but I was beginning to crack.

Monday 20th August - Increase in care package
As a treat we all went to the local farm shop for breakfast, before I drove Viv and John back to Stourbridge. Alan was still experiencing tummy pains. The

social worker at the Marie Curie Hospice called to confirm a doubling of Alan's care package. The morning shift would increase from one to one and a half hours.

Lunch and teatime shifts would increase from thirty to forty-five minutes. Bedtime would be one hour instead of thirty minutes. So, for four hours a day, two carers would help Alan. The rest of the day and through the night, his needs were my responsibility. I fell asleep quickly and was out cold when Alan buzzed me via the intercom at 1am because he was too hot.

Tuesday 21st August - Wheelchair adaptations

The morning was manic because I overslept till 9:15am. It was never a quick exercise winching Alan in his wheelchair into the back of the WAV, but I had to do it quickly or we would be late for the appointment at the wheelchair centre for his tray to be fitted.

Later in the day, I found a meeting with one of the directors of my old firm uninspiring. Without doubt, even though we would have to live off savings, I would not be returning to work.

Wednesday 22nd August - Finally, a bed available at Stoke Hospital

Our recently hired cleaner arrived and whizzed around the house while I got on with other things. The manager of our care company called to say future shifts were being increased to four and a half hours a day. I didn't tell her I thought we were only due to have four hours. After a few calls, Stoke Hospital confirmed a bed was available for Alan's PEG operation! After giving Alan one of his favourite meals, avocado and prawns, I packed his bag and winched him into the WAV. We collected mum and set off for Stoke.

When I was sure Alan was settled in his room, I told him I loved him and departed for the hotel at which mum and I were staying. Mum kept coughing in her sleep and was babbling on about potty training baby boys, so the night of undisturbed sleep I needed didn't happen.

Thursday 23rd August - "Ouch"

Alan looked odd in his hospital gown ready for his operation when we visited him at 10am. Mum and I left Alan with the nurses, did a bit of shopping and made pots at the Wedgewood factory. Mum opted to stay in our room while I went back to the hospital. Bleary eyed Alan muttered, "I feel like I have been kicked in the stomach by a horse."

When the nurse showed me how to flush the PEG and clean the stoma site, I recorded it, for fear I would forget something important. Alan shouted, "Ouch" while I practised the flushing process under the watchful eye of the nurse. His joke made me flinch and even more nervous, but I was glad he was his usual impish self.

"The TV's not working," mum announced when I returned to the hotel. On investigation, I established she'd been fiddling with the remote-control batteries and had put them in the wrong way round. Mum did more talking in her sleep, but I managed to get a better night, relieved that Alan was well.

Friday 24th August - Home from hospital
Back at the hospital, a nurse explained the care I needed to take of Alan's stoma site, and I had another practice at flushing. For fear of being strangled by me, Alan restrained himself from more practical jokes! After lunch at the hospital, a nurse reset Alan's ventilator pressure to level sixteen. Mum chatted away about all sorts in the passenger seat on the way home. My heart fluttered every time I exchanged smiles with Alan whenever I saw him in the rear-view mirror.

We arrived home just before the carers turned up. After they left us, Alan and I indulged in a fish and chip supper and watched several episodes of *Frasier*. Bliss! Before going to bed I set up Alan's Army Post Race Picnic event on Facebook. The 10k race was sixteen days away. Urgh!

Saturday 25th August - Lot of effort, not much joy
Three times in the night Alan woke me. At one point he had cold feet, at another it was a mask issue and at 3am he had a painful hip. My alarm rang at 6:30am so I could wake Alan before the carers arrived. Despite the rain I managed to run just over six miles.

Alan got agitated trying to work the joystick on his power chair. It was heart-breaking seeing how much effort it took him to move his fingers less than an inch. Alan's voice was weaker than usual. I hoped it was due to tiredness but a little part of me feared losing his voice would be the next big change, and one that would severely affect his ability to stay positive.

Sunday 26th August - Brotherly love
It was raining outside so Viv, John, Alan and I spent a relaxing morning indoors. Kevin visited with Sue and Tyler. I cried when I told Kevin that, every night, Alan said to me, "Thank you for looking after me today." I was grateful for the comforting hug Kevin gave me, but it made me realise how much I missed having hugs from Alan.

Monday 27th August - Lazy bank holiday
Alan and I had what some people would call a 'duvet day'. I slobbed around in

my pyjamas and we watched more episodes of *Frasier*. Kevin arrived again, this time just with Tyler, and the Alexa device he'd forgotten to bring the day before. He explained how the device worked. I worried Alexa would not understand Alan when his mouth was covered by the full mask of the ventilator.

Tuesday 28th August - My time out
Two ex-Shirley Golf Club members, Iris and Pat, visited Alan. Flushing Alan's PEG tube was difficult, so I contacted my friend Wendy, who had been doing it for Mel for many years. I felt lucky to have other families affected by MND to whom I could refer.

Joking with Alan during the evening I said, "I bet you enjoy a break from me every time I go out."

Giggling, he replied, "Yes, a break is good, but I am always pleased to see you come home." My heart took a little leap.

Wednesday 29th August - Pressure sore
District nurse, Roz, discovered a pressure sore on Alan's toe so applied a waterproof dressing. He'd previously had an allergic reaction to Micropore tape, so we agreed I would keep an eye on this wound and would call her back if things got worse.

My friend, Jo arrived for a quick lunch out with me, while the carers were with Alan. I felt tearful when she offered to go away with me when Alan went into respite. When we were both single, we regularly took holidays together. How life had changed since then.

Thursday 30th August - More PEG care skills and kit to master
Our local PEG nurse, Jane, arrived to show me how to rotate Alan's PEG tube, and to check on my newfound flushing skills. Jane showed me how to clean the stoma site, then how to push the tube a little way into Alan's tummy, turn it 360°, and pull back into position. This procedure was necessary to stop the disk inside Alan's tummy becoming embedded into his stomach wall. It was to be undertaken at least once a week. Jane stressed nothing but tap water be used to flush the tube - Perrier water, tea, coffee, wine or beer were not to be used for flushing but could be administered via the tube any time Alan wanted!

The team from ACT arrived and set up Alan's Eyegaze equipment. It was a brilliant bit of kit, that enabled Alan to direct his eyes across a screen and either select predetermined sentences, or spell out words, questions, or statements. The standard electronic voice sounded like the one Professor Stephen Hawking had but would soon be replaced by the simulated voice Alan had already created in the model talker software. Setting the Eyegaze screen to the right height was tricky but critical. It was difficult initially for Alan to keep focus on what he was doing, but practice, by both of us, would make perfect.

Friday 31st August - Wearing mask in public
At Alan's old office a retirement party was taking place for Norma. Alan was happy being amongst his old workmates and I enjoyed looking at the handsome photographs of him in Norma's retirement scrapbook. I wished I had met him many years before 2006.

At 6:15pm Alan and I met friends Alison and Adrian at our local pub. There was not a lot of space for Alan's electric wheelchair, which caused the management some embarrassment. I was proud of Alan for wearing his breathing mask in public.

SEPTEMBER 2018

Saturday 1st September - Timing of carer shifts

Over lunch at a local garden centre, my friend Chris asked me, "What are your plans after Alan dies?"

Nibbling at my food, I told her, "If I feel I can, I will go to the places Al and I had on the bucket list. Also, I would like to go to Germany to see the girl I met in Vietnam."

Our night-time carers arrived an hour before they were expected, just as we were in the middle of watching a film. Alan preferred 9.30pm to 8.30pm so I called the care company manager to request the later time. I didn't hold out much hope.

Sunday 2nd September - Mistakes and punishment

Alan justifiably got angry with me when I accidentally left him off the ventilator when the phone rang. For my sins I made myself do a run that included a lot of uphill sections. My legs had been twitching for four days. I had tripped up a few times too and I could hear odd noises in my head. Was my own health slipping?

Monday 3rd September - Any doubts?

Alan had been experiencing an extremely dry mouth and the nebuliser machine had been rattling, so I left a message for Marie at Stoke Hospital to contact me.

While watching Noel Edmonds and his wife in a programme called *Eight go rallying to Saigon*, Noel said he and his wife were best friends. Alan turned to me and asked, "Am I your best friend?" I was surprised he even doubted it for a second. Later, out of the blue, he declared, "I love you." I had never been in any doubt about that.

Tuesday 4th September - Am I paranoid?

Stocks of waterproof dressings, spray to put on skin prior to applying dressings and spray for removing waterproof dressings, turned up with Eric, the district nurse. We had grown fond of Eric. He was always cheerful and as he left the house he often asked me how I was feeling, which I appreciated. Alan and I watched some *Frasier* episodes before I did some housework. When the carers arrived at lunchtime I popped out to get a little relief. Everything had felt chaotic lately.

The twitches in my legs kept coming. Tiredness, lack of certain vitamins and low electrolytes all showed up as causes for leg twitches on the internet. The idea I might have MND too plagued my mind. I felt scared and vulnerable. Who would look after me if I had it? I took a video of my calf muscles in case people, in particular my GP, might think I was paranoid.

Thursday 6th September - Money transfers

Twice in the night Alan woke me up because of issues with his breathing mask. In the morning Alan asked, "Please would you transfer £2,000 from my bank account to the Alans's Army JustGiving page, with a note that funds are from sale of Morris." At the same time, he asked me to make transfers to each of his family members. He wanted them to have gifts from him during his lifetime so he could learn what benefit they got from the funds.

Friday 7th September - Wheelchair adjustments

There were a lot of changes needed to Alan's wheelchair when we reached the service centre. The right-hand arm rest was changed to one that included a gutter, because Alan's arm was perpetually falling off the flat rest. Secondly, the technician took away the recently attached tray which Alan hated and enabled the joystick to be controlled by the fingertips of Alan's left hand. Finally, he fixed the problem with the attendant control gear stick at the back of the chair - the one I used to steer from the rear.

In Solihull we bought Alan some Hotter shoes with Velcro straps and no laces. The carers would be pleased. We managed to get home just in time for Eric to change the dressing on Alan's toe. He also checked out another sore that had developed on Alan's stomach due to a reaction to the Micropore tape used to hold his feeding tube in place.

At 7pm we arrived at the Limes Hotel in Earlswood for the surprise retirement party for Norma. One of the guests spent ages telling me how much she respected me, both as a businesswoman and for what I was doing for Alan. Flattered, I responded with, "I am only doing what any person would do for their poorly husband." I was horrified when she told me, "I have heard of people who have walked away from partners diagnosed with MND."

Sunday 9th September - 10k day

Viv, John, Tom, Ben and Claire, all arrived yesterday and got up with me at 6am. We arrived at the rendezvous car park in Stratford-upon-Avon and connected up with the rest of Alan's Army: Christine and Chris Woolley, Simon and Rachel Beacham, Paul and Jo Blount (all from Alan's work place). Alan's family members: Viv, Tom, Ben, Matthew, Suzanne, Helen, Richard. My ex work colleagues: Helen and Vikki, and Vikki's friend Susie. My friends: Angela Jebson, Jane McTigue and Sue Garfitt. Andrea Norris, wife of the man who built our wet room. Karen - a friend of one of the runners and Steve, our neighbour. Unfortunately, three of our runners had dropped out for medical reasons.

The official representative from MND association took a team photograph with the large MND banner in front of us and the handmade banner created by Alan's cousin Christine, held behind us. We were flying the flag for MND big time! I invited a stranger wearing an MND vest to join us. After leaving Alan in the safe hands of family members who were not running, we made our way to the start line.

It was sunny and windy. At the start line, I felt nervous and excited and took loads of photographs because I doubted I'd ever run this far again in my life. The first couple of kilometres I ran with Jane. When she pressed on without me, I didn't feel bad. I was the oldest runner in the Alan's Army. For a while I ran alongside a lady from Stratford-upon-Avon athletic club.

The Greenway section and the last 1km or so through the town of Stratford-upon-Avon, was flat and familiar to me. As I ran towards the finish line, I could see our friends and family cheering me from the side lines. Alan was there in his chair. Tears filled my eyes. The lady from Stratford-upon-Avon athletic club gave me a £5 donation as I crossed the finish line, just before I crumbled into the arms of my friend Christine.

My goal before the race was not to finish last out of the 1200 runners. My best 10k run in training had taken one hour and thirty-seven minutes. I wasn't last and ran a personal best time of one hour and twenty minutes! We had a party at the Village Hall in Wilmcote afterwards, thanks to Rachel and Simon.

I was very proud of the Army. Every member had finished the race. Many had never done any running prior to joining our group. Between us we raised over £17,000 for MND Association. The day would have been perfect but it ended with Alan choking on a drink back at the house. A stark reminder of why we had all done the race in the first place.

Monday 10th September - Sisters are losing their brother
Viv, John, Pauline, Simon, Alan and I took a trip to Hidcote Gardens. Interestingly, when Viv and I were separated from the rest of the group, she told me, "Your position is worse than mine. You have been with Alan every day for twelve years."

I told her, "I could not conceive of losing a brother who had been in my life for sixty years."

On a Facebook MND group, I read a piece by a daughter whose mum was in the final stages of the illness. She had taken delivery of a Just in Case box. Her mum was choking and coughing a lot. It all sounded terrible and unsettled me.

I accepted an offer made by our MND regional contact to speak to a group of health professionals at the QE Hospital later in the year.

AUTHOR'S NOTE
A Just in Case box contains a set of essential controlled drugs which need to be readily available to manage specific symptoms at a person's end of life.

Tuesday 11th September - More problems with bottom
Eric arrived to check Alan's toe - it was healing. Thankfully, the sore on his tummy was almost better too. Julie, our Macmillan nurse, called. "I will arrange for you to meet a psychologist at the Marie Curie Hospice to help you both with your emotional well-being. Also, I will arrange for you to meet a ventilation nurse to discuss using a saline nebuliser to provide moisture to Alan's mouth."

Viv, John and I did work on the garden in the pouring rain. Frustratingly mum refused physical rehabilitation when the asthma nurse recommended it, so the only other option was to go on steroid tablets.

Alan was in a lot of pain due to the weight of his body on his now bare 'sit bones' in his bottom. Viv became tearful after she and I had to get him out of his chair using the hoist to give him some relief. Matthew, Alan's nephew called to question Alan about some money that had unexpectedly turned up in his account. Alan confirmed it was not a mistake. Niece Helen also called for the same reason. Alan got a lot of satisfaction learning their plans for his gifts.

Wednesday 12th September - Bottom problems solved!
We said goodbye to Viv and John and cancelled our meeting with the psychologist because Alan was still in discomfort. There was good news from the ventilation nurse who visited us from Stoke - Alan's CO2 levels had reduced further. She confirmed it was okay to increase his daily dose of Oramorph.

While the floor levelling screed was drying in the hall, ahead of tiles being fitted, Alan was confined to his bedroom. The manager of our care company called to confirm five hours care a day had been approved.

The laxative drugs I had been giving Alan for several days finally worked. He had two bowel movements, both in his pad! We would now have to consider reducing the drug dose, so he did not go too far the other way. I could foresee we were heading for a rollercoaster ride when it came to managing bowel movements. Pauline called to discuss unexpected funds in her bank account and became emotional when talking to Alan.

Tuesday 13th September - Alan's ex-wife
We had a technical problem when three people from ACT came to set up the Eyegaze system. Without success, they tried to link the commands from Eyegaze to the TV and light switches so Alan could be as independent as possible. Another visit would be necessary.

Alan's brother-in-law, Simon, called to ask me how I felt about Alan's ex-wife, coming to visit Alan. Unbeknown to us, Pauline and Simon had remained in touch with Janet. I felt okay about her visiting. In fact, I quite welcomed meeting the only other woman in the world to whom Alan had been married. When I broached the subject with Alan we agreed to proceed with just one condition. I called Simon to say Janet could visit, as long as she didn't mind if I sat in on the meeting. Later Viv called to thank Alan for her unexpected gift.

Friday 14th September - Care package agreed
Alan's foot was still not right, so the district nurse came and changed his dressing. Later that day we gave Amy, one of the carers, a bottle of wine as it was her last shift with us before going off to begin her training as a nurse. Andy and Jo came to visit. To make life easier for me, we all had a fish and chip supper. It was Friday after all!

Saturday 15th September - No more cuddles from Alan
During the night I got cramp in my right calf. Just as I was nodding back off to sleep Alan's buzzer went off. Alan needed me to adjust his bedclothes, as he was too hot. When I gave him a cuddle he said, "I feel sad because I cannot cuddle you back."

The melancholy that swept over me prevented me from returning to sleep. At 3am I wrote on Facebook about missing the days, just six short months ago, when Alan used to be able to stand and hug me.

After the morning carers shift was over, Alan and I watched several episodes of *Frasier*.

"Al, I am getting a lot of twitching in my legs," I raised gingerly.

"You should see the GP," he suggested, "and, if necessary, get some private tests done."

I didn't tell him how scared I was that I might have MND.

Mum's flat was in a mess when I popped round. There was food and water everywhere. She rambled on about a lot of rain getting into the flat, and about strangers asking her lots of questions. There had been no rain for days and her flat had another one above it so was unlikely to get flooded. I was pretty sure she had imagined the people. Eventually I discovered she had attempted to defrost the freezer compartment of her fridge and had got into a muddle. As I tidied up the mess I felt stress washing over me. I felt bad that I could not do more for her.

AUTHOR'S NOTE
Before Alan became ill, we had a healthy relationship and were a tactile couple. We especially enjoyed cuddling up on the settee during evenings and sleeping in a spoon position at night. Sexual intimacy felt different after diagnosis and eventually it reduced to hand holding and hugging only.
mariecurie.org.uk/help/support/terminal-illness/wellbeing/sexuality

Monday 17th September - Good meeting with Macmillan nurse
We had a long meeting with Julie, Macmillan nurse and a doctor from the Marie Curie Hospice.

Subjects covered were...

- Finding a different dressing to stop Alan's nose getting so sore under the ventilation mask
- The need for Alan's legs to be elevated to reduce swelling
- The need for arms to be elevated sometimes, again to reduce swelling
- Trying some different drugs to help Alan with his bowel problems
- Use of Lorazepam as a relaxant
- Trying a mouth spray to help with dryness
- The sore toe that was not getting better

I didn't dare ask Alan how much he worried about the last item on the list, because I had heard his father had died from MRSA following complications from a sore.

Eric took photographs of the sore on Alan's toe before applying a new dressing. If the sore did not improve over the coming weeks, the podiatrist would be called in to examine the wound.

AUTHOR'S NOTE
Methicillin-resistant Staphylococcus aureus (MRSA) is an infection caused by Staphylococcus (staph) bacteria. This type of bacteria was resistant to many different antibiotics.

Tuesday 18th September - Another young football player gets MND

As a new district nurse arrived to undertake an examination, I thought, never in the history of mankind has a big toe had so much attention.

At the wheelchair centre, the fault that had developed with the attendant control joystick was fixed. We also tried a different arm gutter as the recent one did not provide sufficient support.

On our way home I bought some of Alan's favourite sausages - pork and chestnut - and heard on the radio a second young football player had been diagnosed with MND. He was only twenty-nine.

When I looked at the secretions coming off Alan's chest, via the cough assist machine, I was shocked to see what looked like blood. I chose not to mention it to him but would remain observant over the coming days.

Thursday 20th September - Condition progressing too fast

Twitching in my legs woke me up several times in the night. At 5:30am I woke with twitches in my left hand and torso too. It was time to see my GP.

"I have been thinking about my condition getting worse," Alan said, "I feel like time is closing in on me." He added "I want to get all the financial affairs sorted out." I comforted him as best I could, but I too was worried how fast the disease was getting hold of him.

Friday 21st September - CHC meeting is like a full MOT

During the night I woke several times, my mind racing. I made a list of things to discuss with Alan, including the forthcoming meeting with his ex-wife, my physical health and our recent meetings at the Marie Curie Hospice.

Alan was a rational man. Talking things through with him always put my mind at rest. We decided he still had many 'roles' to perform. Firstly, he could be chief researcher, looking into things we might do, such as visiting National Trust properties, going to sports events or attending concerts. Secondly, as always, he was to be "the voice of reason", helping me keep a balanced view in stressful situations. We also joked about him being called *Director of Hazel*, because I wanted him to crack the whip to make sure I kept on top of all the tasks on my ever increasing *To Do* list.

Later, we had a comprehensive meeting at our house about Alan's continuing health care (CHC) plan. In addition to the social worker from the Marie Curie Hospice and the manager from our care company, other professionals attended. During the long session we talked about Alan's balance, behaviour, cognition, mental health, communication ability, mobility, nutrition, skin, continence, breathing, medicines and whether his condition had brought about an 'altered state.' By the end of it I felt like Alan had gone through a full MOT!

The assessment demonstrated that some extra hours of care were needed so that I could have time to collect medicines, do shopping and chores. It was suggested that Alan have a week respite in the Marie Curie Hospice to give me a proper break.

During the afternoon we did a FaceTime call to Alan's sister because his mum was staying with her for her ninety sixth birthday.

Pam, Vice-Captain of the ladies' section at our golf club, popped in. The posters of Alan to be used for her captain's charity day were excellent.

Late afternoon, our neighbours popped round for beers with Alan while I took mum shopping. I suggested she have a short stay in a residential home - a sort of holiday - to check it out. Even when I explained I had to focus on Alan, she was still totally against the idea.

After a severe choking episode Alan said, "It was just saliva going down the wrong way." It was a worrying sign. I wasn't sure what could be done to stop it happening.

Saturday 22nd September - TV issues and an unusual rash
A 'viral rash' was spotted on Alan's back and chest by our evening carer. It wasn't itching and Alan didn't have a fever. We were not using any new products or drugs, so the conclusion was that it was probably a reaction to the new vest tops he was wearing.

Monday 24th September - GP not concerned
Alan sat to me in his wheelchair as I talked about my muscle twitches and weakness in my right arm, to our GP. To reassure me, the GP explained, there were 13,000 patients at this clinic and the odds of me also having MND were extremely low. He suggested, it might be a trapped nerve in your neck. To enable MND to be ruled out, he referred me to a neurologist in the Multiple Sclerosis department of Warwick Hospital for an MRI. If necessary the same nerve conduction test that Alan had, would have to be done too.

On the way back from the surgery *Time to Say Goodbye* by Andrea Bocelli and Sarah Brightman came on the radio. I burst into tears.

Tuesday 25th September - Not good to sit around in poo

I had to help Sadie clean up Alan because the other carer had not arrived and Alan had a soiled pad. He said that it had happened some time ago. Sadie chastised him, "You should have got it seen to earlier because poo can create sores."

Wednesday 26th September - Deep conversation with Alan

While I was giving him his morning hug Alan said, "I'm finding it hard to keep up a brave face."

"Oh Al, you don't need to do that. Everyone knows what you are dealing with is tough."

"I didn't mind opening up to you or my sisters, but I don't want to do so to anyone else," Alan said as I drove him into the lounge. He added, "It upsets me seeing other couples doing the things we are unable to. I am going crazy being in the house so much."

We agreed that I would research things we might do, and he could take up his research manager role once the Eyegaze system was up and running.

Christina and Simon came round and stayed with Alan while I met up with my friend Teresa for a heart to heart while walking around Knowle Park. The park had become a favourite place to walk around together if either of us needed a friendly ear.

Thursday 27th September - Meeting the former Mrs Carter

Sitting in our conservatory, listening to Alan and Janet reminiscing about their lives together in Leeds, made me feel mildly jealous. They used to do long distance runs together - something I had never managed to achieve - and clearly had a good social life. For the umpteenth time, I wished that I had met Alan when we were both younger, so that we could have had more time together. I was beginning to feel cheated by life.

At the Lymphoedema Clinic, the nurse checked Alan's blood pressure, pulse and temperature, which were all fine. She gave us some arm exercises to do to help reduce fluid retention and ordered some compression gauntlets. Alan was already wearing compression stockings which were troublesome to put on, so the nurse also ordered a special slip bag to help fit the gauntlets more easily. More work for our poor carers.

My nephew Martyn and his two children arrived around 4pm.

Tyler was a natural young carer - taking great care when feeding Alan crumpets. Later, he helped me cut up some kitchen roll to make swabs for cleaning Alan's stoma site.

In bed I noticed a change in my twitches. The 'fluttering' was in my right knee and right buttock. Bizarre.

On Facebook I wrote: *"Escaping from the house between carer visits feels like bunking off school. It's amazing how much fun you can have just wheeling the power chair in the back of the Caddy, packing the pee bottle, turning up the radio, setting the air con to a delicious sixteen degrees and driving off to the GPs, the hospice, or the chemist! Alan is the main person keeping me from drowning in sorrow. Not that I go around moping, quite the opposite, it's just that some days a little knife twists in my heart reminding me this beautiful man will leave one day, and none of us will see his smile again.*

It's been a beautiful day today and I don't want to spoil it - so here is my final thought. No matter how tough stuff is, there is always someone who is worse off. We have a lovely home, great friends and family. We are not broken and we have each other. Life is good."

Friday 28th September - Wheelchair breakdown and great golf on TV
We listened to one of our favourite sporting events, the Ryder Cup, as I drove Alan to the dental surgery. After our check-ups, the wheels on Alan's wheelchair jammed on the kerb stone near the car and the engine stubbornly refused to start. Outwardly I showed no panic. Inside I was worried because we had none of Alan's usual equipment or medicines with us. I called the emergency technical team. They talked me through the unlocking process. Phew!

Eric, our district nurse, changed the dressing on Alan's right toe. Good news - the sore was shrinking at last! We celebrated by watching riveting Ryder Cup matches on TV.

Saturday 29th September - Are my feelings changing?
Alan woke me in the middle of the night to adjust his ventilation mask. In the morning we watched Ryder cup matches with Jo and Andy, and more matches later with Dawn from the golf club and her husband, Tony.

At bedtime, Alan noticed I did not say, "I love you too" after he told me he loved me. I cried when he said, "I don't like to think that you may not love me anymore."

I looked him in the eye and promised, "No matter what Alan, I will never stop loving you." But something had changed deep down inside. Part of me had died.

Sunday 30th September - Worried about my mum

"I've seen your brother Kevin dressed as a gorilla and in tears," mum announced when I visited her. Later her care company phoned me to say that mum had called an ambulance because Kevin was having chest pains. The paramedics arrived and found that Kevin wasn't there. Her vital signs were okay, so they left. I explained to the carer that mum often hallucinated, and I wondered how many strange calls 999 were received from people living with dementia.

After a visit from our friend Christine, we did a FaceTime call with Alan's sister, Viv. Then we enjoyed watching Europe beat USA on the last day of the Ryder Cup!

Monday 1st October - First 'meal' down the PEG tube

Whlle carers were showering Alan, I noticed he had no strength in his voice and could not breathe well whilst off the ventilator. The respiratory team in Stoke suggested we use a second hosepipe between the mask and the ventilator machine, joined by a connector. This effectively gave us eight feet of tube instead of four feet. The extended tube meant the ventilator could stay on the trolley outside the wet room, and the mask could be left on Alans's face until such time as it needed to be removed temporarily for teeth cleaning. The mask could be replaced immediately he struggled for air. Ingenious!

Our speech and language therapist checked Alan's swallowing. "It's weak I am afraid. From here on I suggest you feed Alan through his PEG tube as much as possible." I was nervous at first but managed to flush the tube, deliver the high protein Fortisip drink and re-flush the tube without incident.

Before she left the therapist reminded us that we needed to download Alan's simulated voice from model talker so he could use the Eyegaze technology. I took Alan to the GP practice for his flu and pneumonia jabs. Within hours of having my flu jab I looked like a spotty dog. The side effect was a small price to pay to ensure flu would not stop me caring for Alan.

A phone call from CHC confirmed that an extra four hours care per week had been approved so that I could undertake chores away from the house between carer visits. Alan was not himself most of the day. I suspected he was having bowel problems again but chose not to press him.

Wednesday 3rd October - A lot of new kit needed and fun things to do

We had a long and productive meeting with Lesley, our physiotherapist, and Fiona, our OT, who then ordered:

- A special pillow to support Alan's weak neck
- A new sling for the hoist, with an integrated neck support
- A 'tilt in space' shower chair on wheels wlth supporting head rest
- Wedges and special blow-up 'repose' boots to support Alan's legs in bed, to reduce risk of bedsores
- A further wrist splint, this time for his left hand

The waterproof, tilting chair on wheels would mean that Alan could be hoisted onto it from his bed. Then wheeled through the kitchen to the wet room, showered and shaved in it, dried off and dressed in it, before being wheeled back to the bedroom. He could then be transferred to his electric wheelchair.

Lesley suggested that we elevate Alan's legs as often as possible during the day to reduce swelling, and that we contact the wheelchair technician for new supports to be put on the lower half of the wheelchair, to stop Alan's knees flopping outwards.

At mum's flat, her cleaner had news for me. "Your mum was found wandering in the corridor wearing her dressing gown saying she thought she was in hospital."

Clearly her dementia was taking a new turn. I had no idea how I was going to help her. I took mum and Alan to the doctor's surgery. Alan had his routine blood test to check Riluzole was not damaging his liver or kidneys.

While examining mum, her GP asked me how I was coping with Alan's deteriorating physical health, at the same time as looking after mum with her deteriorating mental health. By the time I had finished telling him all the plates I was spinning, and in how many different directions I was pulled, he knew how hard things were for me.

During the afternoon, Alan opened up to our psychologist, Morgan.

"I am fed up being told I am inspirational. I don't want to be a hero. I want friends to know how hard it is for Hazel to look after me, and how frustrating it is for me not being able to help around the house."

Morgan pointed out, "Friends won't see what's going on behind the scenes. It's up to you to let them know."

I loved having Morgan's support.

"You have to find ways to have fun and practice mindfulness. Be aware of your surroundings - what's happening in the here and now," she said, "And notice sounds, sights, smells, tastes and how you feel."

Morgan suggested just sitting holding hands might be all we need to do sometimes.

Finally, she talked about the stages of grief:

- Shock/denial
- Anger (better out than in)
- Sadness (moving on)

- Acceptance

When we got home, we created a list of fun things to do:

- A daily 'walk' after lunch
- Going to the movies
- Visiting National Trust properties
- Spending time in our garden
- Spending time in our conservatory
  (where we could practice mindfulness)

Thursday 4th October - Unexplained fall

Mum's cleaner called to say she had found mum half-dressed on the floor in her flat. The GP had come and had ordered an ambulance. He wanted mum to have a head scan, as her fall was unexplained and could have caused a head injury.

When I arrived at mum's flat, I checked the care company file and was shocked to see that no carer had arrived that morning. The care company were left in no doubt about my feelings when I called them and demanded an investigation. I couldn't leave Alan alone for long, so my sister Clare came over and waited for the ambulance with mum.

When the carers arrived for their shift with Alan, I popped back to mum's to relieve my sister. It was 5pm and still no ambulance. Mum tried to convince the paramedics that she was okay but her blood pressure was high. The paramedics thought she might have a water infection or dehydration issues because she was confused. Eventually mum agreed to go to hospital.

Once Alan was tucked up in bed, I looked back at some old videos of him taken in our early days. They made me smile and cry.

Friday 5th October - A full on day – phew

When the carers arrived at 6:30am, I put on some happy music to try to create a fun atmosphere for Alan. Terese told us she had resigned and was going to a new agency. It was disappointing news. She was one the carers we rated highly. A phone call to Solihull Hospital confirmed that mum was stable but was being kept in for observations.

District nurse, Eric discovered that Alan had some skin damage to his bottom caused by the continence pads. Pro Shield cream was to be used every day as a barrier. To help get more care for mum, or get some respite care for Alan, Eric suggested I explain recent events to the social worker at the Marie Curie

Hospice. When I called her, she was very sympathetic to my situation and promised to see what could be done to help.

Despite the respiratory team at Stoke Hospital guiding me through adjusting Alan's ventilation machine, the battery would not hold its charge. An engineer would have to come out. While talking to the team, Alan requested I be trained on how to increase the ventilator pressure because he felt he was not getting a big enough breath. He was already at level seventeen. Twenty-one was the highest pressure setting. I feared his breathing muscles were deteriorating too fast.

My sister, Clare and I visited a local nursing home to see if it would be suitable for mum. The weekly costs were horrendous, so the idea was abandoned. Simon and Rachel Beacham together with their daughter, came for dinner. It was pleased I had made dessert the night before because the day had been extremely busy and stressful. They were dismayed to learn how much Alan's voice had deteriorated.

Saturday 6th October - Mum appeared to be okay
My sister, Rowena, came to see Alan and talk about mum.
While out shopping I bought a portable Yamaha keyboard. Alan suspected I would never master using it. My plan was to learn how to play it in secret, and surprise him one day. After finding a sitter for Alan, I went to see mum in hospital. She was dressed and looked well but was confused and verbose. Nursing staff told me they were checking out her bladder.

Sunday 7th October - Inflatable boots
Alan and I went shopping for new pyjamas for him because he was not getting out of bed every day anymore. 'Duvet days' were encouraged by our health team and saved all the hassle of the morning routine.

To protect Alan's toes from blanket pressure while he was wearing his inflated boots, I fashioned foot guards from cardboard and foam. Had he been in a white padded suit, he would have looked like an astronaut!
My sister Clare called following her visit to mum in hospital. There was no new news.

Monday 8th October - High heart rate
My brother Kevin went to visit mum in hospital in the morning and Alan and I went in the afternoon. She was being sick and didn't look at all well. The nurse said they were transferring her to the heart and ventilation ward as her heart rate was still over one hundred!

Tuesday 9th October - Call that respite time!?

Alan woke me twice in the night - first because his mask needed adjusting and secondly because he was too hot. Surprisingly, a carer arrived at 9:30am to sit with Alan for four hours, so I could get some respite. Neither social services nor the care agency had informed us that my respite time would start today, so I had nothing planned.

Luckily, I had hired a carpet cleaning machine which I took to mum's flat and used to clean all her carpets. While I had the machine, I also cleaned some carpets in our house too. No rest for the wicked, I thought. Then I thought how silly the saying was. I had no time to be wicked!
Alan's ventilator mask needed a lot of adjustments at bedtime which increased our stress levels and made us both tense.

Wednesday 10th October - Park benches and sweet treats

During the night Alan called for me. He had a lot of lower back pain. He usually slept with the head and knees raised but had slumped down the bed somehow. It was hard work heaving him back into position to improve his posture.

Niles finally married Daphne in *Frasier*! Alan and I had somehow managed to miss the episode containing Niles's proposal, which was frustrating as we had been waiting for that moment for a long time.

I set about cleaning the remaining carpets in our house and then returned the machine during the afternoon. It was an unusually hot, autumn day, so I took Alan for a 'stroll' in the park, trying hard to contain my tears as I read the heartfelt tributes to lost loved ones on the park benches.

Frustratingly, my appointment with the neurologist for 17th October was postponed by the hospital.

A nurse told me at the hospital that mum's ultrasound had revealed gall stones caused by a build-up of cholesterol. Mum also had a cyst on her liver and one on her kidney. Listening to mum ramble on absentmindedly and seeing her fiddling with the cannula that was drip feeding her antibiotics, made me feel low.

At the supermarket I bought a steak pie for dinner, and a sweet pastry treat for me. I ate the treat on my way home while I thought about the biscuits and chocolate that I'd already eaten that day. My consumption of rubbish food was out of control. These indulgences felt like my only pleasures in life. The problem was that consuming them made me feel bad about myself.

Thursday 11th October - Shocking photo

Alan was too hot in the night, so I adjusted his bed clothes. These disturbed nights' sleep made getting up at 6.30am, to wake Alan before the carers arrived, tough. Eric, the district nurse, took photographs of Alan's bottom. He and I were shocked because it looked like that of a baboon. I felt very sorry for Alan. He had always been meticulous about personal care, without being vain.

Two couples from the golf club, Carol and John and Joy and Peter, had early evening drinks with us. I could see Peter was upset at seeing Alan's decline.

Friday 12th October - Clandestine care felt like fun

The sore on Alan's heel was repairing at last. Thank goodness for inflatable moon boots!

I collected a referral letter from the GP so that I could see a private consultant about my twitches. It took two inexperienced carers with low confidence one and a half hours, instead of an hour, to do Alan's lunchtime care. I was not happy with the care company. Clare called me to say our mum thought she was coming home today (but it was not true).

Alan and I got VIP treatment when being shown to the wheelchair seating area ready for the concert by ELO. I was impressed with the friendliness of the staff at the Birmingham Arena.

We had cancelled the bedtime carers because we knew we would not be home in time. Instead, against care company rules, we privately arranged for one of the most experienced carers to help me put Alan to bed. I felt like a child behaving badly arranging clandestine care. It was nice getting Alan ready for bed after several months of leaving this task to the care workers. The carer would not accept any payment or a gift even though it was very late.

Sunday 14th October - A new way to enjoy books

Having spent most of Saturday resting and catching up with some TV, today started off as it normally did at 6:30am. Mum looked a lot better when I visited her, but I could still not understand her ramblings. The nurse suggested that the fall and infections had impacted on mum's dementia.

Alan and I went out in search of a portable CD player and headphones so he could listen to audio books kindly loaned to us by a member of the golf club. In the pre-MND days Alan loved reading, especially books about World War I and II, but turning the pages of a normal book, or using the Kindle, was not possible now he had lost the use of his arms. Back at home, I ordered a set of headphones so I could tinkle on my electric keyboard without disturbing Alan.

Monday 15th October - Unbearable worry

With my referral letter in hand I arranged to see Dr Thomas - the same neurologist at BMI Hospital, Coventry, who had diagnosed Alan's MND. The thought that I might have something similar was unbearably worrying. Having spotted my latest Facebook ramblings, Fiona, our OT dropped me a note, "I do hope you will write a book because your public notes show real insight about life with MND."

Tuesday 16th October - Slightly less worried

My frustration with the quality of our carers reached its limit. One turned up late for the 6:30am shift and neither knew what they were doing. I could see the shock on their faces when I gave them a piece of my mind. There was nothing I could do to stop Alan deteriorating day by day, but I could do something about the quality of his care. Unfortunately, the system was sending social carers whereas Alan had complex medical needs around the cough assist machine and PEG flushing and cleaning. Such support cannot be provided on the cheap.

We managed to get Alan's left side gutter arm rest fitted at the wheelchair centre before having a picnic in a local park on the way to visit mum. It was strange sitting in a hospital ward with lots of bed-ridden people, while Alan, who was paralysed and would die immediately without his ventilator, looked well and handsome sitting in his wheelchair!

Dr Thomas gave me the same thorough examination he had given to Alan back in November 2017. I showed him the videos of my twitching legs. He suspected I might have benign cramp fasciculation syndrome, or a trapped nerve or Spondylitis. He arranged for me to have blood tests, an electromyography (EMG) and neck scan. I came away from the hospital slightly less worried.

Wednesday 17th October - Turning a negative into a positive

Alan surprised me during the morning when he said, "You have a wonderful head, neck and back." He probably had a lot of time to study me as I beavered around him. Lucky for me he never noticed my lumps and bumps, wrinkles and the grey hairs that had started to appear!

At the hospital, I insisted the social worker did not approve mum's release home unless a care package was in place.

"What are your fears?" Morgan asked at our third session with her. Most of her tissue box was used up when I explained.

"I fear letting go of Alan, even though I know I have to. I'm worried I will have an emotional meltdown from the pain of grief after he dies."

Looking forlorn Alan shared, "I worry about leaving Hazel alone, and about becoming totally paralysed."

At one point we discussed how negative we both felt about the looming one year anniversary of the MND diagnosis. With her encouragement, we decided that we needed to turn 21st November into a positive day. Because of Alan's disabilities our options were limited. We settled on having lunch at a favourite restaurant. Morgan approved. We arranged our next session with her on the anniversary of diagnosis day so she could help us through it.

Thursday 18th October - Joy from giving
Unusually, this week we didn't have a visit from our cleaner, so I set about hoovering and dusting the house. When the carers arrived for the teatime shift, Alan needed to have his pad changed and bottom cleaned. Normally that would be okay but Alan's sister, Pauline, her husband Simon and Alan's mum arrived in the middle of the process, so everything was a bit chaotic for a while.

Pauline told Alan what she had done with the money he had given her, and we learned what other members of the family had bought. It gave Alan tremendous satisfaction hearing these stories. Pauline and I spent some time looking at possible places to stay for a mini break with Alan. Our plumber, who had known Alan for many years, arrived to service our boiler. He was staggered when he saw how much Alan had deteriorated in twelve months.

Friday 19th October - No thought for wheelchair users
A different district nurse came to check Alan's toe.

Helen, Alan's niece, arrived with her son Tom at around 11am. Simon, Pauline, Helen, Tom and I took Alan out in his wheelchair for some fresh air. We were horrified to see how restrictive the entrance was into the local park. A fixed bar was not an obstacle for people on foot, but it prevented access by Alan's wheelchair! I felt an instant urge to write to the council about the lack of thought for people who use wheelchairs.

The hospital social worker called to say mum was being sent home next week with a care package of four care calls per day. I requested the same care company as Alan had as I did not trust the previous company, and it would make my life easier.

When the carers came for the teatime shift, Alan needed to be cleaned up again - second big bowel evacuation of the day! At bedtime Pauline gave me a big hug saying, "I don't know how you cope."

Saturday 20th October - Pondering on my legacy and my future value

After a cooked breakfast Simon, Pauline and Alan's mum departed, leaving Alan and I to catch up with *Frasier*, *Strictly Come Dancing* and *Strictly it Takes Two*. As always, we assessed the dancers and guessed the scores of the judges. It made me feel down thinking in years to come I'd be watching these shows alone.

My sister, Rowena sent me a text saying mum's behaviour had got worse, and mum had a severe headache. I felt helpless because there was nothing I could do. During the evening I spent time deleting work contacts from my mobile phone. I felt disappointed that there was nothing tangible to show for all my years of work - no lasting or meaningful legacy.

Sunday 21st October – Nice, but tiring visits from family

Alan's cousin from York, Eric, his daughter Gill and her daughter, Jemma, came to visit. It was lovely to see them, but exhausting having a toddler running around while I was trying to keep an eye on all of Alan's equipment, etc.

Monday 22nd October - Mum almost home

At the last minute there was a hiccup with mum's care package, so she had to stay in hospital.

In an article I read that people who only have money are poor. For some time, I had considered myself to be 'rich'. I had a wonderful husband, a lovely home, financial stability, fabulous family and friends, good job and my health. But soon that would change. Alan would be gone. The thought was too painful.

Tuesday 23rd October - When you don't have kids, your husband is your world

Neil from the golf club sat with Alan during the afternoon so that I could play in the Annual Charity Golf Day. A huge number of ladies at the club wanted an update on Alan. Their kind words were nice, but it was hard relaying our latest news repeatedly, especially when the lump in my throat got stuck.

One of my regular playing partners told me her husband needed to see a neurologist because he had issues with his vision. Like me, she had no children, so her husband was her world too.

I discovered there were still issues with mum's care package when I visited her in hospital.

Wednesday 24th October - Alan 'speaks'!

There was great excitement when the ACT team managed to get Alan's model talker voice working through the Eyegaze technology! All the hours spent months ago recording Alan's voice paid off. When the machine 'spoke', you could hear Alan's soft Sunderland lilt.

A customised stand was needed to hold the Eyegaze screen near to Alan. He now needed to remain patient as he learned how to create sentences using his eyes to activate his voice.

Nephews Ben and Tom arrived and, after being fed, set to work clearing the unruly hedge at the back of the garden. Alan's job was to supervise while resting in the conservatory. The PEG nurse suggested we try steroid cream to treat the over granulation (crustiness) I had discovered around Alan's stoma site. A common problem apparently.

Thursday 25th October - Mum home and upsetting YouTube films

Mum was released from hospital. Our care company could only supply one carer at 5:30pm, so once again I had to lend a hand with Alan. At 8:30pm I went to mum's flat to help her get ready for bed.

Tears fell as I watched a YouTube video called "ALS love story." A girl talked about her friend who had been paralysed by the disease and was PEG fed, breathed through a tube in her throat and needed a lot of care. The silence, after years of listening to the breathing machine, was weird when the girl's friend died. One day, that would be my story.

Unusually, I had twitches in my left knee and right hamstring. My right hand felt weak too which worried me because I would need it to type my book. Four lots of friends had to cancel visiting Alan because they had colds. He liked a variety of visitors for entertainment, or did he just enjoy a rest from me?

Friday 26th October - No hugs available

The district nurse was happy with how Alan's sores were improving. She did, however, suggest we obtain a proper cage to protect Alan's feet from the weight of his duvet. At mum's flat the social worker discussed fitting sensors so that mum's movement, or lack of it, could be detected.

Alan and I watched various dramas. He appeared very relaxed about life. He joked a lot. When I bought him a glass of wine, he called it "whine". When he needed a pee, he gave clear instructions to reduce risk of mishaps. The first one was, "Release the tension" meaning to stretch open his elasticated waistband. When he was done, he sang the line "Shake it off" from the Taylor

Swift song, meaning to remove all drips. Finally, "Put it away" - well that's obvious I hope!

In my wedding speech I had said, "Not a day goes by without Alan making me laugh." Today was like old times. I hugged him and my heart swelled with love for him. I told Alan about my increased areas of twitching. Looking glum he said, "I feel unhappy that I cannot give you a hug anymore." My heart broke.

Sunday 28th October - Sad chat and pee bottle incident
The carers made mistakes when using the pee bottle which resulted in pee going over Alan. He was in a low mood all afternoon.

"Tell me what's on your mind Al?"

"I am angry at having piss thrown over me."

Facebook post: *"Been a bad day today. We both hit a low spot. Normally one of us is up, but today was different - maybe because we are approaching the one year anniversary since Al's diagnosis - memories of that very difficult day are hard to suppress. We will find a way to celebrate beating MND for twelve months on 21st November, but we both know reaching that date means there is less future to look forward to.*

We had a good chat this morning, shared our fears and frustrations, and shed some tears. Alan is sad because his dignity has been taken away, as has his ability to hold me when I find things all too much. His head flops to one side now as his neck muscles are weakening. He can still move his head a little, but fears the day (which is not far away) when he will be completely paralysed. I hate seeing him suffer and dread the day he is no longer with me - the day the breathing machine falls silent, and the cheerful carers and district nurses stop turning up. We both find it hard not being able to cook meals together, cuddle up on the sofa, walk hand in hand - and letting go of the plans we had for our retirement is painful.

We talked today about getting away for a week - just the two of us - somewhere in the country with a cosy fire and lovely views. I have commenced the search for a cosy retreat, with a ceiling hoist (so no need for carers) - a place where we can recharge our batteries, ready to fight on.

As I think about these last 12 months, I can see we have done a pretty good job of keeping our double chins up and making great memories. But behind the smiles and laughter, we are lost in a maze with no knowledge of how, or when, we will reach the end. We know for sure one of us is not going to make it out.

The other expects to be bruised, battered and scarred when she emerges from the exit without her best friend, her true soul mate and the most remarkable man she has ever known."

At bedtime, my feelings come out in a poem.

WHEN THE TIME COMES
When the time comes,
Will she stand tall?
Remember the love she had,
Or bend and buckle,
From the pain of it all?

Will she summon up the strength,
To face the world?
Or wither
As a pale future begins?

Will she smile, and hug, and tell stories,
Of the days before he went?
Or will she fall silent,
Lost in thought,
Broken, brittle, bent?

He can't hold her anymore,
Or wipe away her tears.
He has his own battles,
Fighting his internal fears.

He's got strength and courage too,
But his body is lifeless,
Before he is dead,
Before his last words are said,
Before he takes his last breath,
Before his shadow falls no more.

How will they cope with his remaining days?
Days so bittersweet,
Nights so alone?

When the time comes,
Too soon no doubt,
Will they say all they must,
Will they get their words out?

Will they be as one together,
On this final journey?
Or is this path too tough?
The path they shouldn't have to take,
The one that's steep and rough.
They, and we, will know all this,
And more,
When the time comes.

Monday 29th October - Could Whitby come up trumps?

At mum's flat, I explained my circumstances and Alan's illness, to the lady fitting the sensors. Later that day she wrote to me saying she had looked at my JustGiving link and had donated, because her mum-in-law had died from MND two years ago.

Mum's carer did not have time to dry her hair, so I did. For a brief moment I lost myself in thought as I styled the delicate pale strawberry blonde hair. When mum asked how Alan was, I chose my response carefully. I didn't want to trouble her, or for her to think I would not have any time for her.

Alan and I both sobbed when I read out the huge number of comments to my latest Facebook post. We both gained courage from knowing we had so many people rooting for us.

When searching for a December break, I discovered a company called Disabled Access Holidays. Two cottages in Whitby had profile beds, wet rooms and electronic ceiling hoists! I was beginning to feel optimistic.

As I cleared out documents, photographs, emails and contacts from my work laptop, I felt nothing. None of it mattered. The only thing I cared about was Alan's happiness and comfort during whatever time he had left.

Tuesday 30th October - Jane's invaluable help

Alan had a full day of visitors, so I could have some downtime. Jane, bereavement counsellor at the Marie Curie Hospice, listened calmly as I unloaded my feelings.

"I feel angry towards Alan occasionally. Then I feel angry at myself for not spending all my time with him. I am worried about my own health. I'm eating too much rubbish. I don't know how I will cope with mum's deterioration at the same time as Alan's, and I feeling frustrated at not being able to make plans."

"You are dealing with a lot of loss and change," said Jane. "Self-care is important. You should not feel guilty about taking time out for yourself." Her wastepaper bin filled up with soggy tissues as we discussed how I thought life for me would be at the end of Alan's life, and after he died.

Jane pointed out, "You are losing your husband as well as losing your work identity, and you have no control over anything." She told me, "When you look back in years to come, you will not believe how much you handled and coped with."

As we walked in the park near the hospice Teresa told me she worried about intruding into our lives. I assured her it was okay to ring any time.

I ate two chocolate bars as I wandered around Marks & Spencer's looking for some vests for Alan. Mum had been complaining about a pain in her jaw, but the dentist could not see any reason for it, so I took mum home and gave her some painkillers.

After a welcome massage and posture realignment session from my therapist, I resumed my search for our December holiday cottage and a care agency in Whitby.

By this stage the night-time routine took an hour and included:

- Turn on pressure relieving mattress
- Remove Alan's ventilation mask
- Administer medicines
- Put hoist sling under Alan and hoist him onto bed
- Remove shoes and trousers and check pad for soiling - clean up as required
- Do leg exercises
- Hoist Alan off bed onto commode/shower chair
- Move Alan to wet room
- Put towel behind Alan's back to help lean him forward
- Clean up Alan and empty/clean commode pan
- Clean Alan's teeth
- Wash Alan's face and hands

- Remove tee shirt and put in laundry bin
- Put on pyjama top
- Wheel shower chair to kitchen
- Use cough assist machine
- Wheel shower chair to bedroom
- Put hoist sling under Alan and hoist him onto bed
- Put on pad, underpants, and pyjama bottoms
- Raise head and knee area of bed
- Put on wrist brace
- Put barrier cream on heels (to reduce pressure sore risk)
- Put on blow-up leg supports
- Put on lip salve
- Turn on ventilator and humidifier machines
- Secure full mask to Alans's face
- Move power chair to kitchen and plug in battery charger
- Plug in ventilation machine charger
- Plug in hoist charger

AUTHOR'S NOTE

The morning routine was largely the same as above but in reverse. However, it took up to two hours because most days it had the addition of showering, hair washing, shaving, face and body moisturising, twenty minutes of nebulising (to administer drugs to help clear secretions) and feeding Alan his breakfast.

Wednesday 31st October - Two hours up close and personal

At 2:45am Alan woke me with the alarm. "I cannot move my head anymore." Sadness crept over me. He had dreaded becoming fully paralysed. That day had now come. I held him for a long time. By 7am no carers had turned up. I rang the agency. Eventually only one arrived, so I helped her with the two-hour routine. It was not a problem. I felt closer to Alan in the process, literally!

The former Scottish rugby international, Doddie Weir, spoke on TV about his book and the foundation he had set up to raise £1m for MND research. Yvonne and Becky, associated with Alan's workplace, visited. They had recently completed the Chester marathon and had raised £1,000 for MND Association.

Dr Shamu at Coventry Hospital did the same muscle strength tests on me that Dr Thomas had done, before pronouncing, "The condition could be benign, but an EMG will give us further understanding."

AUTHOR'S NOTE

Doddie Weir's foundation has gone on to raise many millions of pounds. Doddie was presented with the Helen Rollason Award at the BBC Sports Personality of the Year Awards in December 2019. He was also awarded an OBE by the late Queen Elizabeth II.

Doddie sadly died in November 2022 at age fifty-two. Since then, his wife and three sons, all under the age of twenty-five, have carried on the work that Doddie started.

NOVEMBER 2018

Thursday 1st November - Useful afternoon tea

We attended an afternoon tea social event, paid for by the local MND Association branch, at a garden centre. It was helpful meeting other families in the same boat as us, in a casual setting. Initially I sat next to Paul, the guy who used to live in South Africa. I liked his attitude. He had many travel plans and was a 'live in the moment' sort of chap. When Paul and Alan started talking about football, I moved away. I spoke with Marie, the Irish lady, whose husband, Parmar, was diagnosed around the same time as Alan. Her feelings about potential loss were similar to mine but she said, "I have a daughter who will give me something to live for after Parmar dies."

Bill gave me useful information about potential holiday venues. He had lived with a slow version of MND for 15 years.

On the night shift, carer Ligita gave Alan some thick wool socks made in her home country of Lithuania. She refused to take any money for them.

Friday 2nd November - Am I being too efficient?

To save me forgetting to rotate Alan's PEG tube weekly, I gave it a rotation every day, but the site was looking sore. Was I being overzealous? Viv and John arrived late afternoon and after a beef stew dinner we all had an early night.

Saturday 3rd November - Another (very) scary moment

The treat of the day was a trip to the movies. After lunch, the four of us set off in the wheelchair adapted vehicle to a cinema near the NEC. Part way through *Bohemian Rapsody* I noticed a beeping sound. At first, I ignored it but then I realised it was coming from the back of Alan's chair.

The battery levels of his ventilator were dangerously low.

Immediately, I pushed Alan out of the cinema with Viv and John following me, not sure what was going on. I had a moment's panic when I realised the car park ticket was not yet validated so I had to run back to the cinema.

After pushing our way into the lift and whizzing past people in the car park, frantically shouting, "We have an emergency," we got Alan into the back of the WAV. I panicked again. We had not paid for the parking! Luckily there was a facility at the barrier.

As I broke the speed limit trying to get home, the ventilator beep changed to a continuous tone - the sort you see in movies when a person flatlines. In the rear-view mirror, I could see Alan's head had rolled to one side. His eyes were closed! Spontaneously, I howled out loud. Had he died? My cry caused him to open his eyes. He told me later, "I shut myself down to conserve energy." Phew!

When we got to the house, I rushed in, grabbed the spare ventilator, and hooked it up to Alan while he was still in the van. Panic over!

Over dinner at the local pub - with a spare battery in tow - Viv thanked me for my quick actions at the cinema. When I put Alan to bed, he thanked me for saving his life. It had been a scary day - the second time I had thought I might lose Alan (the first time being his fall back in May).

The big lesson - never go anywhere without checking the ventilator battery was fully charged, and away carry a spare battery.

Sunday 4th November - Second attempt to see *Bohemian Rhapsody*

Viv and John set off for home after breakfast. Alan and I went back to the NEC cinema to see the rest of the movie. "You can sit in the accessibility box on the first floor," said the lady at the cash desk when I explained what had happened the day before. "There will be no charge, and here is a voucher for two more tickets to see another movie another time." Wow!

The movie was great.

"Some of the song lyrics were too close to home," Alan mentioned as we made our way to the car. I knew he was talking about *Love of my Life* and hugged him tightly.

Monday 5th November – Insights from an old friend

One of the carers did not show up so I helped the other one get Alan up and ready for the day. This set back my plans to shower and wash my own hair. After lunch I did some shopping and met up with an old work friend. He had lost his mum and dad some years ago, had no siblings, no children and no partner. It was useful hearing how he managed his life alone and the attitude he adopted to avoid feeling sorry for himself.

During the evening Alan announced, "I don't think I will be able to swallow for much longer, so can I have some of my favourite foods in the coming days." It was another depressing moment but, as ever, Alan was being practical and thinking ahead.

Wednesday 7th November - "The other side of great love is great pain"

Thinking about going to Lynton during Alan's respite week saddened me. It made me recall the first time I took him to the Valley of the Rocks during our courtship.

When I showed him where I wanted my ashes to be scattered, he said, "I don't want to think about that, but I will do it for you." It was about then that I realised I loved him and wanted to be with him forever.

During the session with Morgan at the Marie Curie Hospice, Alan said, "I want people at my funeral to really experience what it was like to have to cope with what I am going through." He cried a lot. Privately I thought we would have to put people in straitjackets for them to experience MND. "I also want my affairs to be in order so there's nothing for Hazel to worry about after I pass away." We agreed to tackle all outstanding items as soon as possible.

Morgan smiled, "It's good that you are talking to each other honestly and not hiding things from each other."

My heart sank when she said, "The other side of great love, is great pain." I had invested my heart and soul into this relationship. I was already experiencing grief and wondered how much more 'great pain' there was to come. Morgan asked Alan, "How are you feeling?" His answers were more about practical things than about his emotions, but eventually he admitted, "Sadness is my main feeling."

AUTHOR'S NOTE
The video of the conversation I had with Alan in Lynton during our courtship was one of many I watched in private during Alan's illness. These pre-MND videos reminded me of the strong, fit and able person he was, and put into perspective how much loss he was dealing with.

Thursday 8th November - A week's solitude could appeal
Alan rested on his bed while the technician turned his wheelchair upside down to fix some niggling issues. This gave me the chance to research cottages in Devon which would give me a week's solitude while Alan was in respite. My carer's pass arrived. It gave me a free cinema ticket when I went with Alan. I wished I'd ordered one sooner.

Friday 9th November - Two visits to GP and fundraising ideas
My GP confirmed my blood tests showed no muscle damage. He suggested I have physio on my neck before considering surgery.

On my second visit, Mum's GP offered her a procedure involving a camera into her tummy to check for gallstones. She declined and also declined an injection into her knee to ease her pain. I was beginning to think she was losing the ability to decide what was good for her.

Alan's business partner and good friend, Simon Beacham, stayed with him while Simon's wife Rachel, Christina from Alan's office and I went out to dinner. I didn't feel much like going out but was glad I did in the end. During the meal, Rachel very kindly offered for Alan and I to spend Christmas Day with her and Simon and the three of us recalled the day we did the 10k race. We talked about doing a sponsored 'danceathon' fundraising event, or a sponsored straitjacket sit in to show solidarity with Alan.

Back at the house Simon offered to look after Alan one weekend if it would give me a break.

Saturday 10th November – Log jams and fireworks fun
Alan woke me up twice in the night with mask issues and overheating. Straight after breakfast Alan and I met a lady at his bank to sort out changing his accounts into joint names. There was a wheelchair log jam in Marks & Spencer's because too many of us wanted to use one lift. In the end one of the managers escorted three of us through the rooms behind the store so that we could use a service lift. It was not very dignified.

I felt stressed during the afternoon getting ready for our skiing friends to arrive for a fireworks party. When Alan was out of earshot, Bev, Julie, Nina and Sarah, all asked me how I was. My stock answer to such questions had become, "I am dealing with one day at a time." Alan had fun watching Robert and Tristan trying to set off the fireworks, and we all enjoyed a takeaway curry afterwards, to save me cooking.

Sunday 11th November - Remembrance Day
During the night Alan woke me up several times. He was too hot again and had a dry mouth. I gave him some water. Was he developing an infection? Or did his ventilator settings need to be increased to give him more air pressure?

It was hard to get back to sleep. I kept thinking I could hear Alan's alarm going off. At one point I got up, went downstairs thinking he had called me, only to find him sleeping peacefully. A lovely sight.

The morning brought panic because no carers turned up! Two substitutes were hurriedly called in. These carers were grateful when I let them go early and told them I would handle the visits they were due to make to mum, so they could catch up their day.

At 10am we did a FaceTime video with my nephew Darren, and his wife, Suzanne who had cancelled their visit due to having colds. They offered to have mum on Christmas Day, so that Alan and I could have the day to ourselves.

Alan and I watched the TV coverage from Paris commemorating 100 years since the end of World War I. It featured the faces of fallen men being etched into the sand on the beaches of England and Scotland at low tide. When the tide came in the images were washed away. It made me think, Alan's life is gradually being washed away by MND. At 11am, as in previous years, we watched coverage of the annual Remembrance Day service from the Cenotaph in London. I spotted tears on Alan's cheeks. His emotions were nearer to the surface these days.

Monday 12th November - Whitby trip looking possible
We spent the morning working our way through the items on the *Peace of Mind* list. When I realised how much there was to do, I felt frustrated and agitated. I snapped at Alan and later apologised. It was hard dealing with someone else's affairs especially when they, quite rightly, wanted to maintain control.

A care company in Whitby said they could provide a suitable carer for our planned week in Albany Cottage in December. Yippee! Mum's care company called: "We think your mum has another water infection. Also, we are now applying barrier cream to prevent sores."

Alan and I watched some *Frasier* episodes before watching a powerful World War I documentary. I found the enhanced footage disturbing. Alan enjoyed studying both world wars. He had been an Air Cadet and regretted not pursuing a career in the RAF.

While I was getting ready for bed, Alan's ventilator alarm went off. I rushed downstairs in case Alan's mask was out of position. As I entered his room, the alarm stopped. Alan was in a deep sleep and oblivious to everything. Bizarre.

Tuesday 13th November - Surreal night at the golf club
Alan had a bad night. He had periods of laboured breathing which triggered off the ventilator alarm. He also started shouting out and needed me to take the bedclothes off him, except a thin sheet, because he was too hot. I was worried about him. As soon as practicable I called Stoke Hospital. At 11:30am I had a meeting with mum's social worker, to do a full assessment of care needs.

Golfing mates, Peter and John, looked after Alan while I went with my friend Dawn to the annual prize presentation night at Shirley Golf Club. Sitting at the

Captain's Table, I found it difficult to get into the spirit of things. Dawn won several prizes, as did several other ladies on my table. I only picked up a minor prize.

Incoming Lady Captain, Pam, made an announcement. "The charity I am supporting this year is Motor Neurone Disease Association. Alan Carter has always enjoyed his golf and friendships at Shirley Golf club. He was diagnosed with MND a short time ago. I consider that supporting the charity that supports him and Hazel is vitally important, as they provide an exceptional service to all the thousands of people who have succumbed to this debilitating illness."

Having been to around twenty of these annual events, it all seemed surreal hearing the captain talk about my husband's condition as the inspiration for her choice of charity. During the evening several ladies expressed their concern and asked how I was coping.

Driving home, Dawn spoke of the effects of losing her brother when he was nine. She made me promise to call, or text her, any time I needed someone to talk to. "Alan met you for a reason," she told me. "You are a special couple."

Thursday 15th November - Bank bureaucracy
A new district nurse, Ros, came to do an assessment of Alan's neck. She recommended some gentle exercises to reduce the risk of stiffness.

At 2pm Alan and I met the manager of HSBC Bank, who told us he knew two people who had lived with MND. We thought transferring Alan's account into joint names would be a simple exercise, but it became complicated because Alan could not sign any of the documents. The manager needed us to have the Lasting Power of Attorney (LPA) in place or transfer the funds to another account. We couldn't set up a new joint account online either because my passport and driving licence were still in my previous name. The bureaucracy annoyed us, so later Alan asked me to transfer his funds to my Nat West account, leaving HSBC with nothing! At the Nationwide Bank, it was a completely different story. They set up a joint account there and then with Alan's verbal permission!

Simon Beacham came to visit Alan while I made a quick visit to the shops and dropped in some groceries to mum. Once dinner was ready, Simon left. I was tired and got impatient while feeding Alan. He, quite rightly, pulled me up about it which made me feel bad. After catching up with some TV together, I went to bed feeling totally shattered.

Friday 16th November - False alarms and Yorkshire here we come!
This morning's drama came in the form of a phone call from mum's carer. Mum

wanted to stay in bed because she'd had a nosebleed in the night. She'd used her pendant to call for help because she didn't want to disturb me, but had refused to have paramedics come out, because she was afraid to go into hospital again.

When I checked with her, the house manager at mum's retirement home was unaware that she had triggered the alarm. It was all a bit odd because normally I would have been informed of a pendant alarm event. It turned out a kind man in a first floor flat had heard mum's bleeper going off and had looked after her, cancelling the callout.

"I put the bloody towel in the sink to soak," mum said, but there was no evidence of it. In fact, there was no evidence of a nosebleed anywhere. I wondered if she'd simply had a runny nose and mistaken it for blood.

District nurse Eric ordered a bedframe and some foam heel pads following his visit to Alan. My first physio session at a local clinic brought me some relief. All it took was twenty minutes hands on manipulation and some chin tucking exercise that made me look like a chicken!

My friend, Julia and her friend Kevin, popped in for drinks. Kevin worked at a drug company doing a PhD on nerve renewal. He talked about muscles getting damaged through exercise and some not repairing. It got a bit technical for my small brain, when he started talking about misfolded proteins and prions, but it was all very fascinating. As he was leaving, Kevin said, "You are heroes."

That evening we had fun wearing our yellow spotted Children in Need ears but, as always, the programme moved me to tears. Alan asked me to text a much larger donation than usual for him. Before the night ended I booked Albany Cottage in Whitby!

Saturday 17th November - Extra padding to prevent baboon bottom
Our friend Andy dropped off a more substantial cushion for Alan's wheelchair to help prevent bottom sores. He also talked about alternative back and headrest designs. Unfortunately, Andy worked for a different manufacturer to the company who supplied Alan's chair, but at least the discussion gave us some ideas to raise when we had our next wheelchair assessment.

After lunch, Alison and Adrian visited, bringing carrot cake! We were joined by neighbours Heather and Steve. We discussed fundraising ideas including the possibility of a 'straitjacket sit in'.

Alan and I spent the evening being entertained by England playing rugby against Japan, then judging the performances on the live *Strictly Come Dancing* show from Blackpool.

Sunday 18th November - Friends cannot cope sometimes.

Instead of his usual casual clothes, we dressed Alan in a crisp pink shirt and his smart blue waistcoat before I drove him to Shirley Golf Club for the annual ritual of the new Captain's Drive In.

Alan and I had to sit outside by the flagpole, rather than view the event from the usual position on the patio, because there was no wheelchair ramp from the lounge to the patio. As we were going back to the clubhouse, after Mr Captain had successfully struck his first ball into the distance, Tom, one of the junior members Alan used to mentor, saw us and gave Alan a big hug. He proudly told us his handicap was now almost as low as his dad's.

During the afternoon all sorts of people came to chat to Alan. Later, he told me he was hurt that three members he thought were his friends did not talk to him.

"Maybe they find it hard seeing you like this," I suggested.

In truth, I too was disappointed. The club chairman told us that we could put our WAV in any car parking space if the disability ones were full. Almost as soon as we got home around 4pm, our friends Jill and Steve, and Lesley and Roger arrived with food and wine!

Monday 19th November - Adventures

Straight after breakfast, the six of us set off in convoy for Batsford Arboretum, near Bourton on the Hill. It was a cold day. The enormous Redwood trees, Handkerchief trees and large leaf Magnolia trees were stunning. Unfortunately, we were about two weeks late for the best of the autumn colours, but it was still a lovely day out, despite pushing Alan along sometimes difficult paths off piste!

Back home Alan was struggling with his neck. We had not yet got into a proper routine with his exercises - my fault. So that I could experience the feel of the neck brace we had received, I put it on myself. It was obvious it was going to be difficult for Alan to use due to the position of the wheelchair headrest. In future his wheelchair would have to be slightly tipped back to stop his head flopping forward. His core muscles were completely gone, so he could not sit upright.

I reflected on the tips Lesley had given me following her experience of writing and publishing *Finding Joy Beyond Childlessness* - a self-help book containing case studies of people who were involuntarily childless. Her main advice was, "Simply get the writing started."

Tuesday 20th November - Love all around us

Alan sat with his friend Andy at the golf club while I played in a nine-hole Lady Captain's Drive In competition. Just before Pam hit her first ball into the distance as Lady Captain, I picked two numbers from a prize draw sheet. They turned out to be first and second prizes. Alan and I won two bottles of wine. Was it a genuine win or was somebody just being kind? Either way, Alan and I would certainly enjoy the 'whine'.

Everyone applauded when Pam explained in her speech why she had picked MND Association as her charity. Dorothy, who was born 'up north', kept talking to Alan in a northeast accent which amused him. Sue, who had lost her husband, also called Alan, many years previously, held Alan's hands to keep them warm. The feeling of love in the room was palpable.

We watched three episodes of *Frasier* back at home. Alan was laughing out loud so much he was almost in tears. It warmed my heart to see him so much happier. For the last few days Alan had managed to open his bowels several times, but evidence showed it was time to reduce the laxative medicine!

Over supper we agreed it was hard having so many different carers coming in with differing levels of capability. Should we hire a private carer? Jeff, the new Shirley Golf Club Captain, emailed, "How nice it was to see Alan at the club. You are both loved very much." Wow!

Wednesday 21st November - First anniversary of 'D' Day

The day we had been dreading had arrived. To help us consider how far we had come I read out my journal entry from 21st November 2017 and recited the first poem I wrote in those early days. It wasn't long before we were both in tears.

"We hit rock bottom last November," Alan mused. "Ever since we've been trying to climb out of a massive hole. A never-ending climb, with no knowledge of how far away the top is."

My heart ached when he continued, "The last twelve months has been the worst year of my life."

At Baraset Barn, one of our favourite gourmet country pubs, I asked, "What have been the positive highlights of the previous year, Al?"

After glancing briefly at the lunch menu, Alan began with, "The general highlight has been how friends and family have rallied around us."

His detailed highlights were:

- Experiencing Vietnam

- Overcoming the challenge of being in public in the wheelchair
- Being called 'The most beautiful person in the room' by the golf club captain
- Having the support and patience of a loving wife 'without whom I'd be stuffed'
- Riding on the beach buggy in Wales in July
- Getting the WAV (wheelchair adapted vehicle)
- Finding a nice owner for Morris the MGB
- Seeing ELO

Thursday 22nd November - Second trip to Wales

It was a very frosty morning, so there was no messing about when the time came to fill up the WAV with all the bags and equipment we needed for our trip to Homeland Cottage in Grosmont, near Abergavenny. Alan and I followed Viv and John in their car. For some reason satnav directed us via some tiny country lanes.

My head was throbbing by the time we arrived. Was I going down with a cold? The only item I had forgotten was Alan's Carbocisteine medicine, which controlled secretions in his lungs. I was dreading telling him, but he was alright about it when I finally plucked up the courage.

Before dinner, I helped Alan by exercising his arms, apologising for being rusty. Smiling he said, "You are good because you use the full range of movement, unlike the carers." I noted that I needed to give more training to the carers when we returned home. Alan enjoyed a beer and a small glass of red 'whine' with the meal. I didn't drink for fear that my headache would get worse.

It was a challenge doing Alan's night-time ablutions in the tight space of the en suite, and getting him into bed, but with John and Viv's help, we managed. Immediately lights were out I fell asleep but, at 4am, Alan's alarm went off.

Alan complained of a lump in his coccyx region. I took off the bedclothes and attempted to sort things out. I checked his pad as best I could, but I needed help to roll him to properly assess the cause of the discomfort. John and Viv came to the rescue. We discovered there were lumps in the mattress so moving him up the bed was necessary. At home his extended bed and pressure relieving mattress were invaluable, but here we were making do.

It was difficult getting back to sleep. I started reading *A Different Kind of Life*, an autobiography written by Virginia Williams, wife of Frank Williams from the world of Formula One. Frank had become paralysed after a road traffic accident. Virginia's story of caring for him was insightful for me.

Friday 23rd November - Expecting a new arrival

It took two hours to get Alan up, showered, dressed etc and into the kitchen. A lot of headrest adjustments were needed while we wheeled Alan around Monmouth High Street looking for a pub called The Punch House, where we were due to meet Ben and his girlfriend Claire.

Ben and Claire had arrived when I returned from some shopping. There was much excitement - Claire was pregnant! Just after midnight Alan summoned me using his head activated wireless alarm (called a Rondish). His mattress was uncomfortable again. John and I tried a number of options until Alan was comfortable.

Saturday 24th November - Uncomfortably numb

I woke at 6:30am as I needed the loo which was in the en suite in Alan's room. As I crept past his bed, I discovered he was wide awake. "I've been struggling with the mask and trying to raise the alarm using the Rondish device and the ventilator alarms been going off."

"Sorry Al, I didn't hear it." The cottage had more solid walls than our house. Alan's mask was too loose, and he was not getting enough pressure, so I adjusted the settings. I kissed him, apologised again and wearily went back to my room.

Viv, John and I talked about how the loss of strength in Alan's neck made using the Rondish too difficult. We needed a different solution. When I checked on Alan at 11am he was awake. We both agreed this trip had been difficult for various reasons.

"Will you place my arm around your waist so I can hug you?" he requested looking up at me. I held his arm in place.

"I am sorry for causing all this work and stress."

"Al, it's just bad luck and not your fault."

He smiled and said, "I love you, babe." All my stress melted away.

"I love you too, Al."

Out of the blue tender moments were rare these days, but very special.

John and I showered and dressed Alan and moved him to the kitchen. Within minutes Alan announced, "I feel ready to do a poo and want to go on the commode rather than sit in a soiled pad." Just in time John and I quickly got

Alan out of the power chair, onto the bed, pulled down Alan's trousers and knickers, took his pad off, and hoisted him onto the commode chair. A large deposit was made. The smell nearly knocked John and I over.

Alan inspected his stools - an interesting, bizarre, habit he had developed of late. He was particularly proud of the size of this one! I cleaned Alan's bottom, then John and I hoisted him off the commode, onto the bed, dressed him and hoisted him back into his wheelchair. The next job was to open all the doors and windows!

After a quiet day, at 4pm, we set off for Cardiff in search of a baby monitor (as an alternative to the Rondish) and the restaurant where we were due to meet Ben and Tom. In Cardiff, I suddenly realised I had forgotten to bring the pee bottle. Viv solved the problem ingeniously by going to a sports shop and buying a drinks bottle with a screw cap. We were lucky the shop was open. Not many incontinence pads can cope with the aftereffects of drinking beer!

Alan paid for dinner for everyone.

While I was putting his coat on I sensed he was not enjoying himself.

"I feel helpless," he said out of earshot of the others. "You are brave and strong for coming out and facing the world," I replied, followed by, "I am proud of you for not taking the soft option and hiding away." I hoped the concert we were about to see would cheer him up.

Claire, who worked at the Arena, met us at the entrance and took us to the special wheelchair seating area. Australian Pink Floyd were great but my back kept going into spasm so I couldn't get comfortable. I was extremely tired and dropped off a few times despite the volume of the music. The band's last number was *Comfortably Numb* - the song Alan had said he wanted played at his funeral. I held his hand tightly fighting back my tears. It took us until 1:30am to get Alan sorted out and into bed, but it was worth it.

Sunday 25th November - Smelly mess
The new baby monitor did the trick. At 3:43am, Alan called when he needed his mask adjusting and he called again at 7:45am. "I've been awake for ages with discomfort in my hip but did not want to disturb you," he explained. I hadn't slept well so it really wouldn't have mattered if he had called me, but I loved him for his selflessness.

John was fast asleep, so Viv helped me move Alan while I worried about her poorly back. Between us we managed to get Alan from a five out of ten comfort level to a seven out of ten, using multiple pillows and rolled up towels.

By 8:45am we Alan out of bed, washed, dressed and into the kitchen ready for his nebuliser and medicines. Before long Alan was saying he wanted to go on the commode. This time we didn't make it in time. His bowels opened and his pad and trousers were messed up. John and I got Alan onto the bed so that I could clean him up and change his clothes. Once again the smell was overpowering. An hour later we were back in the kitchen ready for breakfast, and once more the bedroom windows were wide open!

Having travelled back to Carter Castle, the carers arrived at 9:30pm and life returned to 'normal'.

Monday 26th November - Weird dream

Alan reported, "I dreamt about being at my retirement party, staggering around holding onto chairs to steady myself." It was the first dream he had about being able bodied since his legs stopped working.

Tuesday 27th November - Awkward questions

Jane asked me a lot of awkward questions at my counselling session, including had I thought what life will be like after Alan dies? What does Alan want for you after he dies? Also, what do you think it will be like at the end of Alan's life? Also, have you been surprised how you have coped so far?

The most interesting question was, "What have you gained in the last twelve months?"

Jane mentioned that people might think I was okay afterwards and that a new widow can sometimes feel like an outsider at the MND group meetings.

As we talked about all the changes I had endured in the previous twelve months, my tears were uncontrollable. Before leaving the hospice I caught up with the social worker and discussed respite care in either January or February.

Alan was pleased with the fleece lined trousers and long thermal socks I had bought him while I was out. I also showed him the gold chain I'd bought as a retirement gift to myself, so I could wear his wedding ring around my neck. Alan was not impressed with the culinary skills of our carers: "There was a right drama trying to make me cheese on toast for lunch."

When there was a quiet moment, I asked Alan one of Jane's suggested questions. "Who do you want with you at the end Al?"

Without hesitation he said, "You, Pauline and Viv and Simon Beacham."

He had obviously thought about it. I found it too difficult to also ask him what he wanted for me after he died. The rest of the day involved making calls, trying to source a specialist tilt in space shower chair to hire in Whitby.

Wednesday 28th November - No more need for excitement

Waiting for our session with the psychologist at the Marie Curie Hospice, we bumped into our physiotherapist, Leslie. "I am retiring," she announced. Oh... That was a shame. She had been such a significant part of our journey, particularly in the early months.

During our session with Morgan, she asked Alan how he felt about end of life, about organ donation and what exciting things he wanted to do while he still could. Alan said, "I've done loads of things as an able-bodied person, I don't feel the need now." He went on to say, "I'm happy and contented with how I'm living my life now." He avoided the end-of-life question. Later he told me he didn't think his organs would be fit for donation. Privately I disagreed.

Morgan asked, "How hard do you think it will be if and when Alan loses his ability to speak?" Neither of us wanted to think about that. Back at the house, we were relieved to discover Alan's statistics were all stable when Marie from Stoke Hospital did her tests. She lengthened the breath duration on his ventilator machine in the hope that it would give Alan a more settled night sleep.

Thursday 29th November - Preparing for Whitby and sad news

I overslept and hadn't heard Alan calling me when the strap on his face mask was cutting into his ear. I hated it when I made mistakes - even ones over which I had no control - and could not apologise enough.

My cold was coming out, so I wore a face covering while dealing with PEG flushing and giving Alan his medicines. I had become a nurse. Amy from MND fundraising called by to collect the cheques in respect of the 10k run sponsorship. She was thrilled to learn the total raised would be in the region of £17,000!

I started packing for Whitby. I had to be super organised now we had so much specialist equipment. Pauline called and gave us the news that Alan's mum was losing interest in life. Alan had not been able to see Joan since June, and the prospects of him seeing her ever again were slipping away.

To ensure that I didn't let Alan down again, I slept in the single room, which was close to the top of the staircase, increasing the chances of me hearing Alan's alarm if it went off.

Friday 30th November - Perfect cottage

With the WAV packed, and Alan installed, I drove to mum's flat. She waved us off just before noon. We arrived in Whitby around 5pm having stopped for toilet breaks and a snack along the way. At Albany Cottage I deposited the bags inside first. Insisting Alan close his eyes, I wheeled him into the living room. He loved the place, in particular the views.

Christie, the private carer I had hired, arrived at 9pm. Between us we got Alan ready for bed in a wet room almost as big as our lounge! Christie was terrific, which was good because I had booked her for every morning and evening of our stay.

It was bliss having an overhead electronic hoist to help us get Alan into his bed. There was a second bed in the room, so for the first time in a long time, we were able to sleep in the same room. Annoyingly, the ventilator noise prevented me getting to sleep, so I moved to the sofa in the lounge next door.

DECEMBER 2018

Saturday 1st December - How have you done all this?

Christie arrived at 8am and, by 10am, Alan was showered, shaved, shampooed and ready for breakfast. As I cooked some eggs, Alan sat looking out at the countryside.

"What are you thinking, Al?"

With tears running down his face, he said, "I don't know how you have done all this. You must really love me."

Something told me it was a good time to ask what he wanted for me after he died.

"I want you to have loads of fun and to go somewhere where you can be pampered."

That made me cry.

We drove into Whitby to pick up provisions and buy some Proshield barrier cream (which I'd forgotten to pack). It was a grey day. We had a picnic, by the harbour, while spotting people dressed up ready for the Krampus run. We had seen one before in Austria so didn't hang around!

On our way back to the cottage we stopped at the Abbey but, unfortunately, it was closed for the winter. I made a mental note to return one day. After a relaxing afternoon back at the cottage, we watched a few episodes of *Game of Thrones* followed by *Strictly Come Dancing*.

Sunday 2nd December - Exploring Whitby

After eating our breakfast eggs, I drove us north to explore the coast. Most of the villages were out of reach because they were down steep hills which I didn't fancy attempting. Back at the cottage we watched more episodes of *Game of Thrones* before a FaceTime video call with Viv. After more video calls with friends, we ate dinner and watched the *Strictly Come Dancing* results show.

Christie and I managed to get Alan through his bedtime routine in just forty minutes! Again, I attempted to sleep in his room. Around midnight Alan needed his mask adjusting. I could not get back to sleep again after that so went upstairs to sleep on a proper bed in a silent room. During the night I popped downstairs a few times to check on Alan, who was sleeping soundly.

Monday 3rd December - Lunch with 2nd cousin, Lindsey

As Christie helped me get Alan up, showered and dressed, Alan said, "I didn't sleep well. My back was painful." He had chosen not to call me because he didn't think I could fix the problem. We met Lindsey at Trenchers and learned about her 10k fell run and progress on their barn conversion. We drank champagne for no particular reason, after eating fish and chips. It was cold and windy, so I wrapped Alan up tightly in a blanket and wheeled him to the end of the pier where we could see the lighthouse.

More *Game of Thrones* episodes were consumed back at the cottage. Alan didn't want any supper. Pauline, Alan's sister, called to say that their mum was in hospital after a fall.

Tuesday 4th December - MND twin and smelliest sprouts

By wrapping a pillow around my head, and using earplugs, I managed to sleep all night in the same room as Alan! After the usual morning routine, we set off to Huntingdon to meet the couple from Doncaster. It was a bit like a blind date because we had only 'met' virtually via an MND Facebook group. James was in his early thirties and was the youngest person we knew who had MND. James was involved in the Sheffield drug trial that Alan had wanted to join. Because James was diagnosed the day after Alan, his wife Stephanie and I decided the men were MND twins. It was extremely useful comparing stories with them about carers and equipment.

Alan's cousin, Eric arrived at the same restaurant around 3pm. The two men chatted while I helped Stephanie get James into their car. Alan was uncomfortable most of the evening because his bowels had opened, and I couldn't clean him up until Christie arrived. It took a lot of wet wipes to sort out Alan. At times like this I really appreciated the help and professionalism of carer workers.

After lights out I went to sleep quickly, despite the rich smell of digested sprouts in the air from the dinner I had given Alan the night before!

Wednesday 5th December - Jolting me back to reality

Alan's bowels had opened up again in the night which meant more cleaning up for Christie and me before we could move him from the bed. Viv called to say their mum had improved. With the rain beating down outside, I felt sorry that our break would soon be over. I had enjoyed getting away from everything and everyone and feeling so free.

On the MND support group Facebook page, two women posted stories about their husbands passing away. It was hard to know what message to type in support, and harder still thinking one day I would write such a post. Alan looked so well generally it was sometimes hard to believe he was ill at all. Most days I forgot he had a life limiting condition. But every so often something jolted me back to reality.

With Christie's help Alan was tucked up in bed by 10pm. I decided to sleep upstairs hoping the baby monitor had enough range. Alan woke me four times in the night. I needed to do arm, leg and mask adjustments and try to work out why his hip was hurting too.

He became irritable when I struggled to get the mask right, barking, "I know it keeps me alive but it's uncomfortable."

I responded with, "I don't know what to say to that."

Feeling stressed and exhausted, I continued, "Alan, I am tired and need to sleep."

Tears streaming down my face, I left the room for a minute, hating MND, the world and myself.

Thursday 6th December - MND is horrible, but so is cancer
Alan woke me again just before 7am. By the time Christie arrived, Alan and I were both shattered. During breakfast Alan had a choking episode. I had to quickly pull him forward in his chair and tap his back, but it didn't work. I tried other options, including using the suction machine and eventually his breathing settled. "That was a bad one," Alan commented. Apparently he had sneezed and that had caused a blockage in his nose mask which we always used when he was eating. When things settled down I gave him some coffee. While he sucked at the straw I thought, what would I have done if he had died? Tears pricked my eyes. Who would I call first? The thoughts had to be quickly pushed out of my mind or the floodgates would have opened.

I wrote out some Christmas cards. Last year Alan had shared the task, now could not. We finally finished off series one of *Game of Thrones*. I disagreed with Alan when he said, "I don't feel this trip has given either of us the kind of rest we were hoping for." We both agreed MND was horrible and was spoiling things. To stop him falling into self-pity, I said "Cancer is horrible too." We talked about the difference between wanting to die and not wanting to live like this.

Then Alan came out with, "I want you to be able to rest more, babe."

"Nice idea Al, but how is that possible?" I added. "I want to be a good carer, but I make too many mistakes."

Ever the man of reason, Alan said, "No one would be good all the time."

Friday 7th December - We will be back

We gave Christie a thank you gift after the final morning shift. She said, "You have been no trouble. I have enjoyed the week." Oh, how I wanted to take her home with us!

Just as I was hastily packing up the WAV the cottage owner arrived cheerily saying, "You don't have to rush to vacate."

Moving bags into place I told him we had a five-hour journey ahead of us and needed to be home by 4pm.

"Has it been worth it?" he asked.

I told him, "Yes".

The cottage owner asked Alan's age. I told him sixty-four and that Alan was diagnosed with MND a year ago.

I volunteered, "If Alan is alive this time next year, we will be back." Then my throat tightened. It was the first time I had said anything like that.

Despite Alan sitting in the back of the WAV while I drove, we managed several conversations on our journey home. We talked about where we might holiday next, and who we might ask to join us.

"How do you feel about me writing a book about all this, Al?"

"I want people to know what this is like," he said, "For me and for you."

Finally, we mulled over ideas for the book title. Our pet name for MND, the *Mean Nasty Disease*, was a contender. Or, maybe, *Uncomfortably Numb*.

We arrived home just before 4pm. Before long the house was a mess - bags and equipment everywhere. I was very tired and had no enthusiasm for sorting everything out. Carers turned up at 4:30pm and our old pattern of life began again.

Another choking episode happened as the carers were getting Alan ready for bed. I wondered if this was the beginning of a phase. Not being able to eat his

203

favourite foods might weaken Alan's spirit. Alan and I had already dealt with so much change - each phase changed us a little too. How much more could we cope with? When these types of thoughts crept in, I reminded myself of other women, like Wendy, who had been caring for their husbands for many years.

Saturday 8th December - Beautiful people

At the MND annual Christmas lunch at the Crowne Plaza Hotel, Solihull, I sat next to Pat and John who had been married for fifty years. I envied them. Then I felt sorry for her when I learned that Pat was a fundraiser for MND Association because she had lost her sister to the disease.

The local chairman of the Birmingham and Solihull MND group, Roger Leek, thanked all the volunteers. The MP for Erdington gave a speech. I bought ten raffle tickets. It was embarrassing when five of my tickets were picked out. I accepted the first prize, a large teddy bear, but declined the other prizes.

After a quick turnaround back at the house we set off for the Wild West themed ABC Solutions/Aggora Christmas Dinner at a hotel in Alvechurch. While trying to get into the hotel Alan's power chair went into lockdown. After several unsuccessful attempts to get it working, four strapping men carried Alan, in his chair, into the hotel while I called the engineers who guided me though the unlocking procedure. I broke down thinking that last Christmas, Alan had been dancing at this venue.

After Simon Pointon gave his CEO's speech we packed up to leave. Rob, one of the John O'Groats cyclists, stopped me in the lobby. "You can call me any time, day or night," he said, adding, "Nasty things should not happen to beautiful people like you and Alan."

Sunday 9th December - Pâté and tears

The highlight of the day was a visit from Alan's nephew (our best man), Matthew and his wife, Suzanne. They proudly presented pâté they had made using the same recipe Alan used to follow. It made for a nice lunch.

After we had eaten, Alan requested, "Will you give my black down North Face jacket to Matthew please." It was horrible seeing the jacket go as Alan had worn it on several of our ski holidays, but it was good knowing it would stay in the family.

The songs and dances in the *Strictly Come Dancing* semi-finals were so moving. Alan and I both ended up in tears.

Monday 10th December - Practical ideas regarding mum

The Admiral nurse, supporting me with mum was very sympathetic to my situation when I brought her up to date. Her dad had died from MND three years before, aged fifty-one. She knew exactly what I was dealing with and gave me several practical ideas on how to get more care for mum.

Tuesday 11th December - Looking unwell

The whole morning was spent at the wheelchair centre trying to sort out a new headrest. Of all the changes that had happened to Alan's body, his head flopping forward, due to weak neck muscles, was the one that most showed he was unwell.

Wednesday 12th December - Not ready to die

The district nurse arrived to check that Alan's feet were continuing to improve. Our meeting with Morgan was probably our most emotional. Initially we talked about our trip to Whitby and how we wanted Christmas to look and feel. The most poignant thing Alan said was, "I feel like I'm staring down the barrel of a gun." He added, "I'm not ready to die." He also said, "I am worried about the idea of struggling for breath at the end of life."

Once Alan and I stopped crying, Morgan gave us good tips on how to continue to 'check in' with each other every so often. This was our last session with Morgan because she was moving to a new role. We would both miss our honest chats with her, despite the painful realities she gently encouraged us to face. Morgan had given us the 'tools' to keep the dialogue open between ourselves. I was sure there would be days in the future when Alan would hate me asking him, "Is there anything else on your mind?"

I went to bed thinking six years ago Alan proposed. Unusually, we didn't celebrate it in any way this time. In addition to everything else, MND had robbed us of romance.

Thursday 13th December - Feeling the cold

Late morning I took Alan to the annual ABC Solutions Christmas lunch at the Abbey Hotel, in Beoley. I had a relaxing massage and used the spa while Alan ate with his ex-work colleagues. Worryingly, Alan complained of feeling the cold all day.

Friday 14th December - Traditional time with friends

Every year, for many years, Jo, Andy, Alan and I had gone out for a meal together instead of buying Christmas gifts for each other. This year we went to our local pub, The Saracen's Head. A makeshift ramp enabled us to get Alan's wheelchair up into the restaurant. We ate fish and chips. The boys drank beers. Jo and I drank champagne. It was lovely to feel so relaxed.

We giggled at the selfie we took because it looked like Jo and I were holding a sculpture of Alan's head. His black clothing created the illusion he had no body. Ironic really.

Back at our home, Jo told me, "You are wonderful doing what you do." As I burst into tears I said, "Alan's worth it."

Later I confessed to Jo, "I think it will be too hard to stay at Carter Castle after Alan dies." Alan was uncomfortable in his chair most of the day. At teatime the carers hoisted him up to relieve pressure on the sit bones in his bottom. His shoulder blades, hips and bottom were uncomfortable when we put him to bed and nothing we did made him feel better. His hands and legs had been cold at different times throughout the day too.

Saturday 15th December - Antibiotics needed
During the night, Alan was either too hot, too cold, uncomfortable or needed mask adjustments. The carers could not manage the cough assist machine during the morning shift, so I had to do it. It took several attempts to draw up the secretions, which exhausted Alan.

When one of our ski buddies, Robert, arrived to sit with Alan so I could do some Christmas shopping, I trained him on how to use the cough assist machine - just in case.

By teatime, Alan appeared to be getting worse. I had been given permission to start him off on the emergency antibiotics we already had if his symptoms worsened. I administered a dose of co-Amoxiclav.

Sunday 16th December - Scared for mum and Alan!
At 9:30am, mum's carers called to let me know mum was not in her flat. The on-call team had arranged for paramedics to come out because she had fallen off a chair. I checked my phone. There were missed calls from the on-call people and paramedics. I found mum in A&E at Heartlands Hospital. An x-ray ruled out any fractures, but she was admitted to the ambulant emergency care ward for a mobility assessment.

Alan had breathing and bowel issues during a visit from some friends. After everyone left I continued writing in the Christmas cards as we caught up with some recorded TV shows. Multi-tasking was normal these days. We did a FaceTime video with Viv, who was impressed with the McEnroe style headband

I had started using to stop Alan's head flopping forward. Viv told us that Alan's mum was also in hospital in Sunderland. Alan dictated a letter for me to handwrite and put inside his mum's Christmas card.

After the bedtime carers cleaned up Alan for the third time today, he became agitated. I gave him 5mls of Oramorph and we did cough assist to try to ease his difficult breathing. "I feel scared," he said and agreed I should call the GP and the ventilation unit to see what else I could try. I, too, was scared. His breathing was getting worse.

Monday 17th December – Couldn't bring himself to say "MND."
At 7:30am I called the care agency because no one had arrived for the 6.30am shift. Pauline and Simon arrived at 11am and underwent cough assist machine training. I left about noon for my nerve conduction and EMG tests at Coventry Hospital. Checking the readings the clinician announced, "You have not got it." I noted he did not say MND, as if the words themselves were somehow too unbearable to utter.

Relieved but also sorrowful, thinking Alan had been told he had got "It", I stopped at mum's flat and found that she was back from hospital. She was confused and her handbag contained a box of antibiotic tablets - probably for a water infection. I needed to get home, to relieve Pauline and Simon, so I couldn't stay long. I texted mum's care agency, our family and mum's cleaner so everyone was in the loop about her latest incident.

Our GP called to discuss Alan's medicines. He prescribed another box of co-Amoxiclav. "If they don't work, the next step will be treatment in hospital." Oh no! I wrapped up all the gifts I had bought for the carers and handed out the first lot that night. After the bedtime carers left, Alan needed the cough assist machine. This time some phlegm came off his chest.

AUTHOR'S NOTE
Several months later I found out many people in the health services dreaded getting motor neurone disease more than any other neurological condition.

Tuesday 18th December - Kind words from a friend - harsh words from mum
It felt good to catch up with Teresa in Solihull. During a long parting hug, she whispered, "Look after yourself. I care for you my friend." I dashed back to my car, tears streaming down my face. Around 3pm I popped in to see mum. She was angry and aggressive towards me. I reminded myself she was not herself due to the water infection. But it was hard not to be affected by the tone of her voice and hurtful comments.

It was very difficult getting Alan secretion's up at bedtime. Multiple attempts with the cough assist machine were stressful and exhausting for both of us. Not long after I'd gone to bed Alan called me for more cough assistance. We were successful after several attempts. I eventually got to sleep around 2am.

Wednesday 19th December - "I don't mean to be dramatic, but ...."

My alarm went off at 7:50am. No sign of any carers again. I chased the agency raising my concerns about punctuality. At 8:47am carers arrived. The usual district nurse visit took place. Our friends Carol and Graham who were due at 10am arrived at 10:30am with their grandson George. Graham kindly helped get the back garden fence replaced.

Our ex-carer, Terese, was due at 11:30am but in the end did not arrive, which was fine by us as the day had already turned haywire.

My friend Christine Cooper arrived at 12:30pm with sandwiches, home-made mince pies, crumpets and Christmas gifts. Mum's carers called saying mum's behaviour is very erratic and recommended the GP be called out. Alan's business partner Simon was due to visit but had to cancel. I was relieved. The day had been busy enough.

"It's not fair. We are missing all of the things we normally do at this time of year," Alan said as we watched the Lions' Santa sleigh slowly make its way past our door.

I called Stoke Hospital about the difficulties we were having getting Alan's secretions up. Alan needed the cough assist machine again as soon as he was in bed. From 10pm to 11pm we tried to clear his lungs. He became very agitated. We agreed it was time I called 111. The call handler was very good. Once he had taken Alan's medical details and understood his symptoms, he agreed an ambulance should be called.

In the still of the night, while waiting for the paramedics Alan said, "I don't mean to be dramatic, but if this is it, the last twelve years have been the happiest of my life." Tears fell from his eyes as he added, "I have never loved someone as much as I have loved you." It took all my strength to hold back my tears.

Paramedics confirmed Alan's blood pressure was high - 200/124. (A normal blood pressure level is less than 120/80 mmHg). His oxygen saturation was low. By 3am we were in the rapid response unit at Coventry Hospital. Alan's blood pressure was 170/125. Blood tests were taken. Results showed signs of an infection. I heard someone mention sepsis. Two large phials of blood were taken. Antibiotics were administered.

Even though the lights were piercingly bright and, I could hear repetitive beeps and people moaning in pain everywhere, I felt strangely calm. My Fitbit showed my heart rate was sixty-one. Earlier in the evening, Alan's had been eighty-two!

Alan was wheeled to the X-ray department and parked next to a lady with severely swollen, ulcerated legs. While Alan was having an X-ray, screens were put up in front of me and the swollen legged lady. Through a gap in the screen, I saw a trolley being wheeled past with a blanket over what I assumed was a dead body. I shuddered.

Thursday 20th December - Suction begins

Alan was moved to a private cubicle where a different doctor came and checked him over. Alan's blood pressure was 178/112. Listening to Alan's chest he declared "It's clear."

SEPSIS 6 PATHWAY in big orange letters leapt off the page on the doctor's clipboard. I had to ask what we were dealing with, and he replied that he wanted to check the X-ray and blood test before he could be sure.

At 4:45am, Alan's blood pressure went up to 193/117. At 5am, it was down to 162/106. At 5:30am, it was up again to 171/112. A doctor confirmed to Alan the X-ray was clear, but there was a slight infection in the blood. The respiratory team would examine Alan when they came on duty.

Alan's blood pressure and other vital signs were checked hourly, so neither of us got any sleep.

At 10:45am, Holly, a non-invasive ventilator physio, explained Alan would be transferred to Ward 30 for full observations of his lungs, swallow, etc. She suspected Alan's throat muscles were weakening, and aspiration was taking place. In other words, liquids and food particles were getting into his windpipe. From Alan's records, she could see Alan had seen their respiratory consultant, Dr Ali, in February. She discussed a possible course of treatment. It would be important to get the right balance between using drugs to dry up saliva production and managing secretions.

I dashed home to make up an overnight bag for Alan and, briefly, saw mum. She appeared a little calmer but was behaving like a child. There were no packs of her usual tablets in the house because the chemist was unaware she had been discharged from hospital. I had to make an emergency trip to the pharmacist to sort that out.

When I reached Ward 30, Alan was resting in the last bed on the left, by the window. Holly arrived and tried clearing Alan's chest. She asked if it was okay to transfer Alan's ventilation care from Stoke Hospital to Coventry Hospital. This would mean that there would be a follow-up visit once Alan was discharged and meetings every three months to check on his progress. It seemed like a good idea.

Later, Holly had to do a lot of torturous suction to get Alan's excess secretions out. I could hardly watch as she put the tube down Alan's throat, and he gagged. Before I said goodnight to Alan, I carefully fed him a cottage pie dinner. Driving home, shockingly, I momentarily dropped off to sleep at the wheel.

Friday 21ˢᵗ December - A lot of tears

The manager of mum's retirement home called. "An ambulance is coming in four hours to take your mum to Solihull hospital." The GP had initiated the admission because he was worried about mum's kidney function test results.

When I reached Alan, I established he had gone through a lot of tough attempts to clear his airways. He looked well but sounded different. The tubes down his nose and throat affected his voice. I did his PEG flush and made him more comfortable. I left messages for Viv and Pauline, to call me, and spoke to his niece, Helen.

Before I left Alan, he managed to use the bedpan, which was some achievement, because he was laid flat on the bed during the process.

Saturday 22ⁿᵈ December - Alan may never see his mum again

My youngest brother Michael and I grieved while talking about Alan. A telephone call with my friend Angela resulted in a generous offer to call her any time of day or night. My golfing friend Dawn offered for me to join her and her family for dinner. I declined as I wanted to be with Alan. At mum's flat I picked up some clothes and drove to Solihull Hospital. She looked much brighter but was still babbling about strange things.

At Coventry Hospital Alan reported that he'd had more physio on his chest. He appeared a lot brighter. His blood pressure was still high though - 175/110 - but the hospital had stopped using a nebuliser. I gave him his dinner, flushed his PEG and gave him a shave.

Pauline phoned. She and Viv had visited their mum yesterday and were worried as she was not looking well. "I have resigned myself to the possibility I will never see my mum again," Alan sighed.

Sunday 23rd December - Alan's mum seriously ill
My sister Rowena called. I brought her up to date with our news. I visited mum in Solihull Hospital. There was no change in her condition. Alan's sister Viv, and her husband John, arrived at our house with cake, Christmas pudding and food for the 30th of December. Viv told me that their mum had been diagnosed with inoperable cancer. I didn't know what to say and worried how Alan would take the grim news.

Alan looked well when Viv and I reached him. He chatted about his day then asked how his mum was. Viv explained the situation. He appeared to cope well with the dismal news. It was good to learn that Alan's condition was improving. His blood pressure was down to 156/98 - the lowest it had been since coming into hospital. He'd had two lots of cough assist treatments during the day and needed another one which I did for him.

As we walked out of the ward, Viv said she thought Alan looked low. I went back to him. He said he was all right. I got the impression he was relieved that he was less likely now to predecease his mum. Back at the house I posted the photographs we'd taken in Whitby on Facebook. My niece-in-law, Suzanne, called and invited me to go to her house on Christmas Day. It was a kind offer but no matter what, I wanted to be with Alan. Before going to bed I watched *Brief Encounter*. A good old-fashioned tearjerker that helped me let go of my emotions.

Monday 24th December - Best Christmas present!
I woke up before the alarm, my mind full of random, colliding thoughts:

- How will we go about moving my mum to a care home?
- What should I wear today?
- How did Alan cope after we left him, following the news about his mum?

I sent a supportive text to Viv because I suspected her emotions were in turmoil. I could not imagine how she must be feeling losing both her mum and her only brother. During the morning my brother Kevin phoned. We had a nice chat which included reminiscing about going carol singing when we were children. Coventry Hospital phoned late morning with the surprising news that Alan was being discharged. What a Christmas present!

Before I went to visit Alan, Simon, Alan's business partner, arrived. Oddly, he asked me, "Are you about to break?" He told me that when he was splitting up from his first wife, Alan was also splitting up from a long-term relationship. Apparently the two of them had supported each other emotionally. Simon gave me a bag of gifts for Alan.

I gave chocolates and sweets to the staff at the hospital. They gave me a bundle of drugs for Alan, and his personal items. Once we were settled in Carter Castle, I updated Facebook readers and prepared vegetables for Christmas Day, feeling delighted Alan was home.

Tuesday 25th December - Extra special Christmas

Our carers arrived and before long Alan was up, dressed and had eaten breakfast without any dramas. Before the day got too busy, I filmed a poignant video for Facebook of Alan wishing everyone a Happy Christmas, his message ended with, "Don't put off important plans, because you don't know what's around the corner."

Later in the morning, Alan became tearful seeing pictures of his great nephews on WhatsApp. "I love you babe," he said, and got an extra-long, tearful hug in return. We visited mum in hospital before dropping off gifts at my sister's house. When we were back home we did a FaceTime call with our friends, Jo and Andy.

I opened our cards and showed them to Alan. We got emotional as I opened our gifts from family and friends. Alan's work colleague, Christina had bought us a Lord and Lady title. Another work colleague, Vikki gave us one of the homemade tiered cake stands from her wedding to Steve Carter!

Pauline gave us a 'tree' made from packets of our favourite sweets - M and M's! Alan's cousin, Christine had made me a beautifully bound journal. (I used it to keep my daily notes going forward). By the time we did a FaceTime call with Alan's sisters, Viv and Pauline, I was overcome with emotion.

We opened our presents to each other later in the day. Apparently several people had offered to help Alan. Christina, from Alan's office, had bought me a beautiful grey and cream sweater on behalf of Alan and Simon had bought a card and written Alan's words in it. I opened Alan's gifts for him. First, there was a pair of fleece lined trousers. Instead of a fly zip they had a special drop front panel to make it easier to use the pee bottle when he was in his wheelchair.

I also gave him two of his favourite tops from Rohan. My final gift made him cry. I had adopted a tiger for him. The certificate came with a tiny stuffed toy tiger. The toy became his constant companion, right up to the end of his life - it even made its way into his coffin.

Wednesday 26th December - Relaxing with friends
Alan had a bad night. I got up to adjust his mask twice but apparently there were other times he had called me, but I hadn't heard him. Our friends Jo and Andy arrived at 10:30am for coffee, mince pies, prosecco and nibbles. We spent a lazy afternoon catching up with TV and relaxing after Jo and Andy left. Doing nothing was a rare treat for me.

My sister, Rowena phoned, "I tried to visit mum in hospital, but the ward is in lockdown - one of the patients has something contagious!"

Thursday 27th December - A new, unwelcome, phase
I'd only been in bed an hour or so when Alan called me. His chest was blocked and he needed the cough assist machine. At 1:30am, I called 999 because I could not clear his chest. By 2:30am we were in Coventry Hospital, Resuscitation Ward, having gone through rapid assessment. We waited for several hours, listening to patients in other beds moaning in pain.

Initially, Alan's blood pressure was 172/104. Pulse 73. Oxygen saturation 92%. Sugar levels 6.1. The doctor struggled to find a vein so he could take blood samples. In the end ultrasound equipment was used to help get the needle in. At 6:30am, Alan's blood pressure was 153/105 and oxygen saturation was at 93%. One of the doctors suggested an increase in the Carbocisteine drug.

At 10am, we were back in the ward Alan had left on Christmas Eve. It was a relief when the doctor and Holly, the respiratory physio, said there were no signs of infection. It was suspected the issue was the further weakening of the breathing muscles. The doctor suggested alternative medicines be delivered via an automatic pump and called for a palliative consultant to visit us from the nearby Myton Hospice.

Julie, our Macmillan nurse, called me. Somehow she knew what was going on. I was shocked when she suggested, "Alan can choose to come off the non-invasive ventilator if he wants to." Was he so ill, that he might give up the fight now? My mind settled when Alan declared, "I want to stay on the ventilator. I am not ready to die yet."

Julie and I discussed the idea of Alan being moved to the Marie Curie Hospice for symptom control. This was subject to bed availability and the doctors at both the Marie Curie Hospice and Myton Hospice agreeing a plan.

Later Holly had some success using the cough assist machine. Then she came back and did some suction. It was always tough watching the invasive procedure, but it was the most effective way of clearing lungs. To distract him, at one point, I mentioned that it was a dreary day outside. He replied with, "But you brighten up the inside."

Holly explained to us that Alan could be put on a pump - technically called a driver - which would deliver a continuous trickle of medicines into him. She also explained that controlling symptoms with drugs might give a better quality of life, rather than using the risky procedure of suction tubes down into airways. I began to feel a creepy sensation of doom slowly drawing over us.

While eating dessert, Alan said, "My swallowing is getting harder. Also, over the last couple of weeks I have lost spatial awareness of my hands and feet. I'm becoming comfortably numb, like in the Pink Floyd song." I really did not know what to say.

On and off during the afternoon I dozed. By 6pm I realised it was best if I went home. I gave Alan his dinner. I felt scared and concerned driving home. I called my friend Jo but there was no answer. Later I sent texts to family and friends. Simon and Christina from Alan's office both responded. Alan's sister, Viv, called. We had a long chat, concluding that Alan was entering a new, unwelcome phase.

Friday 28th December - A glimpse of my future
It was agreed at a meeting with mum's social worker at her hospital, that the best place for mum was a care home. I concurred. During my visit to Alan, Holly talked about drug options. She suggested glycopyrronium (glyco), administered via a needle under the skin attached to a syringe driver. Also, Atropine drops, usually used for eyes, had proven to be effective at decreasing saliva production.

Worryingly, Alan's temperature was up at 38.4C so he was given Tramadol. His blood pressure was still high at 169/90. Oxygen saturation was at 94%. In an attempt to make Alan feel better about the idea of going to the local hospice, rather than the Marie Curie Hospice where we already knew a lot of the staff, Holly explained that several nurses at Myton Hospice had experience of MND patients using non-invasive ventilators.

On my way home I called Alan's cousin, Christine, to bring her up to speed and thank her for the personalised journal she had made. Carter Castle felt empty and lifeless without Alan. It was eerily quiet. My heart sank when it dawned on me the house would be like this after Alan died.

Saturday 29th December - Myton good but Kevin's not so good.

First thing I sent out updates of Alan's condition to friends and family via WhatsApp and texts. Several positive messages and phone calls came back. Simon Beacham was particularly concerned so we made a plan for him to visit Alan later in the day. My neighbours John, Sue and Andy all caught me as I was leaving for Coventry. With a lump in my throat, I explained the current situation. Before reaching the hospital I dropped into Myton Hospice to arrange a tour.

Alan's blood pressure was still high - 169/80 and his temperature was still up at 38.4C when I finally reached him. I relayed all the messages we had received while giving him his lunch, doing his PEG flush, cleaning his teeth and giving him a shave. My brother Kevin and his wife visited after lunch. Sue and I compared notes about our respective poorly mums. Kevin also mentioned his kidney function was down to 25% as a result of chronic disease. So many people were ill all at once!

When Simon and Rachel arrived to visit Alan, I walked to the car park with Kevin and Sue. Kevin had been part of my life for sixty years. Thinking he might die felt awful but helped me appreciate better how Viv and Pauline might be feeling. The receptionist at Myton Hospice told me someone in her family had MND when she learned why I was visiting. I felt sorry for her but had long since stopped being shocked at how many people I discovered were affected by what I had once thought was a rare condition.

Myton Hospice was smaller than the Marie Curie Hospice but just as warm and welcoming. On my way back to the car park I chatted with an Irish lady who had been visiting an inpatient - a cousin in his eighties. She said she had visited a lot of care homes but was extremely impressed with Myton. She also knew somebody with MND!

I had an amusing telephone call with my friend Carol when I got home. We compared notes regarding our respective mother's behaviour and tried to find humour in the idea we might end up like them in our old age. I decided I wanted to end up like Alan - graceful and full of gratitude, even when facing end of life.

Sunday 30th December - Is this it?

I woke up twice in the night. First time I went back to sleep quickly but, at 3:30am, I was more alert, so I updated my journal. My head was less painful, but I felt I was going down with a cold. My leg twitches told me that I was lacking in sleep and getting stressed. Momentarily, I thought about going for a run, then thought it might be best to conserve energy.

Instead, I finished writing a poem that I'd started the day before.

IS THIS IT?

Is this it - is this the end?
Am I soon to lose my one true friend?
A million thoughts run around my head,
As you lie still and failing in your hospital bed.
Will you know when the end is near?
Will you still speak, be able to hear?
Every day tougher than the last,
With your decline moving so fast.
How do you feel inside your head?
Are you worried you might soon be dead?
A million thoughts running around my head,
As you lie imprisoned in your hospital bed.
The pillows prop up your beautiful face,
Your body broken but full of grace.
Your temperatures up but you feel the cold,
You still look handsome, but has your soul been sold?
My precious man, they cannot mend,
Is this it - is this the end?

It was normal these days to feel like I was living on a knife edge. My fears at their deepest in the early hours of the morning, as the town slept and the house was quiet. I remembered a friend telling me once that I had 'good instincts'. What were my instincts telling me at this time? Logic told me Alan was in danger. The signs were there. An inability to cough, high temperature, weak swallowing muscles and a referral to a palliative care consultant. But my gut told me Alan had more life left in him and that he could pull through this. Yes, he was not well and less comfortable than usual, but I was sure getting him to the hospice was the right thing to do. Professional care and a more private environment would be positive for him. I just needed to keep his spirits up and make him comfortable with the idea of going to Myton instead of coming home.

Monday 31st December - Surviving 2018

My latest message on a Facebook MND support group drew several positive responses from complete strangers. Over breakfast, Alan's brother-in-law, John talked of his feelings about missing out on experiences he and Alan had planned for their retirement. I was beginning to feel low when the phone suddenly rang. For a split second we all froze. Luckily it was Stoke Hospital calling about the delivery of a suction machine. The idea, that I might have to do what the hospital had been doing for Alan, scared me to death. Whether I liked it or not Nurse Carter had to get on with it.

I drove to the hospital around 11:30am, followed by Viv and John. Alan was tired - a legacy from the previous day's rigorous physiotherapy. Alan's temperature was still up at 38.3C, but his blood pressure had gone down to 147/86. Thankfully, his saturation level was good. The doctor extracted some blood but struggled to insert a cannula for delivering antibiotics.

Shortly after giving Alan his lunch he was moved to a private room. Nurses feared he may have an infection. We all had to wear masks to prevent us catching it. Ski friends, Bev and Malcolm, came to visit at 3pm. Malcolm made funny quips when another doctor also failed to introduce a cannula. In the end two anaesthetists were successful using an ultrasound machine to find the elusive vein.

Bev took a photograph of Alan and I holding up a New Year's message for me to post on Facebook. Alone at home, I did what Alan and I always did on New Year's Eve - watched the Graham Norton show followed by a Madness concert. Then I listened to Big Ben tolling midnight and watched the Jools Holland Show.

I was glad Alan had survived 2018. No one knew how much of 2019 he would see. What I knew was I loved him with every inch of me. I would do everything possible to help him enjoy 2019, stay safe, be comfortable and feel loved.

The invisible monster had thrown us all sorts of curved balls during the year, and Alan had defied death at least three times!

It was a tough year on many levels.
Our lives had changed completely.
Our privacy had become non-existent.
Our home had become a place of constant comings and goings.

I had become more of a nurse and a PA, than wife and companion.

As the New Year arrived, I thought it's going to be hard to have hope that Alan will make it to the end of 2019. He was very poorly.

I resolved to try to be the 'glass half full' person I used to be before MND came along, but also I knew I would have to be a realist too.

I wanted, with all my heart, for Alan to make it to our 5th wedding anniversary - 14th June - and to his sixty fifth birthday on 21st June.

My role was to keep him safe and well and keep his morale up, so he had the best possible chance of making it through another year.

If he lived to December 2019 he would defy the diagnosis we'd had back in 2017.

First, I needed him to get over his infection and become well enough to come home.

PART 5 - END OF LIFE

JANUARY 2019

Tuesday 1st January - Uneventful New Year's Day

At the hospital I gave Alan a shave, cut his finger and toenails and flushed his PEG tube. A physio gave Alan some breathing exercise to practise and told him off. "You must ask for help any time instead of waiting until you are really suffering before alerting the nurses." Typical Alan.

Alan's saturation levels were good at 96%. His temperature was 38.3C so more paracetamol was given. A cheery nurse, called Sam, noticed Alan's left knee was hot and swollen. When I saw her later, she confided, "I had a good chat with Alan earlier, he's a good listener and wise."

After giving Alan his dinner, I visited mum at her hospital. She appeared confused. Annoyingly, a junior nurse had filled in mum's CHC document incorrectly, so mum could not be allowed home until a complex needs discharge nurse was engaged. While Alan's work colleague Christina visited him, I spent the evening at home catching up on administration.

Wednesday 2nd January - Perfect stranger

Pauline and Simon were already at the hospital by the time I arrived - we were all hoping Alan would leave the hospital today. He looked very tired while I fed him his lunch. He explained, "Physios needed to work on me in the middle of the night to clear my lung."

Two different physios were working on Alan's chest when we returned. He gagged and I winced as the suction tube went down his throat. Three people from the palliative care team turned up. The doctor confirmed that the respiratory consultant was treating Alan for an infection. The blood tests showed that there was some inflammation too, and Alan needed to stay for three more days.

The doctor talked of using Carbocisteine to help thin secretions and using patches if secretions became too excessive. Other drugs would be administered via a syringe, in a pump driver. The doctor said that he would arrange for a speech and language therapist to check Alan's ability to swallow. He explained that in the hospice Alan would have access to the hospital team as well. If he were to get a further infection Alan would need to stay at the hospital for suitable antibiotics to be administered.

The cough assist machine settings were changed to automatic, rather than patient-initiated breathing, because Alan had lost the ability to form a cough.

After Pauline and Simon left, Alan could not settle. His secretions had built up again. He had a couple of choking episodes too, so the nurses gave him

Lorazepam. "I want to go back to the life I had pre-MND," Alan pleaded. I would have given my right arm to make that happen.

Alan was tired and depressed when nurse Sam came in. She told me, "Alan was my perfect stranger when I needed some personal advice." As ever, Alan was the voice of reason. Sam did her best to cheer Alan up. I left around 8:30pm. In my car, in the hospital car park, emotion overcame me. I gripped the steering wheel and screamed until my throat was sore. Within moments of arriving home, I grabbed a bottle of wine, knocked on my neighbour's door and poured out my heart. Sue and Alex were my perfect strangers when I needed them.

Saturday 5th January - Breaking a golden rule
My mood was low all morning. Even a visit to Tamworth to see nephew Darren, his wife Suzanne and their twins did not cheer me up. I could not stop myself talking about Alan. I tried hard not to cry for fear of upsetting their twins. In happier times, Alan and I had enjoyed being with these small children. At mum's hospital, I pulled myself together and started to formulate a plan to move her into a care home and to sell her flat.

Alan told me, "I had a bad night. The mask kept slipping off, but I could not make the call button work." He mentioned that, "At one point the physiotherapist accidentally left off my ventilator mask." I knew that would have been torture for him. Additionally, he would not have been able to speak loud enough to alert anyone to the danger, when he was off the mask. "A nurse was slow changing my mask too." All this would have caused him distress. I felt angry for not being there. I reported the critical incidents to the nurse in charge. I stressed the importance of regular checks on Alan and explained that his life depended on him being on the mask!

It was clear Alan felt low when he asked, "Why me?" and spoke of, "Hoping for the best but planning for the worst." I felt numb and could not think what to say to cheer him up. On checking his charts, I could see he was on Erythromycin antibiotics.

After I had given Alan a shave, we made ourselves even more morose by watching Les Misérables on iPlayer. Before leaving around 8:30pm I set up the baby monitor I had brought in from home and put the call button next to Alan's head.

My sister sent a text about her visit to mum in hospital. Sleep was impossible. If I wasn't coughing I was crying. I couldn't remember when life had last felt this grim. Was it when I broke up with my ex-husband in 1989, or when I found out I was never going to be a mum in 2005? Alan, breaking one of our three golden rules today by saying, "Why me?" was revealing his feelings. At the beginning of our MND journey we had decided unanswerable questions were taboo (because they unbalanced your mindset). Becoming angry and wallowing in self-pity was also taboo. I assumed Alan must be feeling fed up, scared, unhappy and angry. I felt impotent, of no use to him anymore.

Later that night, I considered calling a friend but didn't want to be a pest. Should I call the Samaritans? What was the point? There was nothing anyone could say or do to make my situation better.

AUTHOR'S NOTE

In hindsight, I should have ensured all hospital staff involved with Alan's care were briefed, confident and competent with the specialist equipment Alan needed. Wrongly, I had assumed they would understand the need for a person with MND to be always on the NIV mask.

Sunday 6th January - Samaritan to the rescue

In the early hours of the morning I dialled the number for the Samaritans. "I used to be a Samaritan many years ago," I blurted out. "I am not suicidal. I'm not looking for answers, I just need someone to listen," which the lady did brilliantly. She empathised well and suggested I acknowledge that, what I was going through, was tough.

I posted a message on Facebook, pouring out my feelings and sent texts to those who were not on Facebook. I was drowning and needed support. In no time at all there were a lot of responses on Facebook. Alan's sister, Viv, kindly offered to travel down from Cumbria to be with me. The cold I had developed was bad, so I stayed at home in my pyjamas all day.

When Andy from the golf club was visiting Alan, he held up his phone so I could do a video call with Alan. My voice was almost non-existent, so it was difficult conversing. Simon Beacham called me saying, "Alan had a different look in his eye." I wasn't sure what Simon meant - I assumed Alan must have looked anxious. During a conversation with the care agency about CHC, the manager said various carers had asked after Alan's welfare.

Monday 7th January - Is 'symptom management' code for end of life?

At the hospital Alan said, "I don't know if I'm close to the end, but I cannot taste anything." I didn't know if that was a sign or not but he was being fed by PEG now so that might have something to do with it.

A nurse explained why Alan was going to a hospice. "Symptom management, respite and access to complementary therapy would all be available at Myton." I kept getting the feeling they knew something we didn't. I wondered if it was all code for end of life.

During a telephone chat with Vikki, who knew Alan through his work, I learned that after his diagnosis, Alan had told her, "I will be in good hands with Hazel as my carer." No pressure then!

Tuesday 8th January - Mum is being lost too
Jane, the bereavement counsellor at the Marie Curie Hospice asked, "Have you noticed any changes in Alan?" Initially saying no, I then thought to myself, is he more tired? His mood had certainly changed. I felt calmer when she offered, "Alan is probably happy just to be with you. There was much strength coming from the love you have for each other." My newfound state of mind enabled me to decide that while Alan was in the hospice, his life should be as wonderful as possible and we must enjoy whatever time he had left.

At Solihull Hospital, I met the complex needs discharge nurse. We discussed mum's care needs, and the fact that mum appeared to be in her own world most of the time. In her view, mum needed to be in a residential home. While texting my siblings to update them I felt unhappy. I had been so busy worrying about losing Alan that I hadn't realised I was 'losing' mum too.

At Shirley Golf Club over lunch, one lady asked, "Are you okay now?" Inside I thought to myself, I will never be okay again. I was disappointed to discover that Alan had not moved into the Myton Hospice because there was a delay in the cough assist machine training.

Alan's notes showed he had been through a lot of physio and suction during the day. He confessed, "I am envious of others in the ward because they can take a stroll around the hospital and grounds, but I cannot." I hoped his forthcoming surprise visitors would lift his spirits. Alan struggled to swallow the dinner I fed him. We didn't discuss it. Enjoying food was one of Alan's last remaining pleasures. He told me a nurse and physio from Myton had visited him and started him on the drug glycopyrronium (glyco).

Viv and Tom's surprise arrival at the hospital definitely cheered up Alan. Later, at the house, Tom asked several questions about MND. I called up the MND Association website on my computer to aid his understanding.

Wednesday 9th January - Preparing to move to Myton
In a distressing phone call with mum's social worker, I learned that mum was

refusing to go into a residential care home, so the hospital was looking for what they called a 'step down bed'. In other words, they were preparing for her to go back to living at home. It was hard for me not to blow my top!

Martin, from our golf club, called. "After sitting in a long queue at the hospital car park, I spent two hours with Alan. All was well." The queues were still bad later. Alan was having physio and using the cough assist machine when I arrived. Viv gave Alan his dinner and Tom and I helped Alan with his leg exercises. We might not be as attractive as some of the nurses, but it was nice for Alan to have family handling his care needs. Maybe, one day, I would surprise Alan by wearing a nurse's uniform!

The day shift nurses, including Sam, came to say goodbye to Alan.

Back at the house, Tom was curious about the world tour Alan had done before I met him. We looked through the two large albums Alan had created of the trip. It was nice seeing his beaming smile shining out from the old photographs.

We spent a few minutes chatting about the forthcoming Burns Night MND event and how selfless and strong Alan had been. After such an emotional day and too much prosecco, my normal ability to contain my emotions was non-existent, and the flood gates opened.

Thursday 10th January - "Am I going to die?"
Viv stayed with Alan at the hospital while Tom and I personalised Alan's room at the hospice. With fairy lights up above the bed, beers on the side table and photos of Alan and I on another table, the large room looked homely. When the ambulance eventually arrived, I wanted to hug Alan, but, frustratingly the team of nurses asked me to step away until they had made him comfortable in his bed.

Alone at last with Alan, he said, "I have been feeling tight in my chest, but Dr Ali said it was probably because I have been using the nose mask a lot, which puts extra strain on my muscles." I suspected Alan was scared it was something else.

Viv and Tom joined us and a few minutes later a huge team of nurses and physios gathered around Alan's bed so that Holly, the hospital physiotherapist, could train them on using the cough assist and suction machines. Viv and Tom left. Soon after, a female doctor, accompanied by two nurses, carefully asked questions about Alan's breathing, sleeping, toilet habits, eating, etc. She took time to learn about us as a couple before saying, "It's impressive how you two have dealt with your situation."

224

Looking up at the doctor, Alan asked, "Am I going to die?" My heart sank.

The doctor asked, "Do you want to die?"

Alan replied with an emphatic "No!"

"Your love for each other will see you through," the doctor assured him, "You will not die until you are ready to, or if you get a bad infection." She went on, "You can stop using the ventilator or the feeding tube if everything becomes too much and you want to go." She also said, "Everything is your call - you are the boss. The hospital can do no more for you now."

There it was, the brutal truth. If Alan wanted to stop living like this, he could. The doctor confirmed Alan could stay at the hospice while his symptoms were 'being managed,' and I could stay overnight in his room any time I wanted to.

Alan was not himself for the rest of the day. He kept worrying and saying, "I think I am at the end of the line." At one point he said, "It's not fair - out of sixty-seven million people I had to be one of the few who get MND." I chose not to remind him of the self-imposed 'no self-pity' rule. He had been through a lot and was tired. My composure was slipping so I kissed him and left him to rest.

When I returned to Alan, watching *Gavin and Stacey* on TV lifted our spirits. I fed Alan his supper becoming aware how nice his room was compared to the hospital ward. It felt like a place where he could get better, not die. The fairy lights were a great idea.

Friday 11th January - Comprehensive meeting with a doctor
Alan's mood was low. He'd had a bad night's sleep because the ventilator mask was not right, but he had not called anyone. It was a positive sign when he announced, "I have been thinking about ways of getting out of here so I can watch the Ashes in the summer."

One of the doctors visited with a couple of nurses. Before long it was agreed to reduce the dose of some of Alan's medicines, to take him off blood pressure tablets and bring in a huge soft blue seat, known as the Amelia Chair, for him to relax in.

Late morning, I had to leave to sort out mum's care funding paperwork and visit her in hospital. I made a video of the bizarre conversation I had with mum in the hope the social worker would see it as evidence mum was not capable of looking after herself. Mum accepted that she could not go back to her own home but didn't seem to understand why. Alan and I were watching more *Gavin and Stacey* when nurse Sam arrived unexpectedly.

Saturday 12th January - Alan's mindset improving

Teresa's husband, Phil called advising me that Teresa's dad had passed away. Teresa and I had often shared stories about watching our loved one's struggling to breathe. I knew she would be glad that he was now at peace but incredibly heartbroken that he was gone. Tom, from the golf club, reported that Alan had eaten a hearty lunch and they'd had a good laugh together.

Mum's hospital social worker called following an email I had sent airing my fears about mum's placement. It annoyed me how often she asked me, "How is Alan doing?" She was being nice to me but deep down I felt she was working against me over mum. I popped around to mum's flat. It had not been cleaned properly, but I had no strength for petty battles, so I took payment around to the cleaner.

After posting a sympathy card to Teresa, I set off for the hospice and was delighted to find that Alan was in a good mood. "I am determined to get better and come home," he declared. Hoorah! Alan insisted I still go on my forthcoming ski holiday. I insisted I would only go if we did a FaceTime video chat every day, and I would come home immediately if his condition worsened. We agreed and settled down for the final episode of *Gavin and Stacey*.

Sunday 13th January - Getting the balance right

During the morning, my brother Kevin and his wife Sue visited Alan, as did Simon Beacham and his daughter, Maddie. By the time I got to him, Alan looked well. He'd had a shower and had been accepting routine PEG feeds. He was yawning a lot which made me think I should start reducing the numbers of visitors he had.

We had a telephone call from Viv telling us Joan, Alan's mum, was very unwell. I tried to cheer Viv up by telling her how Alan's condition had improved. Deep down, I suspected Joan did not have long left.

AUTHOR'S NOTE

It was difficult getting the balance right in respect of the number of visitors Alan had. He needed, and enjoyed the company of others, but too much stimulus from the outside world made him tired.

Monday 14th January - Balloons, blue cheese and strawberries

After sorting a blown fuse on the tumble dryer, I surprised Alan by arriving with balloons, blue cheese (to go with the red wine already in his room), and fresh strawberries. Unfortunately, he'd had another bad night due to mask issues. Alan explained he had met with one of the pastoral team members and they had discussed Alan's beliefs. Alan told the pastor that he did not believe in God but thought each of us had a god within us. Interesting.

For the first time I stayed overnight on a camp bed in Alan's room. The ventilation machine was noisy, as was the constant whirr of the pressured air mattress, so getting to sleep was a challenge. However, I was able to assist Alan when he needed help, which meant he had a better night. As always, our day ended with Alan thanking me for looking after him and us telling each other, "I love you." Alan had survived another day, for which I was grateful.

Tuesday 15th January - Two poorly people almost home

En route to the opticians for a routine check-up, I received a call from mum's social worker. She confirmed my worst fear - mum was being moved to a place called Alexander House, where she would stay for six weeks while being prepared for her return to her own home. When I arrived at Alexander House I found mum looking lost, sitting alone in the lounge. I arranged for her to have a shower while I unpacked her suitcase.

There was a huge traffic jam on the A46 which delayed me getting to Alan's hospice. Smiling, Alan announced, "I have seen three doctors today and they are all happy with my progress." He cheerfully talked about returning to Carter Castle soon. Although I still felt stressed, for the first time in ages my mood lifted a little.

Wednesday 16th January - Uncertainty about mum's placement

My head was throbbing when I woke. When would I learn that drinking red wine, instead of eating a healthy dinner, was not a good idea! A work contact of Alan's called Abigail visited me, bringing a lovely ceramic angel.

At the monthly MND meeting at Marie Curie Hospice, a chaplain, sisters Carol and Sue, and our OT, Fiona, hosted a brainstorming session about what we did to help ourselves cope with our situations. I found it helpful.

Mum was sitting in her room holding Ben, the toy dog, when I arrived. I set up a CD player and organised a commode chair for her room. I didn't want her to pee or poo herself or to find herself lost in the corridor in the middle of the night because she could not find the bathroom.

Unusually, mum gave me a hug after I cut her fringe. Suddenly an Irish lady stopped outside mum's door. After a few minutes of chatting to each other, mum went off with the stranger. I don't think either of them knew where they were going. After I had sewed labels onto mum's clothes to reduce the risk of them going missing in the laundry, I went in search of mum and her Irish kidnapper. In the dining room, I found mum staring at a plate of half-eaten egg and chips, next to a man who was not talking to her. The Irish lady was sitting on her own at the next table. Odd.

It was awful having to leave mum in a place that I wasn't sure about. Staff appeared scarce and no one was talking with the residents or encouraging them to engage with each other. Fundamentally, I disagreed with the idea of mum being rehabilitated for home living, but I had to give this place, and mum, a chance.

Twenty-five miles later I found Alan watching TV. He noticed I was stressed. "Turn off the TV and tell me how life outside these four walls is?" I felt better after sharing some of my concerns with Alan. With Alan's input, I worked on his tax return spreadsheet and tidied up some of the photo folders on his laptop. Back home, I still felt stressed and still had a headache. Around 2am I sent out some texts. My golfing friend Dawn replied straight away. She was stressed too because both her parents were ill. I felt less alone, but sorry for Dawn.

Thursday 17th January - Preparing to leave Alan
The extra strength paracetamol I had taken in the night contained caffeine, so I only managed a few hours' sleep. Big mistake. While packing for my ski trip I swatted away unhelpful thoughts about being on the slopes without Alan before they gathered pace.

Mum's room was in a mess when I reached her. The chest of drawers was somehow toppled over. "I fell because the floor was wet," she muttered. I could smell urine and deduced she had missed the commode. There was an uneaten cooked meal on a tray and a cold cup of milky tea. Whoops, I had forgotten to tell the home mum only drank black tea. As I gave her a hug, she cried, saying, "Alan's dead." I reassured her that Alan was fine and took her to see a nurse for a check-up. This place did not feel right. I was not happy.

At the hospice, Alan talked about his visits from Simon Beacham and Carol and John. In preparation for my week away, I filled up Alan's social diary with visitors then trained the night nurse on how to adjust and change Alan's ventilator mask. I then gave her a list of important telephone numbers to call if necessary. Alan and I parted with smiles on our faces because there had been talk of him being discharged on 28th January!

Friday 18th January - Keeping bad news from Alan

Just as I was about to vent my concerns in an email to mum's social worker, Alexander House called. "Mum was found on the floor in her room and is on her way to Heartlands Hospital for assessment." My stress levels were high. I needed to 'put on my own oxygen mask' as my friend Teresa had recently told me. So, I called my brothers and sisters, and asked for their help with mum.

A new social worker rang me. "I will be handling things for your mum from now on." Would this one be more helpful than the last? The hospital A&E department confirmed mum's head scan was okay. After a hectic morning I eventually reached Alan late afternoon. It was a lovely surprise to see him, in his wheelchair, chatting with his old friend Dave from Leeds.

Later Alan told me, "When Dave first arrived neither of us could speak because we were crying so much." He cried when I showed him the album I had ordered showing our life over the last twelve months and said, "I cannot thank you enough for the things you have done for me."

"Have a good time with the gang," he whispered while we were hugging.

Looking him in the eye and holding his face, my parting comment was, "I want you to stay well now the hospital has mended your body and the hospice has mended your mind." I cried all the way back to my car. It was going to be hard not seeing him for a week.

There was a message from Viv on my phone. Pauline answered when I called back. "Mam is close to death." I had been dreading this happening at this time. We agreed not to tell Alan.

AUTHOR'S NOTE

When you are the primary carer for a loved one, you tend to think you have to do everything for them. You feel guilty if you put yourself first, but you must, or you risk carer burnout.

During Alan's illness, I discovered it was okay to have a break and let family members and friends keep an eye on him. Most people were willing to help and were very capable. It was however difficult to enjoy 'me time' even when Alan insisted I carry on with my life.

Saturday 19th January - Time to reflect

There were a lot of noisy teenage girls in the queue for check-in at 9am at Birmingham Airport. One of them told me they were off to the Bellevue Hotel in Obergurgl. How spooky, that was where I had celebrated my 60th birthday with Alan and *The Ski Gang* just two years earlier.

Before boarding I texted everyone saying they must contact me if Alan's or mum's condition suddenly deteriorated. To ease the guilt I felt, I reminded myself that Alan had insisted I go on this trip and I needed to recharge as matters could get worse in the months to come.

Alexander House called to inform me that mum had returned from hospital at 7pm the previous evening. I arranged for them to make her a special afternoon tea as it was her birthday.

Normally on take-off, Alan would take my hand and smile brightly at me until we were safely in the air. Alone on this flight, I gazed out of the window and tears rolled down my cheeks. Alan was now severely paralysed. His travelling days were over and he would never be able to initiate holding my hand again. In the flight magazine, there was an article about Corpus, a company that used artificial intelligence to create a replica of a deceased person. If it were not for the fact they probably charged a fortune, I would have called them and asked them to make me an 'Alan' to have in my life forever.

It took four train trips, expertly and efficiently woven together by the tour company, to get from Geneva to Wengen. As soon as I arrived at the Silberhorn Hotel, I did a FaceTime video call with Alan. After dinner with *The Ski Gang*, I walked around the lively town. It was Men's Downhill competition day. There were après ski parties everywhere and medal ceremonies for the winners. Alan would have loved it.

AUTHOR'S NOTE
To give myself peace of mind I had booked a succession of visitors for Alan and arranged to check in on him, via them, whenever I could.

Sunday 20th January - Feeling for Stephanie
I managed to ski several runs including a difficult black and various easy blues. At one point I ended up flat on my back when exiting a chairlift. Luckily Robert was there to haul me up. The mountain air was crisp, the white snow dazzled in the sunshine and the cloudless sky was deep blue. The mighty Eiger towered above us in all its glory. It was a perfect day for skiing but, it felt weird being in the mountains, when Alan was hundreds of miles away, lying in a hospice bed.

On a train back to our resort, John spoke of his frustration that Alan, who had always looked after himself and who did not smoke or drink excessively, could no longer ski and would soon be lost to us all. During a FaceTime video with

Alan, via our friends Teresa and Phil, he told me he had not slept well because of difficulty swallowing. My initial instinct was to head to the airport.

I had a text from my friend Stephanie in Doncaster saying that her husband, James (Alan's 'MND twin') had fallen down the stairs, cracked his head badly and was in intensive care. I could only imagine how she must be feeling. I had dreaded the idea of Alan having a major fall, back in the days when his legs were weak.

Monday 21st January - Top of Europe and sad news
Before breakfast I called Teresa for reassurance about Alan's swallowing problems.

After breakfast I confided in Julie and Sarah. "I feel in limbo because I cannot plan anything." We talked about how things would be different after Alan passed away. "I don't want that day to come," was my response. Instead of skiing, I joined Sarah and Julie on the train trip to the Top of Europe. We travelled up through the tunnels in the Eiger and eventually emerged at the station 11,337 feet (3464 metres) above sea level.

The three of us did a tour of the ice caves before moving out onto the viewing platform. As we surveyed the mountains I explained that I had seen a Brocken Spectre once. At that exact moment, a Brocken Spectre appeared in the clouds! We were astounded and stood in silence until its short life ended. We bought Lindt chocolates in the highest chocolate shop in Europe. It would have been rude not to!

Stephanie texted, "James has got some hypoxic brain issues and there is nothing anyone can do." Oh no! Apres-ski back in Wengen went on without me as I walked around the village in contemplation.

AUTHOR'S NOTE
Named after the German mountain upon which it was first seen, a Brocken Spectre is an optical illusion that appears when a low sun is behind a climber who is looking downwards at clouds. The sun creates a shadow of the climber in the clouds and is often surrounded by a circular rainbow, called a glory.

Sometimes only lasting a few seconds, it is also called an anti-corona.

Tuesday 22nd January - Writing in the snow
We stopped for warm drinks outside a mountain hut after skiing runs of varying difficulty. I used my ski pole to inscribe 'Hazel and Alan' in the snow. I did a FaceTime call with Alan. He was saddened by Stephanie's news.

Wednesday 23rd January - Dying well with dignity

The only ski run down from a high mountain top restaurant in Grindelwald, was via a black run. I took a deep breath, begged Robert to stay close behind me and tipped myself over the precipice. Lucky for me the run was number fourteen. Alan would have been proud of me. I managed to ski to the bottom without killing myself!

On a FaceTime video, via the phone of our brother-in-law John, Alan told me he'd had another bad night. My question, "Shall I come home?" was met with an emphatic, "No." After a quick post dinner drink with the gang, I watched a film called *We Need to Talk About Dying*. It pointed out that we are all slowly dying, and people need to think about dying from life, not dying from a disease. It said, hospices are places to live and hospitals are for reversible conditions. It urged people to think of a hospice as a place to complete a life.

The film helped me realise my job was to help Alan be content that he had lived a good life and to help him die well, with dignity.

Thursday 24th January - Weird premonition

During the night, I dreamt Alan was in a casket of water which was being violently shaken and he was drowning. Horrible!

Without John, our trusted 'sweeper' bringing up the rear, I felt uneasy as the mist covered the upper slopes. I decided Alan needed me to come home in one piece and I should not risk falling due to poor visibility. So, I left the gang and took the train down to Wengen.

Alan started to choke during a FaceTime video via our brother-in-law, Simon. It was scary not being there to help. When settled he explained, "They couldn't get my night mask right. I swore at the nurses. I was so agitated. In the end they left me on my day mask and gave me Lorazepam." I thought of the dream I'd had and wondered if I was psychic?

A leg massage before dinner was a welcome treat. Some of us played cards, listening to old albums the barman played on a real turntable. Again, I thought how much Alan would have loved being with us.

Friday 25th January - A life concludes

In the morning I skied with Bev and John. At one point, I gingerly skied part of the black run used for the men's downhill race.

A text arrived from Alan's sisters. Joan had died in the night. When I spoke with Alan via FaceTime video, his two brothers-in-law and my friend, Joanne, were with him. Joan was ninety-seven and had been a terrific mother-in-law to me. It was sad that she had passed on, but it was even more sad that Alan didn't get the chance to spend time with her during her last few months. I couldn't imagine how dreadful he would be feeling. I was returning home in the morning and couldn't wait to hug him. It was noisy in the spa, so I abandoned it and started packing my case.

Saturday 26th January - From the Swiss Alps to Burns Night via the hospice

After a quick breakfast I boarded the 7.33am train out of Wengen. I received a text from my sister-in-law Sue, saying that her uncle had been found dead on the floor by her son. I'm not superstitious, but I worried that a third death might happen. During the train journey to the airport, I texted several friends and eventually found people to take the tickets of the three people who had dropped out of the MND fundraising Burns night.

A huge bunch of flowers, arranged for me by Alan, greeted me when I arrived home around 4pm. Unfortunately, I couldn't spend long with him at the hospice before I had to drive to the Burns Night fundraiser. I sat at a long table with Alan's family, except Viv and Pauline, who had stayed in Sunderland organising Joan's funeral. Before the haggis was piped in and the Scottish country dancing began, I was given the microphone and made an appeal for people to buy raffle tickets.

Sunday 27th January - Best birthday 'gift'

Mum was sitting alone when I arrived about 11am. She complained of having a sore hip. I had a chat with the nurses, helped mum change into some fresh clothes and encouraged her to eat lunch. She had no idea it was her eldest daughter's birthday.

I whizzed over to the hospice, where I was greeted by Alan's niece Helen, her husband Richard and their two boys and Matt and Suzanne, surrounding Alan in his chair. They all sang happy birthday to me and gave me cards and a chocolate cake. It was lovely. Even more lovely was how well Alan looked. I stayed the night with Alan in his room.

Monday 28th January - Difficult choices ahead

Alan had a bad night because of difficulties with his ventilation mask. The hospice chaplain visited. Alan had another interesting conversation about God.

One of the doctors arrived and started some tough conversations. "If you get ill again you could go to a nursing home instead of a hospital," meaning not fighting the infection but allowing death to be managed. He went on, "If you want to come off the ventilator, or when you reach end of life, you could come back to the hospice." The smile on Alan's face vanished, so I suggested we go for a spin in his chair. I arranged a haircut for Alan as I hoped a bit of pampering might help lift his spirits.

Tuesday 29th January - Thinking about Alan's return home
I talked to Jane at the Marie Curie Hospice about Alan and my fears of how I would cope when Alan came home. Most of my friends were telling me, "Look after yourself" which made me worry they could see my reserves were low. Jane asked, "Who is finding it hard to see Alan now?" Alan had spoken with me about people he was disappointed had not seen him in a long time. Jane's question made me realise they probably found it too difficult.

Wednesday 30th January - Forgetfulness
As I pottered about during the day, my friend Teresa called me to check where I was. I'd completely forgotten I was supposed to meet her for coffee!

Thursday 31st January - Planning for Alan's return home
At the hospice, Alan and I met the doctors and a discharge nurse to work out what support we would need once Alan was home.

I noted that:

- Carers would need training on how to feed Alan via the PEG tube
- Alan would need more help with physio and personal care
- Alan's excessive saliva production was now under control but his nose regularly became blocked so would need frequent cleaning
- I would need training on how to use the suction machine
- District nurses would need to be called in when additional injections were necessary
- Careful monitoring of choking would be needed

I was grateful that Julie from Macmillan would still be our palliative care nurse. However, because we lived between two health trust areas, there would be changes to our ventilation specialists. Coventry Hospital and Myton Hospice would be responsible for Alan in future, instead of Stoke and the Marie Curie Hospice.

It was suggested that the care agency provide night sitters because Alan usually needed help with his mask during the night. The drug Midazolam, which is like Lorazepam, could be given if Alan became distressed. I wondered if gin and tonic could also be on prescription for me to take if I became stressed!

The biggest conversation was about what venue Alan wanted to be in at the end of his life. Once decisions were made, including Alan requesting to die at home (rather than a hospice as previously noted), the doctor said she would update the *Respect* form and the Advanced Care Plan.

Our next meeting was with Sue from the ACT team. She came with the long-awaited stand for the Eyegaze device.

Before Simon Beacham went in to visit Alan, I updated him on the day's meetings. He understood that Alan dying at home would be tough on me.

Over dinner with my friend Nina, we agreed that living in a warden-controlled retirement home was a good idea for us single ladies when we could no longer care for ourselves properly. We also agreed we needed to move into one before we lost the mental capacity to make new friendships or make such a decision for ourselves!

February 2019

Friday 1st February - Courage to tackle Coventry Cathedral

The care agency called to say that they would be resuming their service on Monday 4th February, and I had a telephone conversation with Julie, the Macmillan nurse, about support for Alan. Alan was having his exercises when I arrived at Myton. In the communal lounge I chatted with the hospice fundraiser. In a moment of madness, I signed up to abseil down the face of Coventry Cathedral!

Two ladies from the Access to Technology team were in Alan's room when I returned. It took ages to set up the Eyegaze tracking system. Achieving the right alignment was hard because Alan was propped up in his bed, rather than sitting upright in a chair.

"I recorded my biography this morning, but you are not to listen to it yet," Alan announced. He didn't want to discuss the End-of-Life Care Plan which we had to complete. When Steve and Jill from Surrey arrived, I brought them up to date on all the latest news about Alan, then left the three of them to chat.

On my return, Alan asked me to do a cough assist machine procedure because he had not had one for several hours. After we had cleared his lungs, I fed him his dinner then Jill, Steve and I left him watching a Six Nations match. Back at the house, Jill cooked a home-made fish pie and we opened a bottle of prosecco in celebration of my recent birthday.

Saturday 2nd February - Sense of relief

It was a frosty, sunny morning - perfect for the special treat planned for Alan. Jill and Steve helped me get Alan in his chair into the adapted vehicle. I drove us to Coombe Abbey and another hall in the Coventry area, both of which had been potential venues for our wedding. Alan had not been outside a medical environment since just after Christmas.

Andy and Kulvinder, from the golf club, were at the hospice when we got back. I had forgotten they were coming. Whoops. Alan choked badly on some soup after his visitors left. I worried that his poor swallowing would mean he would have to be fed only by PEG tube from now on. Reflecting on a happy day spent with friends, a sense of relief washed over me. It felt like we were past the worst. Things were looking hopeful again.

Sunday 3rd February - Plans for Carter Castle and Alan's Care Plan

Jill and Steve headed off home and I visited mum. One of the nurses told me mum's cough appeared better. I worried that she was still not eating. At Carter

Castle, my mind drifted to thoughts about what I would change in the house when I lived there alone. No matter what I did, the house would only ever be a house without Alan. It would not feel like home.

It was nice to see Alan was sitting in his chair when I reached him. He was watching an old David Niven movie, which was ironic, because David died from MND. Following Alan's instructions, we tackled the job of completing his End of Life Care Plan document.

"Why have you decided to spend your final days at home?" I asked.

"Because I want to spend as much time with you as possible," he replied. He confirmed he wanted to have his two sisters, me and Simon Beacham around him in his final hours, if it could be arranged. To relieve ourselves of the emotional form filling, we watched episodes of *The Crown* and *Ski Sunday*.

Monday 4th February - Have I 'completed' my life?
Watching a film to 3am left me tired. The morning was spent drinking in the peace and quiet of Carter Castle. Soon Alan would be home and the hubbub of his machinery and carers coming and going would fire up. A lady came to collect one of the devices that had accidentally been left at mum's flat. We had a long, tearful chat because her mother-in-law had MND and a young friend of hers also had the disease. She believed poor sleep was a factor. I hoped not or I was in trouble!

Around noon I reached Alan. He was being fed his lunch and choked a few times. How much longer would he tolerate taking food orally? In a call with the care company manager, I confirmed Alan would be coming home today and learned that CHC had told her not to visit the hospice to assess Alan's needs. Was this a financially driven instruction, I wondered?

Shortly into the journey home Alan said, "The next time I go to hospice, I will not be coming home." In his sadness he had forgotten that his End of Life plan noted he was to die at home.

Once at Carter Castle we watched lots of *Frasier* episodes, until the carers arrived and moved Alan to his bed. "I would like a beer," Alan said. I gave him his first one in eight weeks but was not sure he really enjoyed it.

We listened to the biography Alan had recorded in the hospice. It was pretty matter of fact at the beginning, but towards the end, I could tell Alan was fighting back tears. It was highly emotional listening to his thoughts for my life after he had died, and what he thought of me and his family. We cried together, a lot.

"I feel I have had a good life, Alan. Life without you will never be as good," I declared. He tried to reassure me, but I continued, "I don't want to live into my old age without you. I don't think I could allow myself to be in such a deep relationship again. I would be frightened to love and lose another person. It's all too painful." Alan and I agreed it was best for us to live one day at a time. The care agency called advising a night sitter, Laura, would be arriving at 10pm.

AUTHOR'S NOTE
The idea of having a night sitter in the house was difficult to comprehend, but it was necessary to allow me to get better sleep. Trusting a stranger to care to my standard was hard. Also, I feared I would want to oversee the sitter, which defeated the objective! I had to let go. Good quality sleep was essential when you care for someone's every need around the clock.

Tuesday 5th February - A good friend's promise
Via the listening device, at 5am I could hear Laura repeatedly saying, "What do you need Alan?" As I entered his bedroom Laura reported, "Alan has woken up six times in the night with mask issues." She was an impressive carer. I made my positive feelings about her known to the agency as soon as I could so she could be allocated to us more often (hopefully).

Our new key carer, Scott arrived with Rhea around 7am. Scott had been selected by the agency because his father had died from MND eleven years ago. I wondered if he would find working with Alan too painful, or, if his experience would make him more compassionate. Time would tell.

The usual, long, complex morning routine took place. I then gave Alan his medicines and fed him a protein shake drink via his PEG. I was not yet ready to hand over these last two tasks. Rhea did a respite sit between the morning and lunch time carers.

At the funeral for her father, Teresa hugged me as she exited the church saying, "Thank you for coming. I will be there for you."

Tearfully I replied, "I know."

Mum's mental health nurse said, "We need to find mum somewhere better." Eureka - at last, someone on our side!

Mum was distressed after the meeting, saying, "Mick (my dad) is dying." I hugged her and resisted telling her dad died in 2001. It was a day for hugging.

The district nurse handed me a large plastic box back at the house, with the words JUST IN CASE screaming out from its lid. I quickly hid it away. Alan didn't need to know about it. After he had eaten just a few mouthfuls of the omelette Alan mournfully announced, "I am having trouble swallowing and when I feel cold my jaw aches." I made a note to discuss this new symptom at the next MND support meeting. A male carer turned up to do the overnight shift.

Wednesday 6th February - Stressed - who me?

In Alan's room, I was shocked to find the overnight carer was gone. Alan said, "I saw the carer asleep on the floor when I woke up in the night." I was furious. We agreed I had to inform the agency. Unlike Laura, who brought bottles of Coke and puzzles to help keep herself awake, the male carer clearly did not come with the right attitude or intention. My anger was heightened due to my own guilt at, selfishly, turning off the listening device so I could get a decent rest.

After another choking session during breakfast, Alan allowed me to call the speech and language therapist for advice. During the morning, Alan's jaw became painfully cramped. I gave him the lowest dose of oral morphine permissible and called the district nurse. She arrived within fifteen minutes and said it would be okay to give the maximum dose of morphine every hour. It was all very scary. Alan was distressed and anxious.

The headache I had woken up with, became more intense. It was tempting to try the morphine myself but, instead, I took some extra strength painkillers. I collected Alan's sister Viv from the local train station and updated her on Alan's latest symptoms.

A registrar, who worked with the neurologist Dr Thomas, told me the twitches I had been experiencing were due to benign cramp fasciculation syndrome. "Have you been under any stress lately?" he asked gently. I nearly lost it.

In my head I shouted, *"You want to know about my stress! My husband is dying, my mum is losing her mind, my mother-in-law has just died, I have no income coming in, I am dashing about like a mad person and not getting enough sleep!!!"* I chose not to bite his head off and just said, "A bit."

Alan was much improved when I arrived home. "He's eaten a hearty bowl of my homemade soup," Viv said as we gave Alan his medicines and the Fortisip protein drink via his PEG. While Alan was with his evening carers, Viv and I tried to work out how Alan could attend his mum's funeral in Sunderland. Travelling such a long distance was sure to be painful for him. It was a dilemma. Alan

239

would want to be in attendance, as would I. Until now, we had always found ways to overcome MND's challenges, but things were different now. Our best idea was him staying at a hospice in Sunderland the evening before the funeral, but could we get a room?

Josh, and a new carer called Christie, got Alan ready for bed. I was relieved when it was Laura who arrived for the overnight shift.

Thursday 7th February - Muffled 'final' words
Rhea and Scott arrived at 7am. We had a giggle when I did an old joke on Scott.

"Knock, knock"

"Who's there?"

"Scott."

"Scott who?"

"Scott nothing to do with you."

Boom. Boom!

There were more giggles when we discussed the funny lines in the *Gavin and Stacey* show. It was nice having a bit of fun for a change.

After his shower, Alan started to shiver and his jaw began aching. "My tummy feels upset too," he announced. He chose to go into the lounge and have his wheelchair tilted right back, rather than be put back into bed. Within minutes he was asleep. Three hours later he woke.

Pauline arrived and Alan ate more of the home-made soup. He appeared indecisive and lethargic. He was uncomfortable in his wheelchair, so the next batch of carers used the hoist to lift him off the wheelchair seat and put him back in a different position. When Simon Beacham arrived, Alan listened excitedly as Simon shared his plans for an MND fundraising trip in November to Everest base camp. Alan had always wanted to do such a trip with Simon. I was sorry he now had to be a passive observer instead.

After dinner, carers got Alan ready for bed. He needed the cough assist machine, but the stubborn phlegm would not come up and worryingly, I could hear Alan's chest rattling. He became distressed. The oral morphine I administered did not help so at about 11pm I called the district nurses. "They are about an hour away," I was told.

Pauline, Viv and I tried to calm Alan down and gave him more morphine an hour after the first dose. The district nurse turned up after midnight and administered Midazolam.

Alan continued to be unsettled so I called the district nurse team again. They arrived at 2am. They delved into the stashed away Just in Case emergency drug box and administered Diamorphine and Midazolam.

Alan looked hard into my eyes and said, "If I don't wake up, I love you."

He tried hard to say something else which I could not understand. Frustratingly, the combination of the mask he was wearing and the strong drugs, muffled his final words. I felt sure he was saying something profound that he had rehearsed, just in case, but it was no use. I would never know. Everyone, including Laura, our night sitter, was weeping.

For ages I held Alan and rocked him gently, as if he was a delicate baby. We all stroked his hands. I whispered into his ear, "You have been the best thing in my life. I love you so much. Rest now." His head moved a little and I felt him fighting to stay awake, but the drugs were kicking in. He finally sank into a deep sleep.

Laura set herself to watch over Alan like a guardian angel so that Alan's sisters and I could get some rest. She had strict instructions to wake me if Alan woke.

Friday 8th February - Lazarus returns

Laura called me at 3:15am and again at 4am. Each time Alan went back to sleep quickly once I was with him. At 5am, she called me again. He was more distressed. I gave him oral morphine after talking to the district nurse. "Do you want anything else, Al?" I whispered. He said he was too warm, so I took off the duvet.

"Stay by my side till I fall asleep" he asked. My heart sank as I hugged him. Was this it? Was this the end?

My alarm sounded at 6:30am. I discovered Viv had taken over the vigil when Laura's shift ended. Laura had cancelled the morning carers because it was obvious Alan would not be getting up. I relieved Viv and sat holding Alan's hand, listening to the gentle rhythm of Alan's ventilator in the half light. He looked calm. I felt a mess.

Alan suddenly woke and quickly said, "I feel like Lazarus who returned from the dead!" His brightness was a massive relief to us all. Julie, the nurse from

Macmillan, talked us through drug options and suggested we put Alan on a pending list for a bed at the Marie Curie Hospice. It seemed the time had come.

The GP arrived and discussed options with Alan and me:

Alan could go to hospital for intensive treatment.

Or we could manage symptoms at home, with support from the Marie Curie Hospice

Lastly, Alan could give up. In other words, come off the ventilator. This would have to be managed at a hospital as there could be complications.

I guessed right. Alan chose the Marie Curie Hospice option.

Saturday 9th February - The Elephant in the room

I posted on Facebook:

"Here is a picture of some of the 12-15 medicines Al has to take now he is out of the hospice. All these are administered via the feeding tube he thankfully had fitted in July (because swallowing has become a little bit difficult).

It was great to have him home on Monday, but we had a real fright on Thursday night. After getting Alan into bed his breathing suddenly went haywire and we had to call out medical professionals to give him seriously strong drugs to relieve symptoms and anxiety. It took till after 2 in the morning to calm him down and get him to sleep. I think we all thought is this it, including Alan.

The next morning, he confirmed he had thought he was going to die, and that he now felt like Lazarus. I can safely say I have never been through anything like it in my life. It was really scary, surreal at times and terribly emotional. After the Macmillan nurse, district nurse and GP had visited Alan the following morning, he slept for eight hours. When he woke around 6pm, he had some soup, found out from us what had happened the night before (he couldn't remember any of it) and then got another seven hour's sleep.

I am beginning to think in a former life Alan must have been a cat. Since he has had MND he has had a number of "life threatening" scares. First there was the time I found him flat on his back in the lounge having fallen backwards and cut his head open on the corner of the solid wood coffee table. Then there was the time his ventilator battery packs ran out when we were at the movies. Then there was the emergency admission to hospital on 19th December and again on Boxing Day night. Now this! So whatever else we call him, I think Alan qualifies for the title of Miracle Man.

I do hope his luck holds out because, as I have said before, I need him to stay around for a tad longer.

Massive thanks to our night-time sitter who calmly held me and Alan's sisters together on Thursday night and bless the out of hours district nurses for being there and finally, the drug companies (we always forget to thank) for developing the magic solutions in little bottles the nurses injected. Hopefully next week will be a whole lot less eventful!"

Alan woke saying he was feeling much better in himself. The phone rang. Mum had been taken to hospital with a suspected fractured wrist after a fall at Alexander House. Perhaps now the authorities would realise she most certainly should not live on her own.

Julie, our Macmillan nurse, called. Now that Alan appeared out of danger, I asked if she could check if a hospice in Sunderland might accommodate Alan for a night or two at the time of his mum's funeral. We liked Julie a lot. She was professional, reliable, warm hearted and always managed to say what needed to be said, clearly and with compassion.

Viv, Pauline, Alan, and I looked at music options for Joan's funeral. No one raised 'the elephant in the room', whether or not Alan would attend the service. I hoped Alan would choose not to go. I did not want to be the bad person who refused to take him.

Sunday 10th February - Anxiety and fear levels rising

Not long after Pauline left, Viv's husband, John, arrived. We all watched a DVD of the Australian Pink Floyd concert, but I found it difficult to concentrate. My anxiety and fear levels were increasing. Both the GP and Julie had talked about Alan going into a hospice. They had indicated Alan had months, maybe weeks, left to live!

I was confused. Weeks could mean as few as four. Months could mean as many as twelve. How close were we? Why couldn't there be more clarity? Was I missing something obvious? Alan looked well to me, but I was in strange territory. His secretions appeared to be under control. Maybe his recent breathing and swallowing issues were indicators his end of life was imminent? Was there worse to come? Would we be able to successfully manage his anxiety levels?

Deep down in my heart I believed Alan had more than four weeks left in him. I prayed he would make it to his sixty fifth birthday on 21st June.

Monday 11th February – No room at the inn

Viv and John looked after Alan while I visited mum. She was being given arm exercises in the lounge and recognised me straight away.

Julie called about hospice beds in Sunderland. When our friends Jo and Andy arrived, I told Alan, "Sorry Al, there were no beds available on the dates we need them." I hoped the cheerful natures and philosophical thinking of these friends might help soften the blow.

Friday 12th February - A splash of red

In Doncaster, the crematorium was full of about 200 people. Stephanie was only in her thirties and had been left with three children when James (Alan's MND twin) had died in tragic circumstances. James was a keen Manchester United fan, so Stephanie wore a red dress and we were all invited to wear a splash of red too. A lovely idea.

At the end of the service the curtains remained open. We were all allowed to file past the coffin, paying our respects to James in our own private way. Another lovely idea. Instead of going to the wake, where I would have felt odd, I indulged in a KFC meal followed by a Gregg's cake on my way home. My eating was out of control again.

Wednesday 13th February - I wanted to scream at the carers

Not long after my alarm went off I heard a panic taking place in Alan's bedroom via the listening device. Downstairs, I discovered that one of the carers had got into a muddle regarding Alan's mask. I stifled the instinct to scream at them but barked, "DON'T YOU REALISE WITHOUT THE MASK ON, ALAN WILL DIE!"

When all was calm later, Alan declared, "I am fed up with being in the lounge." So, I put him in the adapted van, with some old items from the garage. I drove us to the local municipal tip to dispose of the rubbish (not Alan!). It was not the most romantic of outings but the furthest we had ventured for a long time. We agreed that if he was well on Valentine's Day, we would go to Broadway - the location of our blind date on 14th June 2006.

The GP and I had a conversation about the lockjaw issues and problems with Alan's bowel movements. He asked me to make sure the carers kept Alan warm after showering him and allowed me to increase the dose of laxatives. We had just started watching one of our favourite films, Dirty Dancing, when the carers arrived. They took longer than usual to do their job. Standards appeared to be slipping.

As always, once Alan was tucked up in bed, I flushed his PEG tube with water before administering his drugs, and ensured the tube was properly capped off before we said our goodnights.

Thursday 14th February - Our last Valentine's Day?
In a dream, Alan and I were in Broadway where we had our blind date. He asked me to get him up out of his chair and remove his ventilator mask. He asked me to give him a high dose of Lorazepam or morphine so he could die calmly in our favourite place. I woke full of anxiety. My instincts told me this would be an emotional day.

While the carers got Alan out of bed, showered and dressed, I secretly decorated the lounge with fairy lights. When the carers opened a Valentine's card I had left for Alan on his wheelchair I heard them chuckle at my reference to *How do you like your eggs in the morning?*

I cooked Alan an egg in a heart shaped pan, but after just two mouthfuls it became too much for him to swallow. Once lunch was prepared, I took Alan into the lounge for another surprise. I opened a second card I had bought for him. There were tears and hugs. I was sure he, like me, was thinking this would be our last Valentine's Day together.

During lunch, Alan had another swallowing episode. Annoyingly our speech and language therapy specialist had cancelled her visit due today. We didn't go to Broadway. Alan was not well enough. Instead, he sat in the sunshine in his wheelchair outside the front door, while I worked on the lawn. Various neighbours popped over for a chat.

By mid-afternoon Alan was experiencing difficulties with secretions. I added a further Hyoscine patch to the side of his neck to help dry up the excess production. A district nurse gave Alan a dose of glyco. Later, I called the district nurse again and another dose of glyco was administered.

After all the drugs Alan didn't feel like eating dinner so we settled down to watch the DVD of *A Star is Born,* my Valentine's gift to Alan. Carers came at 9.15pm, so the film was abandoned. We were a bit nervous when a new night sitter arrived. She was mature and had a background in nursing so we would see how she performed before allowing ourselves to worry.

Friday 15th February - Balancing drug doses
It was a busy morning, starting with a long telephone chat with a lady in her fifties called Tracey who had been referred to me by a mutual friend. Tracey's husband had died from MND a few years ago. Our friend Adrian arrived, then

his wife Alison an hour or so later. Alan's cousin Kathleen, and her husband Michael arrived, followed later by my sister Clare and David. I somehow managed to juggle everyone, including the carers.

Alan had another choke after lunch. The frequency of choking was worrying. To reduce the dryness Alan felt in his mouth, I was told to decrease the Hyoscine patch on his neck by one quarter per day. I felt I was morphing into a nurse. During the evening a district nurse gave Alan a higher dose of glyco. I hoped it would do the trick.

To wind down from the busy day we watched the remainder of the previous night's movie together. Alan was still not right by bedtime, but I managed to get him calm enough to sleep. I could not sleep.

Saturday 16th February - An emotional conversation
The carers called me while I was getting dressed. "We think there is something wrong with Alan's ventilator. He is complaining of not being able to breathe." When I could not find any faults, Alan agreed some extra oral morphine would relax him. He also agreed not to have a shave or hair wash, so he could remain on the ventilator throughout his morning ablutions.

When we were alone an extremely emotional conversation began with me saying, "I wish I could take all this away from you, Al." We discussed the tricky art of giving enough drugs to dry his excess secretions, without overdrying his mouth. We also discussed the idea of him coming off the ventilator, to end his life on his terms.

I called the Macmillan nurse about fluid retention in Alan's arms. She thought it might be oedema, which could be contributing to the build-up of secretions in Alan's lungs. "I will arrange for Alan's kidney function to be checked," she said, "He may need diuretic drugs."

A district nurse put an iodine dressing on Alan's sore toe. Alan successfully ate a poached egg for breakfast and soup for lunch. At dinner, after just a few mouthfuls of beans, he choked.

Douglas and Pam from the golf club visited. Douglas was doing a charity bike ride in Scotland in April, hoping to raise £5,000 for MND Association. Alan suggested he start practising going up hills soon. We knew the roads around Loch Ness were not flat!

AUTHOR'S NOTE
I deliberately started the difficult conversation about coming off the ventilator

as a measuring stick for Alan's emotional state. I dreaded him choosing such an option, but it was worthwhile bringing it up every so often. Knowing he wanted to carry on living gave me strength to carry on. If he had wanted to die, I would have complied with his wishes.

Sunday 17th February - I'm not a nurse, I'm a carer!
It was clear the two carers doing the morning shift were nervous types, so I supervised. When asked to manage the ventilator, one protested, "I'm not a nurse, I'm a carer!"

I quickly responded, "Nor am I, but I've had to learn how to look after Alan, and all of his equipment and you need to too."

The other carer told me he had nursed his parents and wife to end of life, and he had no kids (like me). His story broke the walls of the dam I had created, sending tears down my cheeks.

Nina and Robert arrived late morning but didn't stay long because I had forgotten they were due!

We were relaxing, watching TV, when Alan remarked, "I think I have only got weeks left." My heart squeezed tight in my chest. "I am worried about the grumblings in my chest, and I am losing my one last remaining pleasure." (He was talking about the loss of eating solid food). A lump in my throat prevented me from replying. So I held him. Then both our dams burst.

Via the magic of modern communications systems (aka FaceTime video calling), sisters Pauline, and Viv and niece Helen, came to Alan's rescue with cheerful chit chat! Late afternoon Alan needed extra glyco to dry up secretions, and another dose early evening. By bedtime he was still anxious so a further injection was administered, his biggest dose of glyco to date. A new night sitter arrived just after 10pm. A bubbly, inquisitive girl.

Monday 18th February - Alternative plan for Joan's funeral
In a briefing to the morning carers, it was agreed, in view of the heavy doses of drugs Alan had been given, I would encourage Alan to have a day in bed. Alan was given a bed bath and was set lying on his side, to relieve pressure on his bottom, which was becoming sore. It took several pillows and rolled up towels to secure him into position. Alan slept beyond lunchtime.

Eric, the district nurse, was confident Alan had some oedema. Stepping out of the front door he said to me, "You can call me anytime," emphasising the word anytime! We liked Eric. A GP and Julie from Macmillan agreed Alan's blood pressure tablets should be stopped and, subject to results of a blood test, anti-depression drugs and diuretic tablets should be started.

After a little gentle persuasion, Alan accepted my idea for celebrating Joan's life here at home on funeral day. Only one carer arrived at teatime, so I helped turn Alan in his bed. He'd had no food all day but I didn't encourage him to eat.

At bedtime, Alan cracked a joke making Laura, our favourite night sitter, and I laugh. The Lorazepam and oral morphine had kicked in. Was he relieved that we no longer planned to make the difficult journey to Sunderland? In some quiet time together, before I retired to bed, I soaked up Alan's happier mood. Holding his hand felt like receiving an injection of warmth which went coursing through me. The familiar tickle in my tummy reminded me of the early days of our courtship. I loved that he was happier and hoped, privately, it was not the sort of euphoria some people get just before they die.

Tuesday 19th February - Shocking leaflets
When I woke, I lay for a while listening to Alan's breathing via the monitor. He was still alive. For the first time in ages a poem popped into my head.

MY HEART BREAKS

As you lie in your bed,
Pillows propping up your head,
I feel for you and my heart breaks.

As your body fades away,
With each passing day,
I feel for you and my heart breaks.

Your eyes still sparkle bright,
You're not giving up the fight,
But there is a limit to your life,
You could pass away any night.

I don't want you to go,
But in my heart I know,
Time is not my friend,
Soon it will be the end.

As I watch you in your sleep,
My pain buried deep,

I feel for you,
And again, my heart breaks.

During my Tuesday respite break, I visited mum. Alan enjoyed his visit from golf club mates, Carol and John, and Joy and Peter but, afterwards, was not quite himself. At bedtime his chest was rattling a lot despite an earlier shot of glyco. He asked me to call for another injection. When I became too tired, Laura sat with Alan. She woke me at 1:15am when the district nurses arrived. Alan was fast asleep but they roused him, offering a minimum dose of Midazolam, which he accepted.

After the nurses had gone I was shocked to discover two leaflets on the kitchen table. One was about registering a death, and another about coping with bereavement. Inside I was like jelly when I hugged Alan tight and gave him a good night kiss. I wanted to stay with him but was too tired. Back in bed I cried myself to sleep.

Wednesday 20th February - End of life started
In the kitchen, I found Laura explaining to the morning shift carers, "Alan does not want to get up."

I sat on Alan's bed and held his hand. The lump in my throat shifted enough for me to say, "You do know I love you don't you?"

Looking very tired he responded, "You know, I love you too."

I called Alan's two sisters to alert them as to Alan's deterioration. Both said they would come as soon as possible. I called Teresa for more immediate local support. District nurses injected more glyco. Teresa and I discussed the scary leaflets in the lounge, keeping one ear on the pace and depth of Alan's breathing in the room next door.

Julie from Macmillan arrived and confirmed Alan's 'end of life' started when he went into Myton Hospice. I was startled. Alan then stated he would prefer not to go to a hospice or hospital at this time. He agreed to have the syringe driver fitted today so that glyco could be given automatically. Julie arranged for blood tests to assess Alan's kidney function, to be sure a bigger dose of his water retention tablets was safe. Also, she said it was to, "Check the extent of any heart failure which might be causing the fluid build-up." Heart failure!!!?

Julie recommended limiting Alan's daily fluid intake to 1.2 litres and confirmed it was okay to use Lorazepam for anxiety and Oramorph for breathlessness.

Because the glyco in the syringe driver would help dry up secretions, it would be necessary to reduce the Hyoscine patch on Alan's neck gradually. Julie promised to arrange for the psychotherapist from the Marie Curie Hospice to contact me, and indicated a home visit might be possible. In a daze I wrote everything down. By now, I was incapable of retaining even the simplest information.

The lunchtime carers could only get Alan washed and dressed when the district nurses had fitted the syringe driver. After Pauline arrived, I distracted myself by bagging up some garden waste and driving to the tip. It was closed. I'd missed it by four minutes! Other distractions were, collecting clothes from mum's flat, picking up some medicines from the chemist and buying food. I felt like running away. Then John and Viv had arrived. I still felt wretched but forced myself to eat.

Thursday 21st February - Feeling lifeless

My first task of the day was to explain to the morning carer team how carefully they needed to move Alan now he had a syringe driver attached to him. Viv and I both agreed it was hard to accept how poorly Alan was now. Alan's old friend, David from Leeds, spent a few hours with him. Afterwards, Alan said, "It was hard to say goodbye to David, knowing I may never see him again."

At 2pm Eric, the district nurse, arrived to fill up the driver. That would be a daily event from here on. While Pauline was preparing dinner, her husband, Simon arrived. Alan and John watched *Sunderland Till I Die*. Despite it being a cheerful film about the glory days of the football team everyone supported, Alan ate only a small amount of dinner and declined a sip of wine. I sensed something was wrong.

One of the carers came to me while Alan was in the wet room.

"Alan says he feels lifeless." I immediately went and hugged Alan.

"You okay, Al? Shall we have a proper chat when you are in bed?"

He agreed.

"As well as feeling lifeless, I felt nauseous after the lunchtime PEG feed."

"Okay," I said. "You are probably tired."

He agreed we should call the district nurse if he felt the same in the morning. We lost ourselves in a Fred and Rose West documentary until the night sitter arrived. She was one of the day carers we'd had several months previously but, now, she was heavily pregnant. I hoped Alan would not need lifting and turning in the night!

Once Alan was in bed, there was a sombre atmosphere around the house. Alan had told me several months back he wanted his two sisters and his best friend Simon Beacham, to be around him when he passed away. I feared that while Pauline and Viv were at the house Alan might let go of life and slip silently away.

Friday 22nd February - Doing my bit to help the Marie Curie Hospice
Alan did not want to go into his wheelchair after his morning wet room ritual, so was put back onto his bed. The carers were too chatty around Alan. I wanted to bite their heads off but, instead, asked them to work more quietly around Alan. He needed calmness, not a catalogue of their personal lives. Stress was creeping up on me again.

At lunchtime Alan went into his chair. Later, Kevin helped me move Alan back into his bed, because he was uncomfortable in the wheelchair. We could both see Alan had little or no muscle left. Seven year old Tyler did a brilliant job acting as waiter, taking dishes of nibbles around to everyone. He was good with Alan too. He would make a wonderful carer.

I was grateful it was a mild, sunny day while I was doing a fundraising slot, wearing a huge yellow Marie Curie daffodil hat, outside a supermarket in our neighbouring village. Several people chatted about their experience of the hospice as they stuffed notes and coins into the collection can. One lady had a sister-in-law with MND, so we swapped mobile numbers. It was rewarding and fun doing something to help the hospice.

Not long after I arrived home I began to feel quite stressed. I walked to the local shops to help calm myself down. During the evening, I pottered around the house while Alan rested. Suddenly I heard the ventilator alarm ringing. A carer had left Alan's mask off after giving him some water. It made me angry and doubt whether anyone could look after Alan the way I did.

To help me calm down again I listened to some music in bed. My stress levels rose again when the night sitter called saying Alan had soiled his pad. The two of us rolled Alan from side to side so we could remove the soiled pad. We cleaned him and wiped the sheets as best we could. We lifted him off the bed so we could put on clean sheets, then got him into fresh pyjamas. It was about midnight when I finally turned out my light.

Saturday 23rd February - New fence and no more Riluzole
Alan had a good night's sleep but still elected to stay in bed after he was

dressed. Pauline and Simon left and our neighbour, a jeweller, popped round to advise me about replacing the lost stone in my engagement ring. He and John started erecting the new fence panels between our respective gardens.

Joanne and Andy arrived with flowers and flapjacks. Andy became the third man working on the fence panels. The freshly painted, red cedar panels were a great contrast to the bright green shrubs and created a nice new view from Alan's bedroom!

Despite using thickener in Alan's drinks, he had three choking episodes. He complained of feeling there was something stuck in his throat. On one occasion I had to slap his back. "Ouch, you are being too rough," he complained. Tears formed as I hugged him.

"I'm sorry Al. I don't want you to die because I didn't work hard enough to save your life." His back and shoulders felt knobbly under my hands. The muscles had gone. No wonder my slaps had felt rough - there was nothing left to protect his skeleton.

When the carers were doing his arm exercises in the afternoon, I noticed Alan vacantly looking out of the window. What was he thinking? "I want to stop taking the Riluzole tablets," he told me later. This was a big decision. A sign he was no long fighting his battle and had accepted his fate.

Sunday 24th February - Choosing between time with Alan and time with mum
Viv and John departed around 11am. For the first time in several days, Alan and I had the house to ourselves. We giggled a lot as we watched *Cuckoo* and some rugby matches. The social worker called, asking if we were happy with Alan's care agency. She explained an option was to have a Personal Health Budget, which involved hiring, firing and managing carers ourselves. It was not a viable option. I was already spinning too many other plates and we were generally happy with the agency.

Despite the afternoon weather being glorious Alan declined to sit outside or come with me to watch mum having art therapy. Unusually I could not find someone to sit with Alan so, I chose to stay with him, based on the probability mum would outlive Alan. Mum's care home rang to tell me mum had painted a daffodil, a tree and a butterfly. I felt bad because I would have liked to have witnessed that.

AUTHOR'S NOTE
Arranging for someone to be with Alan, when I could not be there, was not just for company, it was essential. Between the hours the carers came, Alan might

need a drink or a pee, moving a little to increase comfort, or an adjustment made to his ventilator mask, in addition to help with life threatening emergencies like an issue with the ventilator.

Monday 25th February - Joan's alternative funeral

As soon as the carers arrived, I explained it was the day of Alan's mum's funeral and that he might not be himself. One carer was flustered because she had overslept. I also suspected she was not happy working with the new carer on her shift. I took her to one side and urged her to calm herself down. While the carers attended to the long morning routine, I set up a shrine in the conservatory - fresh flower heads floating in a pretty bowl of water, with a candle each side of the bowl.

In the conservatory with Alan, I lit the candles. We planned to replicate the entire funeral service, as it happened, in real time in Sunderland. We played the same music, sang the same hymns and I did the same readings. Then Alan and I spent a moment talking about our happy memories of times with Joan, followed by a moment of silence. Then I doused the candles. Afterwards, we sat outside in the sunshine and had a stiff drink. Red wine usually made him choke, but vodka and tonic worked nicely!

The opportunity felt right to raise the topic of where Alan wanted his ashes to be spread. He asked for some to go to Broadway Tower - above the town where we had our first date. I suggested some go to Sunderland (where he was born) and some to the Valley of the Rocks in Lynton (where my ashes would eventually go). Also, some to the Alps (where we had enjoyed skiing) and some to Askham Fell in Cumbria (where the whole Carter family had spent many happy hours walking with him). He liked my ideas.

When Laura arrived for night sitting, I called the district nurses at Alan's request, for a top up of drugs. A grumble had developed in his chest. It had been a stressful day for him.

Tuesday 26th February - Alan's life saved by quick thinking carer

While I was getting dressed for the day, I received a panic call from one of the carers, "The ventilator's not working - Alan's not getting any air!" I threw on a bathrobe and rushed downstairs.

By the time I reached the wet room, the other carer advised the panic was over. He had worked out that the air intake valve, at the back of the ventilator, had sucked in the plastic sheet being used to stop wet room water going onto the electrical device. His initiative had saved Alan's life. Phew!

We were given lots of advice by our speech and language therapist when she arrived to check Alan's choking issues. Amongst other things, she suggested Alan only eat pureed food in future. Eggs were to be boiled or scrambled rather than fried. We were advised to check out the MND Association website for the eating and drinking guide. Smoothies made from soft fruits, bananas, blueberries, etc. would be okay to consume.

The therapist pointed out that choking was a result of something getting stuck in the airway and coughing was a reaction to something that had gone past the airway. She also suggested that, if drinking by a straw became problematic, using a spoon to deliver liquids orally was okay. She suggested Alan's locking jaw was probably due to a drop in his temperature or clenching his teeth at night. She recommended exercises to help keep his jaw mobile.

The regular Tuesday respite carer looked after Alan between breakfast and lunch. During my massage and facial at a clinic in Kenilworth, I became emotional while relaying my story to the beautician. For the first time I heard myself use words I'd avoided since diagnosis, words such as 'terminal' and 'dying.'

Alan's niece Helen, and nephew Matthew arrived in the afternoon. Soon after, nephews Tom and Ben, and Ben's partner Claire arrived. They were all on their way home from Joan's funeral in Sunderland. Ben and Claire announced that they planned to give their daughter (due to be born in July) the middle name Alana - the nearest girl's name to Alan they could think of. Alan and I were moved. We were even more moved when they said had the baby been a boy, he would have been called Alan.

As Helen left she gave me a card to read to Alan. He and I both cried when I read out her memories of time with her Uncle Alan and her affectionate words for him. After watching more TV and having ice cream for dinner, Alan became agitated. He accepted a dose of oral morphine, which settled the feeling that something was in his throat. We shared the happy news, about Alan's expected great niece having Alana as her middle name, with Laura when she arrived for the night shift.

AUTHOR'S NOTE

It was common practice to protect the ventilator, with a waterproof sheet whenever it was near the wet room. The incident above led to the idea of a placing a guard over the ventilator before covering it with the plastic sheet.

Wednesday 27th February - Baby food
Laura reported that Alan did a lot of talking in his sleep and had the usual issues of his mask slipping off. Hmmm, was CO2 building up? While I was visiting mum, the district nurses had changed the position of the syringe driver as a large blister had developed near the incision point. Also, the needle had fallen out - possibly due to carer handling errors, so not all the drug was getting through.

Alan's work colleague Christina visited, just before I gave Alan a horrible looking baby food dinner. Weirdly, as ghastly as it looked, he enjoyed it.

After Christina left, as delicately as possible, I asked the awkward question, "Alan, would you like to dictate private notes to your family members while your voice is still working?" He said he would consider it.

Thursday 28th February - Memories
It was a bleak day outside. The recent beautiful sunshine had vanished. One carer did not arrive, so I started off the morning routine with the one that did. Eventually a second carer turned up, so I left them to it.

For a change, I gave Alan his breakfast and medicines in the lounge rather than in the kitchen. Afterwards I asked, "Is there anything you want done to give you peace of mind?"

"Yes," he replied, "I want to go through my memorabilia boxes." Out of the blue he asked, "What worries you most about being on your own?" A long, emotional conversation followed where I confessed I worried about being heartsick all the time while missing him.

As we watched *Cuckoo* to the end of the series, I started composing a mental list of things I was going to find tough. I could not cope with the idea of Alan being taken away from the house after he died. I imagined myself screaming and hysterically throwing myself to the ground. The thought of watching Alan die was way too painful.

Pauline arrived and stayed with Alan while I attended a speed awareness course. A camera had caught me dashing through Kenilworth on 29th December on my way to Alan in Coventry Hospital. Periodically in the four hour course, I got lost in my own mental memorabilia boxes.

MARCH 2019

Friday 1st March - Sisters

Another unsettled night, alleviated by oral morphine and the care of the night sitter. After Alan's long morning routine, he and I did a FaceTime video with Pam, the Lady Captain of Shirley Golf Club. She had become incredibly supportive of Alan and I since learning so much about MND.

My sister, Rowena came for lunch, in celebration of her birthday (on 2nd March). As a surprise for Ro, I had also arranged for our other sister, Clare, to join us. It was rare for the three of us to have quality time together. Alan sensibly chose to rest in the lounge, rather than suffer our cackling and giggling!

Alan handled watching the video of Joan's funeral well, but it pained me to think the next funeral could be Alan's. Before lights out I set up a new JustGiving page, in aid of Myton Hospice, in respect of the forthcoming leap off the roof of Coventry Cathedral.

Saturday 2nd March - A simpler life

During the night, I overheard Laura trying to understand Alan. He was not coherent even to me. Through a process of elimination, I identified that he wanted his duvet to be put back on. Earlier in the night, he had asked Laura to take it off. Too tired to get up, I let the carers do a basic routine and left Alan to sleep.

Pauline arrived and we watched the BBC clip of John King, a seventy-seven-year-old man from Worcester. He had chosen to end his life by coming off his ventilator at a hospice. It was terribly heartbreaking to watch, but useful preparation, in case Alan made a similar decision.

After buying some flowers, I collected my repaired engagement ring from my neighbour. He talked of being only forty-seven when his wife died, leaving him to bring up their two children. There was an enormous canvas photograph of her on his kitchen wall. What a lovely idea.

Pauline went home armed with the flowers and Alan got up at teatime. Today's conversation was about our new, simpler lifestyle. We agreed we had more time to just be in the moment and be mindful. "Our psychologist would be proud of us," I said, smiling. Alan agreed.

Sunday 3rd March - Fears of catching a cold

The carers had to give Alan a bed bath because he didn't want to get up. Our ex-lodger, Jaki, visited and decided to do the Glow for Myton fundraising event, which I had already entered. It was a fun 5k walk/jog/run around the streets of Coventry at night, wearing bright, fluorescent clothes.

The headache I had woken up with was still going strong when Alan got up at teatime. We relaxed in the lounge, with no lights on, listening to Classic FM but my pain did not subside. In fact, I felt quite ill. I had a tickly cough and my temperature was up. It would be a disaster if I caught a cold. Alan needed care around the clock, which I delivered, with five hours covered by carers. Catching a cold from me could prove fatal to him.

My Coventry Cathedral abseil fundraising page reached £410 and people who had seen my email about it, were arranging to come and support.

Monday 4th March - Prayers and questions with Vicar John

After breakfast Alan and I had a long chat about my fears and what life would be like for me after he died.

"You should go to a sanctuary for pampering and spiritual rejuvenation," he suggested.

"I hope your family will still involve me in family events," I confessed, "I don't want to lose them as well as you."

I told him, "I am worried about seeing them take away your body after you die. I fear I may be overcome with anger or despair."

Finally, "I think I might go to Broadway or Stratford-upon-Avon on the 14th of June each year." He knew why. It was our most special day of the year. On 14th June, we met in Broadway in 2006 and married in Stratford-upon-Avon in 2014. I could feel my chest tighten as my emotions welled up.

Luckily, our friend and retired vicar, John arrived at that moment. I had known him since he became a neighbour at my old house in 2003. With his encouragement, we opened our hearts. Alan confessed to feeling bad about not being there for his mum, when she was dying.

"You were there for your mum when she needed you during her life," John reassured. I liked his suggestion that, "Dying is like having the opportunity to get on an early flight to a nice holiday location." Also, I liked, "There is no point in asking why. It's better for us to ask what is happening and what can we do about it."

John went on, "Deep love like your love leads to deep emotional pain," and "Love is not about taking, it's about giving." John admitted, "I don't have answers for everything and I don't understand everything, but don't be afraid of dying, it's just part of the journey."

John held our hands. As he prayed for us I could hear his breath catching with emotion. He commended Alan, "To go into God's care," and asked God to, "Help him find peace."

As John's prayer continued, I felt my temperature rise and then, I felt myself become calm and peaceful. By the end, John and I were both crying. We left Alan in the lounge and walked into the hall, where John and I hugged and cried some more. He told me he wished he could do more. He agreed to ask Vicar Peter Thomas from St Peter's church in the village, to contact us.

Back in the lounge, Alan started crying.

He remarked, "I think your idea of me dictating private letters to each member of the family is a good one." I took a brief walk, to try to control my emotions. While I was out, the district nurse moved the position of the driver again, into a location I felt was not suitable when Alan was sitting in the wheelchair. Had I been there, I would have pointed that out.

Early evening, I received a phone call from mum's care home. "Yvonne's had a fall and the ambulance is on its way." Our neighbour Alex agreed to sit with Alan until the night-time carers came.

In Heartlands Hospital A&E department, I found mum on a bed in a corridor. She was her usual chatty self but confused. An X-ray showed nothing was broken. When nurses tried to get her onto the loo, she had a dizzy spell. Her blood pressure was high, so they decided to keep her in overnight. I sent a text to my siblings to ask for their help and one to mum's social worker, urging her to find mum a more suitable home.

Tuesday 5th March - Unexpected sadness and joy
It was 3:30am when I got to sleep so, after a brief chat with the carers at 6.30am, I returned to bed for some more rest. Mum was in the elderly person's assessment unit when I returned to the hospital. The sister on duty arranged for me to meet mum's doctor. Peering over his specs he said he liked to look beyond the obvious, and mentioned a syndrome which develops when elderly people fear falling. He gave me tips on how to get mum into the right care home, allowing for her capacity and capability.

When we were alone, Alan and I watched some comedy on TV. Suddenly Alan started to cry. "I don't like watching couples in bed having hugs. I miss us doing that," he said, "And I miss us dancing together, cooking meals together and being able to go on holiday." We agreed we had no choice but to accept the things we could not change but we could change some things. I promised to hug him more while he was on his bed.

"I want you to go on holidays after I die," he announced. I couldn't imagine travelling without him. Where would I go? I would never be able to go to places to which he and I had already been. Who would want to come with me? Would friends be a good enough substitute? These were bridges I would have to cross when the time came. Some unexpected joy came into the day when Sunderland beat Bristol in the Checkatrade Trophy.

Wednesday 6th March - Grateful for being in Solihull Metropolitan Council
Alan got up in the morning but went back to bed at lunchtime. He slept most of the afternoon and got up again at teatime but struggled to get comfortable in his chair. In a telephone conversation, Wendy spoke of her frustration at not being able to get the help she needed for Mel, who had been living with MND for several years. I was grateful we did not come under Birmingham Council, who appeared to offer less support than Solihull Metropolitan Council.

Thursday 7th March - Alarm bells
Alan was tired, so I gave him his morning medicines and he stayed in bed. During a visit from Wokingham based friends, Angela and Dave, we talked about our trip to Vietnam in April 2018, and they talked about Japan. Alan had never expressed an interest in going there but I made a mental note for my 'after Alan dies' bucket list.

Alan started crying while watching TV and mournfully said, "I am worried about how much sleeping I am doing." My mind went into a frenzy of alarm bells, which prevented me from coming up with a helpful response.

Friday 8th March - Reassurance from St Peter's
We had a chaotic morning because Suzanne and Ian from the golf club arrived, shortly followed by the unexpected arrival of Vicar Peter from the local church. I chatted with the vicar in the lounge, while Alan was kept company by our friends in his bedroom. Vicar Peter spoke of the possibility of me 'hitting a wall' after Alan passed away. He made a point of stressing, "The church will be there for you at all times." Just as the vicar was leaving, Eric, the district nurse, arrived to check up on Alan's skin.

Alan stayed in bed until teatime - mainly because sitting in his chair on his muscle-depleted bottom was causing sores. In the afternoon, Alan's breathing became difficult and his throat was sore. Oh no, had he caught my cold? I administered oral morphine and hunted down the throat lozenges.

At teatime, the carers moved Alan to his wheelchair. We decided it was time to watch season three of *Game of Thrones*. Because the pregnant night sitter was unwell, Laura was drafted back in. We liked Laura a lot. She was a model night sitter. She was very trustworthy and had real empathy with both of us. I wondered why we could not have her every night (which she said she would prefer).

Saturday 9th March - No future as an action hero

Jo and Andy arrived for a brief catch up followed by Gina and Ray from the golf club. They came to sit with Alan because I had a rooftop to 'jump' off. Once I had registered with the Myton fundraising team at Coventry Cathedral, I found I was surprisingly calm as I chatted with Simon and Rachel and my ex-boss Martin and his wife. Other friends had kindly showed up to witness me launch myself from the top of the iconic building. Many fellow abseilers looked good in their red Myton tee shirts. I wore my bright blue MND tee shirt with several layers underneath to keep out the cold March breeze. I looked like a miniature Michelin man!

In the holding area, I was given my safety hat and harness and listened to the briefing. The lady in front of me turned out to be a seasoned abseiler. I had only done one, off Table Mountain in Cape Town, with Alan by my side every scary inch of the way. Inside the building my friends Frankie and Ruth, from the *More to Life* group, found me. Their arrival calmed my increasing nervousness.

Climbing up the narrow spiral staircase and negotiating the short sections of metal ladders to the roof was tricky. At the top I was panting hard - probably as much from nerves as from the exertion. A man hooked my waist belt onto a safety line and told me to walk across to my handler. My nerves were out of control as I gingerly moved across the lead roof. Before I had time to think about it, I was hooked up to my descent rope and the safety line was attached to my handler. "Stand on the small board and lean back," the handler instructed. "Take one foot off the board and place it on the wall."

My legs went stiff. I felt like a concrete statue about to fall over (do statues have feelings?). To kill the butterflies fluttering around my stomach, I thought about Alan in his bed and all the other people with MND and the families I had met at Myton. I resisted the urge to look down over my shoulder and took a very deep breath.

Once fully on the wall, gripping hold of my safety rope, as if my life depended on it (and it did), I took tiny tip toe steps down the wall. I felt like I wasn't making any progress, so I started to do mini hops, imagining I was Tom Cruise in Mission Impossible. Part way down the wall I heard a familiar voice shouting for me to wave. I stopped, tentatively turned, looked down, waved at my friend and quickly returned to the correct position.

There was much jubilation when I landed into a pool of helpers. I spotted the seasoned abseiler and mouthed, "Thank you." Friends showed me their photos while my heart rate returned to normal. One video showed a blue blob moving down the wall at the pace of a snail. I decided not to bother auditioning to become an action movie character!

AUTHOR'S NOTE
For younger readers, the Michelin man was a very rotund cartoon character made from Michelin tyres, used in adverts on TV, centuries ago.

Saturday 10th March - Losing two loved ones at the same time
Around 2:30am, the night sitter called me. Alan was complaining of a rattle in his chest. I called the district nurse. Once we adjusted his bed, so he was almost sitting upright, Alan fell asleep. After doses of glyco and Midazolam at 3.30am, I hugged Alan and whispered, "I love you." He just about managed to say, "Thank you for looking after me," before he drifted back to sleep.

As soon as my alarm went off, with Alan sound asleep, I cancelled the morning carers and went back to bed. When I saw Alan at 10am, we agreed to cancel the lunchtime carers too.

Alan insisted I go to my nephew's wedding even if he couldn't. I called Clare. She was pleased I would be spending some quality time with the family. I floated some of my ideas about Alan's funeral with her. Some days it was felt easier to talk about such practical things.

By the time Simon and Rachel arrived around 5pm, Alan was more alert, so I visited mum. She looked wretched sitting alone in the conservatory staring into space. On checking with the staff, I was disappointed they had not yet instigated the change to her medicines, as recommended by the doctor at Heartlands. I went to bed feeling low. I was losing Alan to MND, and mum was disappearing into her dementia.

Monday 11th March - Another illness in the family

During the morning carers shift, I had to give Alan a suppository. He had not opened his bowels for several days. One carer became flustered thinking the shift would overrun. I trimmed Alan's fingernails and trimmed his eyebrows.

Mum's care home called to tell me she was experiencing chest pain and was being taken to hospital for tests. At the same time Sue, my sister-in-law, sent a message advising that Kevin, was going for tests for an autoimmune disease. Superstitious people say, "Things happen in threes." Could it be true?

Again Alex, our neighbour, stayed with Alan, so I could see mum. Eventually, a doctor examined mum and we found out her chest X-ray was clear, and her blood tests were okay. He suspected the issue was her hiatus hernia.

I called my Kevin. "I have high levels of protein in my urine," he said. "The hospital doctor has ordered more tests and a kidney biopsy."

Mum became anxious, thinking she had missed Andrew's wedding. At 7:30pm I had to leave her and relieve Neil, from the golf club, who had followed on from Alex.

During his evening meal Alan choked on some ice cream and brought up some nasty phlegm. When I was giving him some oral morphine, via a small syringe, I noticed the inside wall of his cheek looked rough and ulcerated.

Laura called me just before I went to bed. She needed my help to hoist Alan out of bed and onto a bedpan. After his bowels had opened, we cleaned him up and returned him to his usual sleeping position. It may sound silly, but it was always a relief when Alan produced stools. I returned to bed. Poor Laura had to watch over Alan in a room that did not smell of roses!

AUTHOR'S NOTE

For many months Alan was only able to sleep on his back and getting him comfortable was always a long job. We had to put two pillows under his head and pillows under both of his arms to prevent pain in his shoulders. His hands and wrists were in special braces to prevent his fingers curling inwards. A rolled-up towel was placed on the side of each leg to stop them falling open and protective boots put on his feet to reduce risk of sores.

The head of the bed was raised slightly, as was the knee section of the bed. Rolled up towels were put next to his head to prevent it from falling over, causing pain in his neck.

Tuesday 12th March - Struggling to find words

Only one carer turned up for the morning shift, so I helped her with the full morning routine. We got Alan into the shower chair so he could do a poo over the pan, then we cleaned him up, cleaned his teeth and washed his face. He elected not to have a shower or get dressed but wanted to go back to bed for more sleep. I had to admonish him when he told me, "In the night I feared I was not getting enough air, but I would not let Laura wake you. I wanted you to get a good night's sleep."

He was so selfless.

Our usual respite sitter arrived giving me time to shop for a dress, suitable for Andrew's wedding. Viv and John arrived mid-afternoon. At teatime, the carers lifted Alan out of his wheelchair for a few minutes and put him back down. This simple exercise improved his comfort level from three to eight out of ten. Vicar Peter arrived to discuss readings and hymns for the funeral services and give us his views on Michael Deeley, the local funeral director.

For the second night in a row, the night-time carers were late arriving. Once their work was done, they asked me to see Alan. He was struggling to express himself and was clearly frustrated. I could see his mind searching for the word he wanted to say. It took some time to establish he wanted the waterproof mat under his back to be straightened out. Viv thought maybe Alan was tired, but I suspected he was losing his speech muscles.

While I supervised Laura giving Alan his medicines for the first time, Alan kept talking about the earlier incident. It clearly concerned him. I destracted him with, "Don't forget Ben and Tom are popping in tomorrow after the Sunderland match tonight." The team were just outside the automatic promotion zone to the Championship and the family had high expectations for the play-off matches. In bed I cried. Alan appeared to be entering a new phase in his decline.

Wednesday 13th March - Carers not up to scratch

In the morning, our carers consisted of one who was new to being the leader and another, who was new to doing the morning shift. Between them they got a low rating. After Viv and John left, Alan asked to return to his bed. Sitting for long periods in his wheelchair, even fully raked back, was now very painful.

I had to prepare Alan's ex work colleagues, Norma, Yvonne and Wendy, for what they would see. From their shocked looks it was clear they had not realised Alan had declined so far, so fast. After the girls left, I sent a text to the care agency, "Today's lead carer was not yet ready to be the one in charge."

Thursday 14th March - Review meeting with care agency

On waking, the first thought that came to me was, it's four and three-quarter years since our wedding and, twelve and three quarter years since our blind date.

Before MND came into our lives, I wouldn't count quarter years, but time was running out and every day was precious. Alan had not been himself since his spell in hospital. Over recent weeks, he had needed considerably more drugs to keep his secretions and anxiety under control. I really hoped we would reach our 5th/13th year anniversaries, but my heart was heavy. Every day, Alan was getting weaker.

The morning carers were much better. The manager and assistant manager from the agency came and did a review of Alan's needs and listened to our views on carers. Overall, the standard of carers was high, but Alan's needs were complex now. They responded well to my appeal for competent carers with the right attitude and a consistent team, that could become familiar with Alan's particular requirements.

Mum's social worker called to say that a nursing home the other side of Solihull had agreed to take Yvonne, subject to meeting her. I was invited to check it out on behalf of mum, because mum had 'lost mental capacity'.

The evening carers included a young man who was super competitive. He wanted a top score from us. Some carers did not like the idea of being evaluated. We felt it was necessary as Alan deserved the very best care we could get.

Friday 15th March - Review with Macmillan Nurse

Alan chose to go into his wheelchair, after his usual morning routine, because Julie from Macmillan was due. When she arrived, Julie discussed Alan's medicines, the discomfort in his bottom while sitting in his chair, the change in cognitive ability and whether he should go to the hospice for symptom control or respite.

"The drugs you are taking will slow down your thinking," Julie reassured Alan. It was a great relief because we were aware that 15% of people with MND, like Wendy's Mel, develop frontotemporal dementia.

We also spoke with Julie about John King. He had recently been in the news for having his non-invasive ventilator removed so his life could end. Julie confirmed Alan could come off the ventilator but only in a hospice.

Mum's social worker rang to say that the nursing home had formally offered a place to mum. She assured me it had good reviews. It felt like a take it or leave it offer, but I was relieved that, at last, the authorities believed it was no longer safe for mum to live on her own! During the evening Alan needed a top up of glyco and Midazolam. We watched Comic Relief until the night sitter arrived.

Saturday 16th March - Breathing and sit bone problems

During the night I could hear the night sitter was having difficulty understanding Alan, so I popped downstairs. If Alan's voice stopped working we would all find it extremely hard to understand his needs. Alan went back onto his bed after his shower. During a visit from our friends, Jenny and Nick from Sutton Coldfield, Alan's syringe driver started beeping. Within an hour the district nurse had filled it up.

Extract from my Facebook post:

"How sad am I getting? This morning while the carers were getting Alan ready for the day, and after I had prepared his medicines, I read the T&Cs for Google Chrome before downloading. Some would say I need to get a life!

It's true, life is very different these days. Since 4th February Alan has not been able to leave the house. He is a lot weaker and he finds he has pain now when he is in his wheelchair. If he gets up in the morning, often lunch time or teatime, the discomfort is too much and he needs to be hoisted back onto his bed. About 50% of the week, he chooses to go back onto the bed after he is showered and dressed by the carers in the morning and is only hoisted into the wheelchair later in the day.

The video below [on Facebook] shows what's involved in getting Alan from wheelchair onto his bed. It was filmed in September 2018. Now he cannot move any limbs himself and, instead of struggling for breath, he is on a ventilator 24x7, which further complicates the transfer process. Plus, he now has a 24x7 drug driver (which involves having a line from a pump fixed into his stomach which is constantly pushing in drugs that reduce the amount of fluid accumulating in his lungs, and reduces the anxiety caused by breathlessness). This too creates further challenges for carers when they handle him.

Good news, the ventilation nurse was pleased with his stats yesterday. However, occasionally he needs the district nurses to give him a top up of the driver drugs. Eating and swallowing are now seriously difficult for Alan. Most of his nourishment is in the form of Fortisip drinks delivered via the PEG feeding tube fitted into his tummy (oh yes, that's something else the carers have to be careful not to dislodge).

Overall, Alan is very poorly really but he is a fighter. Alan has got the option to come off the ventilator that is keeping him alive - it's classified as 'treatment'. You may have seen that MND sufferer, John King, took this option recently. Thankfully, Alan told our MacMillan nurse the other day he wants to stick around and see his beloved Sunderland football club get promoted and England win the Ashes. So, if any of you have influence over the managers of these two teams, now is a good time to share Alan's story! I, of course, would like to think he wants to stick around because he loves my wit, charm and company, but that did not feature in what he told our nurse!

Would I swap my new, somewhat limited, life for anything? Not at all. I am however going to have to find something interesting to do while all that football and cricket is going on - it will drive me bonkers reading more T&Cs! Luckily, we both love rugby and there is a very exciting day ahead. Be great if the Irish beat the Welsh and our boys beat the Scots at Twickers so we secure both the Six Nations Trophy and the Calcutta Cup.

Happy weekend everyone. Love the people you are with and do something you have been putting off, because the T&Cs of life contain no guarantees for any of us!"

Despite the need for me to sit Alan forward in his wheelchair every so often, to relieve pressure on his sore bottom, Alan decided to go into the lounge to watch the final Six Nations matches on the larger TV. Don't ask me how, but England managed to throw away a thirty-one-point half time lead over Scotland and lost the tournament.

All afternoon Alan was making a lot of noise on his out-breath. I put the full face night mask on him, to relieve pressure on his weak breathing muscles. My brain went into a spin. Was this the dreaded death rattle? Alan gave a low rating to one of the night-time carers, "She was rough and impatient with me." The other, newer carer was mindful and cleverly came up with some good ideas to aid his comfort.

Sunday 17th March - Going out together
While my sister Clare and her husband were with us, Alan's breathing became troublesome, so I swapped his day nose mask to the nose and mouth night one.

Clare and David looked on in shocked silence. I'd witnessed other visitors look horrified when they saw what Alan had to go through. Alan became tearful as he looked out at the sunshine just before lunch. "It would be a lovely day for a round of golf or a bike ride," he lamented. It was time to try to take him out.

For the first time since 4th February, I packed Alan and his machines, into the VW. In the golf club lounge, a ladies meeting was taking place. I stayed there while Andy looked after Alan in the casual bar. When I eventually took Alan into the lounge afterwards, several ladies made a fuss of him. His voice was quite weak. He could not make himself understood. It was time to leave.

Before going home, I drove to the care home to which mum was going. Due to his weak neck muscles, Alan's head was jostled around in his headrest as I travelled over the unusually bumpy road. While Alan rested in the vehicle, a nurse showed me around the care home. Mum's room would be number fourteen. A good omen I thought, but the place was bland except for a few gaudy mirrors. It made me angry that I had accepted it without seeing it.

On the drive back home, I had to stop driving. Alan was too uncomfortable. Would this be our last trip out together? At home, I broke down. Alan tried to comfort me. "Anyone else would have broken from all the stress you have been under," he said before offering one of his pearls of wisdom, "You should see how mum gets on. She may not even notice the décor if they fuss over her enough."

Alan announced, "I think I could manage the journey to Andrew's wedding, but it will be too much sitting in the chair all the way through the service and reception." Throughout the documentary, about the six wives of Henry VIII, I felt down. As I kissed him goodnight, Alan said, "I have only just realised the enormity of what you have been handling."

Monday 18th March - Moved mum to new care home

Alan had a choking episode while drinking cranberry juice. I collected mum and took her to her new care home. It took ages to do all the paperwork with the manager and the head nurse, but the thoroughness of the Care Plan was impressive. At teatime, mum was taken to the dining room. It was a good time for me to make my exit. At no time did mum ask about Alan. He had slipped from her memory.

At 6pm, I thanked our friend Adrian for staying with Alan for an unexpectedly long time. Alan only ate a little bit of ice cream. His days of taking anything orally were numbered. Mum's move had gone better than I thought but, as I tried to sleep, I wondered how she would be when I next visited her

Tuesday 19th March - Deep conversation

For the first hour of the 6.30am carers shift I had to help because one carer was late. Rhea did her Tuesday respite sit which enabled me to see mum and get to the opticians. The *Do Not Resuscitate* form had to be collected from mum's old care home and delivered to the new one. I found mum sitting in the dining room looking okay. Thank goodness. I put up a TV in mum's room and met the manager. "Your mum does not need a walking frame," she declared. I refuted her statement with, "Mum had several falls in her own home, in hospital and at Alexander House. I think a frame is essential, don't you?" The surprised manager had clearly not been given all the facts.

Before dinner, Alan and I had another deep conversation. Key questions were, where should I live, and should I find a new partner? Alan suggested, "You should sell the house because you will not be able to move on, until you move out." He continued, "You should find someone to share your life with. Someone you can love, who will love you, and who you can rely on." I didn't respond. "I don't like the idea of you being with someone new, but you deserve to be happy again."

To that I did respond. "I think I will be afraid to get emotionally close to another man, but I will consider finding a good man to be my companion."

"My life has been the best these last 12 years," Alan declared. "I am humbled by all the love being shown to me. I'm amazed how many friends I now have, since meeting you." We discussed what I would do with my life. "I feel a bit envious," Alan said looking despondent.

"It might sound good Al, but without you, it will never be the same."

It was during these times of closeness that I felt the most love for Alan. He was so level-headed, wise, thoughtful, humble and generous. He never complained about his illness. He raised a smile for everyone who visited, and he bravely soldiered on when every new twist and turn took more from him. I felt blessed to have found such a man and devastated that I would grow old without him by my side.

Wednesday 20th March - Goodbye Marie

Before the alarm rang I woke with a lot on my mind, including where I would live in the future. I reminded myself I was only supposed to concern myself with the 'here and now'. Worrying about life without Alan would ruin what little time we had left. Alan enjoyed a long visit from golf club member Phil. The two men were from either side of the River Wear. This always made for some good banter.

After lunch Marie, ventilation nurse from Stoke Hospital, arrived. It was her last visit because Alan was under Coventry's care now. We thanked her for her wonderful support. As she stepped out of the house, she said, "You are doing a great job." The tight grip I had on my feelings these days loosened.

Simon Beacham was catching up with Alan when Viv and John arrived. I sent an email to mum's new care home detailing the dates of all of mum's falls. Thank goodness I had my notes to draw from! The bedtime carers were early and got everything done in an hour. They scored highly! Before going to bed I tried on my outfit for Andrew's wedding. My comfort eating had increased my weight. I neither looked, nor felt, good.

Thursday 21st March - Funeral decisions with Alan
At 2:30am, I heard voices via the monitor so went downstairs. Laura was struggling to understand what Alan wanted. Through a process of elimination I worked out that he was too hot. Earlier I had put a blanket over him because he was no longer wearing pyjama bottoms and had accidentally left the heating on high. "I've been having a recurring dream," he mumbled, "about being the custodian of the People's Freedom Charter!" He could still make me laugh, bless him.

Laura reported Alan had not slept well. Alan chose to go into his wheelchair after his usual ablutions, ready for a meeting with the local funeral directors. Michael Deeley facilitated a long chat with Alan, Viv and I about all the practical aspects of Alan's funeral. Michael asked if Alan's body should be at the house rather than at the funeral home, the night before the service. I imagined Alan's coffin in our lounge, and me locking the doors so no one could take him away from me. "No, keep him with you, Michael," I reluctantly uttered.

Michael suggested some options for the wake venue before telling us, "It's extremely helpful meeting the person I will be caring for. I wish more families would do it." Finally, I asked Michael to find out if we could have both John, our friend and retired vicar, and Vicar Peter handle the service.

As soon as Michael left I gave Alan some oral morphine to ease the pain of being in his wheelchair for so long. He fell asleep almost immediately. Pauline arrived just before our psychologist, Morgan. Viv and Pauline left us to share our fears with Morgan. She gave us helpful guidance on the type of mindset we needed to adopt.

While Alan's two sisters stayed with him, I went into Solihull. Teresa gave me a bunch of red roses and we cried as I talked about Alan's funeral arrangements. She suggested, "Why not leave Alan's coffin at the church the night before the service? It's a place of sanctuary." And then, "Not everyone could read at a funeral, but I think, knowing you, you should read the eulogy yourself. It may help you to start to heal." She also reminded me, "At dads funeral, I told you I will be there for you." On parting, Teresa's remarked, "I bless the day *More to Life* brought us together."

Friday 22nd March - Visit to St Peter's Church

Mum was sitting alone in the hall at her care home looking lost and lonely. I checked a list of her possessions with the nurse and paid £50 into mum's personal expenditure account. Mum picked at her lunch which didn't look very appetising. Nothing I did cheered her up.

Alan was in bed when I arrived home. He had developed a grumbling chest and the district nurse had been called in to top up the glyco in his driver. During the teatime carers shift, Pauline, Viv and I visited St Peter's Church. Viv became emotional. She had only just lost her mum, now Alan was very poorly. Personally, I found the church to be a place of peace and tranquillity. Viv prepared dinner while I watched TV, holding hands with Alan. His breathing was fast and shallow. Was this it?

Saturday 23rd March - Lucky for me

During the night I had a headache, an upset tummy and a stiff neck. Andy and Jo arrived bringing a new pressure relieving pillow for Alan to try on his wheelchair which made a lot of difference to his comfort.

Alan and I had quality time together, while Pauline and Viv kindly did some housework. After lunch I went to Myton Hospice to collect my Glow for Myton pack, picked up some groceries and collected some additional Just in Case medications from the chemist.

Worryingly, Pauline and Viv reported that they had called the district nurse for a further top up of glyco. I panicked when I realised I had lost my iPhone. A quick phone call to the supermarket confirmed that somebody had handed it in. Phew!

Sunday 24th March - Lots of parts make up a life

Pauline left just after breakfast. Viv and I spent the morning raking over the lawn and tidying up the back garden, while Alan sat in his wheelchair watching a war film. I poured out my heart to my friend, Christine at a local garden centre. At one point she wisely said, "There are lots of parts that make up a life. Losing someone does not mean the end of all life." We talked about me having a large portrait photograph of Alan made for the house. From my phone we chose one of Alan wearing his black polo neck, in the restaurant on our last ski holiday, in Morzine. (This picture is now on the front cover of this book).

When the carers made a mess of changing over Alan's mask, leaving him gasping for air, I became angry. During the evening, I had to call the district nurse for yet another top up of glyco.

Monday 25th March - Alan's condition deteriorating
My headache refused to go away despite taking two doses of painkillers. Jo and I had an early dinner at a pub. I almost dropped off while driving the car home. Alan was watching England in a football match but said he felt bad - perpetually gagging - and sick. The district nurse administered a glyco top up but could not give an anti-sickness drug because it had not been prescribed!

Tuesday 26th March - Discussion regarding Alan's prescription
Alan chose to stay in bed. Our Macmillan nurse suggested increasing the glyco dose in his driver and stopping the Nystatin Alan was taking to cure his mouth ulcers, because he could be experiencing side effects.

Alan was depressed when I returned from buying a replacement for our broken tumble dryer. I tried to cheer him up, "Tomorrow will be different Al," and by putting *Game of Thrones* on to distract him.

Wednesday 27th March - Accidental overdosing
The two male carers were uncoordinated and disorganised on the morning shift. They took two and a half hours, instead of two, which did not include cleaning up the wet room. One of them said he was going to ask to come off Alan's run. I had to point out to the other one that he said pardon every time someone spoke to him. He agreed to arrange a hearing test. I sent a text to the care agency with our views.

Our Macmillan nurse, Julie, called and clarified what drugs should be given to Alan going forward. She pointed out I had been accidentally overdosing Alan with Furosemide - the fluid retention drug - confusing millilitres with micrograms! I felt awful. I was not a trained nurse, but I had the responsibilities of one.

Patrick, our financial planner, arrived soon after Viv and John left. He brought a book about golfing, a bottle of champagne and some chocolates and confirmed our affairs were in good order. I cried when Patrick said, "When Alan dies, call me," as he left our house. Eric, one of our favourite district nurses arrived, having heard from Julie. He increased the glyco drug in Alan's driver to 600mg. The maximum Alan could have in a day was 1200mg.

Alone in the house, Alan and I watched another episode of *The Crown*. Alan's chest started to grumble. I gave him some Oramorph which left him a bit spaced out and mumbling. For the first time I tried using the Barbara book - the communication aid we had been given months earlier to help me understand what Alan wanted.

Helen, Alan's niece, popped in briefly after working in the area. I organised an injection for Alan because, worryingly, his grumbling chest was no better. Simon Beacham arrived for what was now a regular Wednesday evening catch up. As he left I asked, "Would you like an active part in Alan's funeral service?" Without hesitation he offered to read a poem. By late evening Alan still had grumbles so another district nurse came out to administer more glyco around 11pm.

Thursday 28ᵗʰ March – Carer's complaints
After her night sit, Laura reported that Alan had had a good night. What a relief. At 10:30am, Alan's friend, Kevin and his wife Ness arrived. They stayed with Alan for a couple of hours, giving me time to do chores around the house.

Alan and I were annoyed when a formal letter arrived out of the blue from the care agency, criticising our methods for trying to improve the care Alan received. The agency did not have independent assessors overseeing the work of their carers, so I felt it was up to me, as Alan's principal carer, to find a way to maintain standards. It was not something I relished but I needed to be confident that Alan was being cared for in the way he needed and deserved. Most of the carers were good. I suspected it was one of the less competent ones who had complained.

During the lunchtime carers visit, I checked out West Midlands Golf Club for its suitability for a wake. It was too brightly decorated and business like, so I disregarded it. Val, from our golf club, popped in bringing three lovely cakes. Alan could not have his - too much risk of choking. Alan returned to his bed when the lunchtime carers came. He slept most of the afternoon.

One of the teatime carers told me, "I have witnessed some carers complaining to the agency. I defended you and think you should reply to the letter with your viewpoint." I did not have the energy.

Alan's grumbles returned. Another dose of glyco was given before we returned to watching *Game of Thrones*. If I had been given authority to administer the drugs, I would not have had to keep calling the district nurses.

Friday 29th March - Useful distractions
Julie from Macmillan visited at 10am. After I had poured out my heart to her, she calmly went through Alan's list of medicines to reduce the risk of further mistakes. She arranged for a home visit from the wheelchair OT, to save us going to the wheelchair centre. "I will also arrange for the palliative care doctor from the hospice to visit you next time and we will get a prescription for some anti-sickness drugs to go into the Just in Case box". My stomach turned when she said, "I will visit weekly in future." That meant things were bad.

Just after lunch, I had to call the district nurse team for more glyco. Before they arrived, Alan became maudlin, saying, "I think I am getting close to the end."

I tried to reassure him. "We don't know that Al." My heart was breaking but I smiled and told him, "Sunderland Football Club have not yet been promoted, so you cannot go yet!"

When Eric came to give the glyco dose I sat outside and cried. Eric found me and tried to comfort me, but no words could save me from the pain I was feeling. To take our minds off upsetting thoughts Alan and I watched more *Game of Thrones*. As I gradually refocused myself on living in the moment, I blessed the makers of blockbuster box sets. We became so engrossed in the drama we were surprised when the carers turned up!

While Christina, from Alan's office, sat with Alan, I picked up extra supplies of glyco from a chemist. The extra supplies turned out to be necessary as Alan needed a further dose not long after I returned home.

Saturday 30th March - Calling 111
Laura reported Alan had various issues with his ventilator mask all night and had not slept well. Despite this, Alan chose to go into his wheelchair after his two hour morning routine. While in the lounge watching *The Crown* with Alan, I developed the art of multitasking. One eye on the TV, the other checking emails and Facebook messages! Katie, our speech and language therapist, had responded to my note about Alan no longer eating and only having small sips of liquid. "Unfortunately, I don't think there is much else we can do." I chose

not to tell Alan. I kept a lot more from him these days, which left me feeling isolated.

When the district nurse came to do the daily refill of the syringe driver, it was agreed to increase the driver dose of glyco to 800mgs - a 100% increase on the dose from a week ago. Mid-afternoon, Alan's chest grumbles returned so I called the district nurse team. Instead of giving more glyco as I expected, Eric called Julie at Macmillan's. They both agreed more needed to be done and that I should call 111.

After giving the triage nurse on 111 Alan's case history, symptoms, and temperature reading, she referred the matter up the line. Within minutes, a consultant called back and agreed a GP should examine Alan. At 5:15pm two doctors arrived and checked Alan's vital statistics. His blood pressure was 163/108 (a bit high), his heart rate was 84 (also a bit high), his blood oxygen saturation level was slightly low at 95% and his temperature was okay at 37.5C. It was agreed that some of the antibiotics in the Just in Case box should be used and paracetamol given. The doctors left me with the instruction, "If Alan's temperature goes above 38C, call 111 again."

My own breathing was shallow when I called Myton to cancel my role in the fundraising Glow Run. I also called Malcolm, Alan's friend, to cancel his visit. Once the carers had got Alan back into bed, we watched more *Game of Thrones*, but he was exhausted from the effort of coughing up a lot of fluid and phlegm.

When our brother-in-law, John arrived, we turned off the TV and within minutes Alan was asleep. I sat and watched Alan as he slept until the night sitter arrived. A million questions ran through my mind. Was he coming to the end of his life? How much longer could he go on like this? Should I call in Simon and his two sisters so they could be here, just in case? Would it worry Alan if I did that?

Sunday 31st March - Calling 999
Once again Alan had a bad night. He said he, "Could not get enough air." He slept most of the morning after a bed wash.

Eric reloaded the syringe driver and told me, "I spent most of the night thinking about you and Alan."

My eyes stung from the tears that were trying to get out.

While Alan slept, I quietly did jobs around house and replied to more emails. When the lunchtime carers arrived, I stuck red, white and black tape on the syringe driver tubes to make them easier for the carers to spot.

Our golf club friend, Andy arrived at 2pm to watch an important football match with Alan and John. Disappointingly, Sunderland lost the final by one penalty goal.

"We think you need to come to Alan," one of the carers said as they got Alan ready for bed. He didn't look good. He didn't argue when I suggested I call 111 again.

Laura, our night sitter, arrived while I was speaking to a helpful Scottish clinician at the 111 service. He managed to tweak the system so that the doctor could come out. It was 10:30pm. The doctor phoned me immediately. On hearing my assessment of the situation and reading the file notes, he told me to call 999. Fifteen minutes later an ambulance arrived. The paramedics did all the usual checks and confirmed temperature was up at 38.1C. Blood pressure was high at 150/93. Oxygen levels were low at 90% and pulse was high at 93. Some sort of infection was brewing.

Inside, I was panicking, but on the outside I stayed calm as the paramedics transferred Alan onto a trolley bed, after Laura and I had hoisted Alan off his own bed. Alan only agreed to go to hospital on the basis his condition was reversible. We had already been told by Marie Curie that Alan was on a pending list at the hospice, should he need admittance for symptom control or, if his condition became irreversible. As Alan was put into the ambulance John broke the tension, "Al, this is a bit of an overreaction to Sunderland losing!" Laura insisted on following me to the hospital in her car. John stayed behind to look after the house.

At Warwick Hospital, a nurse read all of Alan's statistics again and set up a drip for liquid paracetamol, sodium chloride and potassium. He also gave a large dose of strong antibiotics. An X-ray was done, together with blood tests, ECG and a sputum sample. I explained that we had been told that, in these situations, oxygen was not to be given because it would weaken muscles and cause carbon dioxide to build up. The nurse agreed.

Alan was admitted to Oken ward. I sent texts to Alan's family to update them and a text to Eric thanking him for all his support. Laura stayed with me and Alan till 3am. When I was sure Alan was settled, I kissed him, walked to the hospital car park, got into my car and broke down. It was 6am.

AUTHOR'S NOTE

The tubes from the syringe driver device to the needle just underneath Alan's skin, were long, transparent and thin. The drug in the tubes was also clear. These factors made it difficult to see the tubes amongst Alan's clothes and bedclothes. This meant the tubes to the driver needle were sometimes accidentally pulled out when carers handled Alan, resulting in less of the drug entering Alan's body. It turned out to be a good idea to put tape markers on the tube to reduce this risk.

APRIL 2019

Monday 1st April - Fearing the worst

By phone, I explained to Julie, at Macmillan, what had happened and hoped she would be able to get a bed at the Marie Curie Hospice, if Alan needed symptom control, or was coming to the end of his life. John asked, "What's your plans for selling Alan's car?" The BMW had been sitting on the drive, unused, for several months. "I don't have time or emotional strength to let it go at the moment," I replied.

Alan was on a bedpan when I reached him. As I helped the nurse clean him up, I noticed the poo was loose. "It's the third movement today." he announced, followed by, "The doctor told me to expect a three to four day stay in this hospital, because there is a large amount of fluid on my left lung. Pneumonia has been mentioned." I offered to give him a shave. He declined, but allowed me to change his nose mask to his full-face mask.

"Is it okay for me to stay with Alan outside normal visiting hours?" I asked the nurse. She approved, but said Alan would be moving to the ward that specialised in respiratory conditions soon.

"I am struggling to cope with everything now," were the first words Alan said when we were installed in Mary Ward. Before I could reply, he added, "I'm not sure if it's worth fighting the fight anymore."

I told him, "We need to find out more about what's happening and what they could do about it."

He surprised me with, "I don't want any visitors - not even Simon Beacham."

I frowned.

"Tell Simon I think my race is almost run."

The two of them had done lots of running together, including the Stratford-upon-Avon marathon. It was not like Alan to give up but, clearly, he was extremely low now. I felt scared.

Simon was dismayed when I called him. "Please tell Alan from me you're not at the end of the race yet." We both agreed not to speak to any of Alan's other ex-work colleagues at this stage. I spoke to Wendy. We agreed to still meet the following day for a brief coffee. I rang everyone who was due to see Alan and cancelled their visits.

"I am feeling sorry for myself," Alan said on my return.

"Oh Al. I know It's tough but remember at the beginning of all this we said we would not do self-pity."

At 9pm, Alan passed another motion and became distressed. "I feel like my body is emptying out," he said, looking glum. I could sense his fear, but I didn't know what to say. Before I left him at 11pm the nurse gave him Lorazepam to help reduce his anxiety.

Tuesday 2nd April - Advanced planning

Rain was pouring down outside when my alarm went off at 8:30am. Wendy arrived just after 10am and handed me two bunches of flowers. I drove us to Stonebridge Golf Club, which had a lovely room suitable for Alan's wake. It felt strange talking to the event manager at this time, but my thinking was simple. Alan may not be in mortal danger, but the more I could do now, the less there would be to do in the distressing days after Alan died.

Unusually, Alan would not talk to me when I first arrived at the hospital at around 2pm. A nurse was taking note of his vital statistics. His blood pressure was normal, as was his temperature and heart rate.

When we were alone, Alan revealed, "I have passed lots of poo but I'm worried that I have not passed any urine." He was still on antibiotics, via a cannula in his hand, as well as the usual drugs, via his syringe driver. "A doctor visited earlier but didn't tell me anything. Then one of the nurses messed up changing over the night mask to the nose one, which is why I am still on the night one." He told me another nurse, who could not hear what he was saying, had simply walked away from him. I noticed a nil by mouth sign above his bed.

A student doctor came and took a lot of notes about Alan's medical history. I asked him outright what was wrong with Alan. Without hesitation he replied, "He's got pneumonia."

A nutritionist arrived and said Alan would be given four Fortisip fortified drinks per day via his PEG at the same time as medicines were administered. Two more doctors arrived later, and confirmed Alan had aspiration pneumonia in his left lung. The pneumonia had been caused by food particles going down his windpipe and was different from viral or bacterial pneumonia. My conscience pricked me. Should I have limited what Alan took orally and used the PEG feeding method more? Alan loved his food, to deprive him would have been cruel.

The nil by mouth directive made sense to me now. I was asked if Alan had an advanced care plan. My mind was all over the place. Did we have one? Was that the same as the *Do not Resuscitate* document? The staff were worried about Alan having diarrhoea and began to talk of moving him to a private room. The prospect exacerbated his low mood.

Before I went home Alan told me, "I am nervous about the night team's ability to cope with my mask issues."

To reduce the risk of nurses getting it wrong, I spoke to the sister in charge, "It's important Alan's mask is regularly checked during the night. Even a small leak will severely reduce the amount of air he will receive."

Wednesday 3rd April - Shock at not finding Alan
My long, deep sleep was only disturbed when the delivery van arrived with the new tumble dryer. My plan, to get to the hospital in time for the 1pm meditation class at the Chapel, was foiled when Vicar Peter turned up unexpectedly. My tears fell as I spoke about life after Alan died, selling the house and mum going into a nursing home. He appeared to be sorrowful too and offered to lead a prayer.

When I reached Mary Ward I couldn't see Alan anywhere. For a split second I feared the worst. Surely the hospital would have called me if anything had happened? "Your man has been moved to the private room at the back of the ward," a fellow visitor told me. Phew! Before going into Alan's room, I quizzed a nurse who confirmed the move was only because of his record of passing stools.

Alan was in a very sorry state when I found him. No one had bothered to make it easier for him to communicate by changing the full mask to the nose only one. His mouth was thick with dried saliva which had crusted around his lips. As I set about making him more comfortable I felt terrible for taking so long to get to the hospital. I rearranged the room, so it was easier to move around his bed. He complained of feeling breathless. Although anger was bubbling up inside me, I calmly asked a nurse to give Alan some Oramorph and if we could see a doctor.

A lady called Hannah told us Alan had aspiration pneumonia, but nothing was growing by way of an infection. "Alan is now allowed sips of liquid by mouth if he wants them," she told me. "We are confident we have the right antibiotics in play." She was not aware of the X-ray that was supposed to be taken of

Alan's tummy to see if he had overflow. She didn't think overflow was the problem but arranged for some of the laxative drugs to be stopped.

After a bit of gentle persuasion, Alan agreed to see Simon Beacham. I made the phone call before Alan changed his mind. Once Simon had been and gone, I set up Netflix on the iPad so we could continue watching *The Crown*. Nothing I did relieved Alan's anxiety. It was 11pm when I left.

AUTHOR'S NOTE
Overflow is caused when the bowels are compacted, and liquid faeces squeezes past the hard stools coming out as a runny brown liquid.

Thursday 4th April - Planning next steps
Immediately on waking up naturally around 8.30am I called Julie at Macmillan so see if she had any influence over Alan's care at Warwick Hospital. In a telephone call with my friend Jill, she suggested leaving Alan's casket in the church after the funeral service. This was because I had confided in her that I couldn't face the idea of going from the church, a place of sanctuary, to a crematorium I'd never been to.

Alan needed me to change his mask and clean his teeth and mouth when I arrived. With me guiding his hand, Alan signed the form transferring ownership of his BMW to me so I could more easily deal with its sale. During a meeting to discuss our options with a registrar and Hannah, we agreed our preferred plan was to transfer Alan to the Marie Curie Hospice for symptom control, once he was well enough.

Alan started talking about the day we first met and wept. I held him for a long time when he declared, "I feel like I have taken a few more steps towards the end of my life." To distract him, I set up a war movie on iPad for him to watch so I could go and compose myself.

As I left the ward a young lady visiting an elderly man asked me about Alan's welfare. I explained he was terminal and needed twenty-four-hour care. She told me she had put her wedding on hold because her grandfather was so ill. Both our lives were on hold.

In the car park I purchased a weekly car parking ticket for £16. It had been costing £9 each trip because I had been staying at the hospital so long. Alan and I watched more of *The Crown* before I had to leave.

Friday 5th April - Ups and downs
In phone calls with Pauline and Viv, I explained Alan was improving slowly but

his spirits were not great. It was good to see Alan had perked up a lot when I arrived at the hospital. I did the usual mask changing and mouth cleaning for him. He agreed for me to go public with the news of his current situation, so I sent emails and texts to all our various friends. Wendy replied saying Mel had fallen because of his weak legs and, she complained about how poor the work of their carers was. Dawn from the golf club texted, saying her mum had passed away. It felt like there was nothing but sad news everywhere.

During the afternoon a nurse took Alan's daily statistics. Everything was looking better.

At 6pm we did a FaceTime video with Viv and John. The conversation was stilted because Alan found it hard to speak - partly from emotion but, also, his voice was weakening.

Around 9pm, I left Alan watching a documentary about the Roman Empire. It amazed me that he still had such a thirst for knowledge and a sharp mind. It was a blessing he had not developed frontotemporal dementia like some people with MND did. Talking to Stephanie in Doncaster about life now she was a young MND widow, gave me a glimpse of what was ahead of me. Sadness and loneliness.

Saturday 6th April - Problems with cannulas
There was a lot to do before I could visit Alan. Alan's car had to be taxed and arrangements needed to be made for people to visit him, including his nephew Tom, which would be a nice surprise.

Alan woke from his sleep when I was cleaning his face and mouth and changing over the masks from the night one to the day one. He told me there had been problems with his cannula, so the intravenous antibiotics had not been topped up. To take his mind off things, I read some of the forty or so replies to my latest Facebook post. Matt, one of the cyclists, had commented, "I would do the Land's End to John O'Groats bike ride all over again if I thought it would make a difference." Alan cried.

Some of the visitors to patients in Mary Ward were beginning to pop their heads into Alan's room, just to say hello, which was nice. During lunch, the sun came out and the sky was blue for the first time in several days. I hoped it was a positive sign.

Alan's antibiotic dose was five hours overdue, and his syringe driver was beeping, so I started chasing up the staff. One nurse tried to get a new cannula into Alan's left foot and then his left arm, without success. At 6:15pm a nurse took Alan's observations, so I mentioned the overdue antibiotics to her, having chased other nurses an hour earlier. Eventually around 8pm, a senior nurse finally got a new cannula into Alan's right wrist. I needed to consume more episodes of *The Crown* with Alan before I felt decompressed.

Sunday 7th April - Imaginary journeys

Waking up early gave me time to water the seeds I'd sprinkled over the bare patches in our lawn and do some special shopping on my way into hospital. The staff, patients and families in Mary Ward all appreciated my gift of an Easter egg each. The man, in the bed opposite Alan's, gave me a box of Milk Tray in return! Bless him.

As I was giving Alan a shave and face wash he reported he had not slept well. I was helping Alan with his leg exercises when our friends, Jo and Andy, visited. After they left I gave Alan his PEG feed, then we watched a film on the iPad. At 4pm, I received a text from Tom - he was in the building. My plan worked. Alan was delighted with the surprise visit from his youngest nephew.

As I was getting Alan ready for bed, he began to weep. "I want to come home." I was not sure we would cope at home given the amount of nursing and personal care he needed. He went on, "I am worried because my chest grumblings have started up again." I let him talk without replying. "To pass time, I sometimes imagine us travelling in a motorhome."

Before MND came along, we were planning trips in our retirement, taking several months touring across various continents, playing golf and skiing. It was incredible he could imagine things he would never be able to do, to help him stay sane during boring days in his 'cell'. I stayed with him till he fell asleep.

Monday 8th April - Move to Marie Curie in the air

Julie at Macmillan phoned. "Marie Curie will have a room for Alan later in the week." While I did the usual morning teeth cleaning, etc., for Alan I gave him the news, hoping it would lift his spirits. A doctor confirmed, that because previous blood test results were good, antibiotics could now be given via the PEG rather than via cannula. Good job we had the PEG!

While Hannah tried to take blood, without success, I thanked her. She looked perplexed. "Julie told me you helped get Alan a place at the Marie Curie." After two further unsuccessful attempts by doctors, eventually a senior nurse was successful prising blood out of Alan.

Tears fell down Alan's face while I was sorting out visitors for later in the week. "I have never had this many good friends in my life before," he sighed.

"You are loved by many, Al. Your situation has bought out the best in people. You would have done the same for them."

Tuesday 9th April - Move to the Marie Curie Hospice

The hospital called me. The hospice had a room available! I dashed over to the hospital. Within an hour, an ambulance crew had arrived and Alan was on his way to the hospice. As I followed the ambulance, tears poured down my cheeks. This time last week, I thought Alan was going to die.

Alan was installed into room nine. Shortly after, Dr Nikki and Dr Andrew arrived and asked Alan about his life and recent events. "I want to go home to die," Alan told them. They explained there were a few more steps before that could happen. Firstly, the strong antibiotics had given him oral thrush, so various drugs would need to be tried. Also, his chest grumblings and bowel movements would need to be stabilised and a social worker would need to check the correct care package was in place before he could go home.

At one point Fiona, our OT, popped in to provide a special call button device for Alan's pillow, which could be activated by his head. Unfortunately, when we tested it later, it was impossible for him to operate.

Simon Beacham arrived around 5:15pm, which released me to attend a meeting at mum's nursing home. The distance between mum and Alan was now just seven or so miles, so travelling between them would be a lot easier than the fifty-mile round trip I had been doing! It was useful meeting the relatives of the other residents and finding out what social activities were planned at mum's care home. She looked very thin and confused but overall she appeared happy, which was a great relief.

I sent texts to friends and family updating them about Alan's new location before returning to the hospice. Alan was watching ladies' international football, England versus Spain, when I reached him. There had been no TV at the hospital to take his mind off his health.

Adam arrived and introduced himself as Alan's night nurse. He was professional and charming - I could tell he and Alan would get on. Adam returned later with a nurse so I could train them both in how to change the various masks attached to Alan's ventilator. He had been using the machine to receive pressurised air for nearly twelve months, twenty-four hours a day for some time. I went to bed around midnight, totally exhausted.

Wednesday 10th April - Last rites offer

I arrived at the hospice and brought in Alan's special tilting shower chair. I found Chaplain Charlie (genuinely, that was his name!) with Alan, discussing the opening hours of the day centre. Alan appeared uninterested.

I noticed from Alan's drug chart he was now on four doses of Oramorph a day, which I hoped would settle down his breathing. Morgan, our psychologist, said she would arrange a referral to Hannah, the social worker. Hannah's help would be key to getting the right care package in place for when Alan returned home. Morgan left us with a note of her hours of work and invited Alan to ask to see her at any time.

Fiona collected the redundant head activated call button. Then Julie, the Macmillan nurse, arrived telling us she had only found out this morning that Alan had been admitted yesterday. Alan told her about his food fantasy - steak and kidney pudding. When I was eating my sandwich, he confessed to having recently dreamt of eating a corned beef and pickle sandwich, and a tuna and cucumber sandwich. That was odd because in all the time I lived with him, he only ever made himself ham and tomato sandwiches!

The day continued to be busy. Vicar Peter, from our church, arrived and offered us the use of the church grounds on 12th May to watch the 100 mile Vélo bike riders pass through the village. After praying with us, he startled me with, "You can call upon me at any time to administer last rites." He continued, pointing to his bag, "I always have everything with me."

Teresa, Phil and I discussed box sets while Phil tried to fix the TV which wasn't working. "You can stay over at ours anytime," Phil offered, "It's far closer than your house."

When I returned from a brief trip to the shops, I could see Alan's position had changed. "They gave me a suppository and an enema," he declared. Around 6pm Alan could feel his bowels grumbling, but only liquid went into the bedpan.

The nurse informed us, "A larger enema will be given tomorrow unless your bowels open naturally." I hoped the threat of such a thing would do the trick!

At the tea station outside Alan's room, a lady taught me how to give a soothing arm massage known as The M technique. I practised it on Alan to try to settle him before I went home. Restless and fretful, I didn't get to sleep before 3am.

Thursday 11th April - The Dignitas option
A heavy frost had formed overnight. It made me fear for the welfare of the seeds in our lawn. It seemed to me that all the things I'd lovingly cared for

lately were struggling to flourish. As an invited guest, I attended the Solihull Safeguarding Adults Board brainstorm at a hotel in Solihull. The Council decision makers were interested in my experiences of dealing with Adult Social Care teams so they could plan their next twelve months resources. I had plenty to tell them!

"Laura, the night sitter, visited today," Alan reported, "and staff tried to shower me using my chair in the en suite."

"How did that work out?" I enquired.

Eyebrows raised, he replied, "It was a bit of a debacle."

Around 1pm, Paul Whelan, from the MND monthly support meetings, rode in on his mobility scooter. We learned he was regularly at the hospice because he was involved in setting up the man shed. The two men chatted merrily about football and golf. Then Paul revealed, "I have already booked my place at Dignitas in Switzerland. I don't want to become a burden to others." Before his diagnosis in 2010, Paul lived in South Africa for twenty-five years. With his MND he had visited four times in the eight years. "My most recent visit was last month, for my son's wedding." I admired his spirit.

Paul told me about the tragic losses he had experienced in his life. Like so many people I'd met with MND, he'd had a successful career and was a charming character, full of passion for life. I was touched when he declared, "I hope when my time comes I'm half the man Alan has been."

Around 4.30pm, I was offered and accepted a massage by one of the therapists. Afterwards, feeling more relaxed, Alan and I watched the last episode of *The Crown*. I trained a new night nurse in how to change Alan's masks and left around 10:45pm, totally exhausted. I became aware that, sadly, this had become a regular part of our routine.

AUTHOR'S NOTE
The staff at the hospice were extremely willing and keen to help Alan, but it was a tricky job showering him in their en suite, which was half the size of ours at home. He was used to the Carter Castle tried and tested slick operation.

Friday 12th April - Bowel issues and oral thrush continue
My head ached and I felt sick when I woke. Was a migraine coming? There was no rush to get to the hospice as Alan's friend Malcolm was visiting. In Alan's study I started looking at what was involved in sorting it out. It felt weird going through his diaries, etc.

At the hospice, Alan said he was not impressed with one of the nurses. "She got my mask changeover wrong and wasn't good at listening to me." (I will call her nurse H).

Dr Andrew visited. "I am happy that secretions are more managed but not happy about continuing bowel movement issues and the thrush in your mouth, Alan."

At 5pm, a small army of carers came in to give Alan a bed wash. Again, Alan was not impressed. They were slow and didn't wash under his arms or back very well. Alan had always been fastidious about personal care, so it frustrated him when he didn't feel completely fresh. Soon afterwards Nurse H came in to do his medicines. I watched her carefully. I could see why Alan did not rate her.

Another new night nurse came in. I ascertained she was fully trained in how to change and adjust the masks before I went home. As I was leaving Alan tried to tell me something, but it was difficult to make it out. "Can it wait till tomorrow, Al?"

He nodded to indicate, 'Yes'.

Saturday 13th April - Tears and emotional declarations
With two days' worth of clothes and my wash bag, I arrived at the hospice around 10:45am, in time for a visit by Douglas from our golf club. He talked about his forthcoming bicycle challenge around Loch Ness and with a smile announced, "The fundraising for MND Association is going well. We could achieve £10,000!"

Alan asked for a bedpan immediately Douglas left. It took three or four carers a long time to hoist him and get the pan under him, then they needed me to hold the pee bottle in the appropriate place. It was Alan's second bowel opening of the day. At last!

When we were alone I asked, "What was it you tried to tell me last night Al?" He said, "I love you very much - to the edge of the known universe and back." I held him and we both cried.

After Alan and I had watched the second day's play from Augusta, Alan's golf club friends, Andy and Kulvinder, arrived so I left the three of them chatting. As I walked Alan's visitors back to reception, they told me they were surprised how chatty Alan was and, "We are playing in a Shirley Golf Club tournament tomorrow - we want to win it for Alan."

286

Alan was crying when I returned, "I am humbled that they took the time to visit me." He still could not believe how popular and loved he was.

We watched the third day's play from The Masters. It was exciting stuff which kept us up until midnight. I settled into the portable camp bed in Alan's room. After telling him I loved him, he responded with what he had said every night for over twelve months, "Thank you for looking after me."

Sunday 14th April - Bath time

It was not easy sleeping on a camp bed with all the machine noises. I stirred at 7:30am feeling cold, pulled up the blanket and dozed until 8:30am. When a nurse arrived to do Alan's medicines, I washed his face, gave him a shave, and cleaned his teeth. I asked the nurse why Alan was on paracetamol but she didn't know. I also mentioned that I had noticed Alan's hands and arms had become puffy.

During Dr Nikki's morning visit, she agreed to stop the paracetamol, increase the water retention tablets and reduce the glyco in the driver. "The persistent thrush in your mouth could be down to an imbalance in your saliva or the fact that your tongue is no longer working effectively." Turning to the nurse she instructed, "Cleaning Alan's mouth using sponges on sticks and descaling his tongue, will be needed from now on."

The next conversation was intense and pivotal.

The doctor asked, "What do you want to happen if you get another infection?"

Alan confirmed, "I don't want to go to hospital."

The doctor said, "In that case you would be treated with antibiotics at home, but you will not get better." She went on, "Your breathing will deteriorate and more Oramorph or Midazolam will be needed."

Finally, "If you are near end of life, and want to come to the hospice to be taken off the ventilation so you can die on your terms, we would give you drugs to ensure you are comfortable throughout the process."

For a moment the world stood still.

Alan looked downcast. "It's good having a plan, rather than just dealing with situations as they arise," he managed to say calmly. Part of me thought Alan had reached a new plateau. Maybe he could go on for some time as he was? We just needed to make sure he was well cared for and people with colds stayed away.

One of the carers announced, "We have a special bath waiting for you if you want it." Still keen to experience life to the full, he accepted.

A large, crane-like contraption was wheeled in. Alan's whole body was wrapped in towels and sheets and lifted up from his bed. With Alan held aloft, the contraption was driven around to an enormous room containing a huge jacuzzi bath. Three nurses and I steadied Alan as the arm of the contraption lowered him (and all the linen), into the water. I washed Alan's hair - giving it the kind of scrubbing he loved - while the nurses turned on the jets. Alan revelled in the sensation of his legs floating in the water.

After his special bath, the crane winched him out and nurses covered him in fresh towels. With water dripping everywhere, the crane, returned Alan to room nine so nurses could dry him and apply moisturiser. "Not a bad way to spend our monthly anniversary," he joked, "Now I know how sheep feel being dipped!"

At lunchtime I walked into town, picked up a Happy Anniversary helium balloon, a newspaper and some lunch. Back at the hospice we watched the final day's play of the golf from Augusta. Tiger Woods won. I nodded off several times while we watched a new drama, before lights went out at 11pm.

Monday 15th April - Planning a continuing care package
During the night, Alan's mask slipped several times so we both had a disturbed night. When the nurse came to do Alan's morning medicines Alan needed to use a bedpan. It was a good time for me to go home to do some chores.

During the afternoon our visitor Adrian shared stories of the cruises he had done with his wife, Alison. Alan was probably too poorly to go on a cruise now, other than in his vivid imagination. The inside of Alan's mouth looked awful despite the drugs being used to clear up the thrush. A swab of his saliva was taken.

The hospice social worker, Hannah and the continuing health care (CHC) nurse popped in. It was agreed that Alan probably needed level three care, whatever that was, but a full assessment would be necessary. The 10pm news included pictures of a terrible fire at Notre Dame Cathedral in Paris. I went home when the programme ended.

Tuesday 16th April - Feelings of impending doom
At Walmley Golf Club, my friend Jo and I played well despite my mind being elsewhere. Part way around the course, I told Jo, "I think I have built a shield around me, to stop feelings getting in or out". I was aware other women with

terminally husbands had done the same. "I have become a bit of a machine, going through the daily routines without feeling anything."

After lunch with Jo, I returned to the hospice, without a prize, but refreshed by the exercise. During the day, Alan had been visited by our friends, Carol and Graham, followed by Kevin, Sue and Tyler. Paul Whelan and Tom had also popped in.

The morning in the open air gave me time to reflect. I opened up to Alan. "Jo has suggested she and I go away in the future."

Once again Alan stressed, "I don't want you to be alone once I pass away."

"I know, Alan, but it's very difficult to imagine wanting to be married again."

He reminded me, "I felt like that before I met you."

"What changed your mind?" I asked.

"I didn't want to lose you, so marriage was the right step."

We both cried. It made me feel unhappy seeing tears in Alan's eyes.

"Let's think about all the wonderful memories we have," I suggested.

"This time last year we were in Vietnam," Alan reflected.

At home, I read more of *With the End in Mind*, a book by palliative care consultant, Kathryn Mannix. A knot built in my gut and the tears fell as I learned about people who had been cared for to the end of their lives in hospices.

Wednesday 17th April - Up and about
The ironing and housework complete, I watered the bare patches of the back lawn. I'd given up trying to salvage the sorry looking, front lawn. In room nine I was surprised to see Alan sitting in a special padded blue chair. The chair was on casters, so I pushed open the double doors, and wheeled him around the water fountain in the garden. It was such a nice day I continued our journey through the main building and out into another garden. Archways of climbing plants created welcome shade over the paths and the scent of spring flowers filled the air.

On our way to the MND support meeting, we stopped at the hospice memorial garden. On a huge stainless steel obelisk, there was a quotation from Marie Curie.

"Nothing in life is to be feared.
It is only to be understood.
Now is the time to understand more,
so that we may fear less"

At the MND support meeting, chaired by Fiona, our OT, we caught up with other families living with the Mean Nasty Disease.

Some families were having issues with care companies, others were considering the option of using the hospice for respite. I explained our positive experience of the hospice in-patient unit and demonstrated the Barbara book, which we were beginning to use, to help us understand Alan's needs. It was odd seeing how much Alan had deteriorated compared to some people who had been diagnosed many years before him. At the end, Mel and Wendy visited Alan because he had retired to room nine during the meeting.

When I went to fetch some water, I found our skiing friends, Bev and John, waiting at the tea station. I had forgotten they were coming! I gave Bev an M technique hand massage while John spoke with Alan. When the nurses came to give Alan his medicines, Bev, John and I went outside where I shared the recent decisions Alan had made regarding next steps.

Thursday 18th April - Andrew's wedding day
All dressed up in a white, pink and pale green dress and a bright pink fascinator, I popped in to see Alan. The last thing I felt like doing was going to a wedding, but I would not let down my nephew and godson, Andrew and bride to be Lauren.

The venue was a lovely purpose-built barn. It was good to be with my family and see Lauren and Andrew looking so happy. Christina Perri sang, *Love You for a Thousand Years*, while Andrew's brother, Callum and I, witnessed the signatures of the newly married couple.

When there was an appropriate moment, I showed Andrew and Lauren a video Alan had made for them. With his now very weak voice, he wished them a long and happy life and apologised for not being with them. When it was over Lauren touched the screen as if to touch Alan's face. Andrew said, "Alan is with us all today."

During the wedding breakfast I sat next to my sister, Rowena. She broke down in tears a few times so I took her outside and asked what was wrong. "It's horrible what's happening to Alan," she wept, "It's just not fair." We both cried.

During the evening reception I caught up with most of my family. The day had been enjoyable, and I was not the emotional wreck I feared I would be, but I left as soon as I could. Driving home I had a strong feeling of wanting to be with Alan - just like in the early days of our courtship, so I diverted to the hospice and surprised him. My love for him was greater than ever.

Friday 19th April - Good Friday
While watering the front lawn I had a good chat with Alison, my neighbour opposite. We agreed to have a night out when the opportunity arose.

Alan was unwell and being checked over by a nurse when I arrived. He complained of feeling weak and having 'something' in his throat. He was flushed and was struggling to breathe. A doctor checked his ears, nose and throat and found his ears were blocked. Another problem was the build up inside his digestive system was putting pressure on his diaphragm.

Andy Gould, from the golf club, patiently waited outside Alan's room. He agreed to obtain some olive oil ear drops from the chemist. Pineapple juice was prescribed as a natural remedy for oral thrush. I stayed overnight at the hospice. I got up at least a dozen times to sort out mask issues for Alan. Without my usual eye mask or earplugs with me, it was a bad night. I could not block out the light and noise.

Saturday 20th April - Fond memories
I delivered Easter eggs to mum and the care home staff. Mum picked at her chocolate egg and chatted away about events from her past. She seemed okay.

Back at the hospice late afternoon, Rowena and her husband Steve had a long wait to see Alan who was having another sheep dip bath. He told me several people had struggled with the ventilator tubing, which was why he was still on his night mask. He had enjoyed seeing Jo and Andy earlier. Totally shattered, I left for home earlier than usual.

Sunday 21st April - Fairy Garden sign
My morning was spent catching up with letters and emails and getting the house ready for Viv and John's visit. At the hospice, Nina and Robert visited. Alan was distressed. The call button we had rigged up by his head was not working and he needed a pee. By the time I found a bottle, it was too late. Whoops!

Nurses changed Alan's pad while Nina and Robert strolled the hospice grounds. Back in room nine they shared details of the South Africa trip with us.

After lunch, I collected Viv and John from the station and John stayed with Alan, while Viv and I walked in the fairy garden. We found a plaque which I liked:

"Every day may not be good, but there is good in every day"

Alan's voice was weak, so I helped him explain to Viv and John the end-of-life decisions. To cheer him up we watched the Heineken Cup rugby semi-final, followed by an old John Wayne movie. The three of us left around 8pm.

Monday 22nd April - Clever new system for hydration

We left for the hospice around 10:45am. By the time we reached Alan, impressively, he was already in his day mask having had his medicines, a wash and so on. Viv and I did some shopping in Solihull. John and Alan were watching a movie, while keeping an eye on the football scores, when we returned.

The Sunderland team were close to a play-off position in League Division One. Their success was helping Alan's mood. Momentarily, I thought about writing to the team manager and asking for a favour for Alan, but then remembered my 'to do' list was already overflowing. Nurse Adam set up a new management system for ensuring Alan was given regular mouth washes and sips of water. He was a top nurse.

Tuesday 23rd April - Florence Nightingale lives

As I was watering the patches of the lawn, I realised I was willing the grass to spring into life. It was a shame I could not sprinkle water on Alan, to return him to full health. "I had a good night," Alan told Viv, John and me, "but my throat is sore. It's been flagged with the doctor when he did his usual assessment of all my symptoms." Alan would not be going home any time soon.

Alan smiled widely as I straightened his bed linen. "What's so amusing?" I asked.

"You look like Florence Nightingale," he grinned, "I love you." It was nice to see he was calmer and brighter than he had been for several weeks. Back at the house, I could not sleep for fretting Alan might die soon. The last time I checked the clock before I dropped off, it was 1.30am.

Wednesday 24th April - Another sad milestone occurs

Around 7am, I woke up with a start. I thought I heard Alan take a deep breath and, then everything went quiet. The dream was preceded by a nightmare where I was trapped by a large volume of incoming water.

A poem started brewing in my mind.

ANOTHER DAY

Another day over,
Another day closer to the end.
Another day when the sun rained down,
And soothed our troubled brows.
Or the rain fell like tears,
And refreshed our weary souls.
Another day when
Your face betrayed you,
Showing a smile when, deep inside,
You were crying.
Another day when
Your vital signs were good,
But really
You are dying.
Each passing day is one more step,
Towards the cliff
From which we will both fall.
The cliff that is
The end of life for you,
And an open book,
With no text for me at all.
A dark gaping ravine,
Too awful to imagine,
Too painful to conceive.
So I don't go there.
I just get through another day,
Knowing the next could be the last.
Tomorrow I will wake,
To face another day,
And make the most of what I've got.
But you, my beloved darling,
One day, will not.

The tree and hedge cutting man arrived and my brother Kevin phoned. He wanted me to meet him at mum's flat so he could collect some items. By mid-morning I felt frazzled. Trusting the tree man to do a good job, I left him at the house and drove to the hospice. At reception, I collected a prize, a large chocolate bunny, Viv had won by successfully guessing its name was Scooter. She chose Scooter because she and John had recently bought a real one!

During the afternoon, the man from the wills company presented us with documents to sign in front of our friend, Christine. It was like a scene from a movie seeing the wills man help Alan sign his name. Indeed, most of the time these days, events felt like scenes in a drama or film. Suddenly my worst fear came true. Alan's voice stopped working. I had got him ready for bed and put his night mask on when he tried to say something, but the words were too garbled to understand.

I grabbed the Barbara book but still could not establish or guess what he wanted. I welled up and hugged him. "Don't panic Al, I am going to stay with you till you fall asleep."

Eventually he managed to say, "What's the matter?" I had assumed he was too hot or too cold or needed a pee bottle but, all along he was concerned about me. I told him some of my fears and held him for a long time afterwards.

Even though I didn't have an overnight bag, I made up the camp bed and tried to sleep, surrounded by the noise from the ventilation machine and air mattress motor, and with an ache in my heart cutting me in two.

Thursday 25th April - Poignant question

It was not a good night's sleep. Several strange dreams came to me. Either Alan or his ventilator alarm woke me, at 1am, 2:15am, 3:30am, 4:45am, and 7:30am. Each time, I adjusted his mask to reduce leaks. When Alan asked me to adjust his mask again at 8:15am, I decided to get up. My head was throbbing. Nurses came in at 8:30am. We agreed to let Alan rest. I had a shower, while nurses gave Alan his medicines.

Near the tea station I met Ellie. I taught her the M Technique massage so she could do it on her mum. At Chaplain Charlie's weekly service in the hospice's Quiet Room, I found the hymns and prayers emotional. Most people attending were in-patients and older than me.

Back in room nine, Ian had finished reading and acting out a short story to entertain Alan. I was impressed that Ian and Sue didn't leave the room or flinch when a nurse came in and gave Alan his medicines via his PEG tube. Around 1:30pm, Alan fell asleep. He didn't stir when the staff came back at 2:30pm to give more drugs. Was he fading away?

At 6pm, Simon Beacham arrived and stayed till just after 8pm. As I walked Simon to reception, he became the first person to ask the question on everyone's mind, "Do you think Alan will make it out of here?" I didn't have an answer. After watching some TV with Alan, I went home, full of fear Alan would never return to Carter Castle.

Friday 26th April - Golfing stories

The doorbell rang, it was the lymphoedema nurse, who was not aware of recent events. "I will update our records," she promised, after I tearfully explained how ill Alan was. "Don't worry Hazel. If you need us in the future, you will be given top priority."

Andy, from the golf club was at the hospice when I arrived, waiting to see Alan, who was being given his medicines and having a wash. Andy's wife Dawn then arrived so the three of us sat and chatted in the Family Room. They noticed my bag full of books and papers and jokingly asked "Are you carrying around an office!" I showed them my two handwritten journals of Alan's life since diagnosis, my blue book full of medical meeting notes and read them some of my poems. Dawn hugged me with tears in her eyes.

My sister Clare and her husband David arrived just after lunch. Every one of our visitors, except Clare, talked about golf. "I will take it up when David retires," Clare promised.

Alan entertained us with tales of how he filled up time when alone in his room. "I imagine myself changing my shoes, preparing my golf clubs and walking up to the first tee," he explained. "I hardly ever make a bad shot these days," he joked, "In fact, I play like a pro!"

I could not resist coming back with, "Well, that's a bit different from when you used to lose your temper at all those duff shots, when we played practice rounds together."

Andy chipped in with, "Several of us at the club have been shocked how you always manage to beat us, Alan."

I met a lady from South Africa called Cathy, at the tea station. We had a good chat.

Alan and I finished one drama and started a new one. Eventually, we exchanged our usual lovely good night messages and I settled down onto the camp bed. When I was writing in my journal, I realised I was now putting down minute by minute detail - every moment was beginning to be important.

Saturday 27th April - Persistent leaks from night mask

All through the night Alan's alarm was triggered because of leaks from his ventilator mask. I had to make adjustments at 12:30am, 1:30am, 2pm, 2:30pm, 3:15am, 3:30am, 3:50am and 4:10am. In the end I had no choice but to disable the alarm, but I still woke up when he called out or the mask whistled as air escaped.

At 5:55am Alan wanted water. At 6:20am he wanted a bedpan. While nurses tended to him, I put on my bathrobe, took a pillow and blanket, and hunkered down on the black leather settee in the Family Room. Twenty minutes later, I was cold and still awake. I closed the blinds and curtains and eventually fell to sleep. When I woke it was 8am, but I was too tired to move so hunkered down again until 9am.

A nurse was doing Alan's medicines when I grabbed my clothes and toiletries from the bedroom. I showered and got dressed in the visitor's wet room. (No one was allowed to use in-patient en suite rooms).

On returning to Alan, he and I agreed we both needed more rest. I put a 'Do not disturb' sign on the door and closed the curtains. Alan slept while I put all the scribbled notes I'd made in the night into my journal. Teresa and I chatted in the Family Room about her father's death, walked around the hospice grounds and sat in the Quiet Room for a few minutes, while Alan slept.

Dr Beverley came to check on Alan. She suggested trying paracetamol and linctus for his throat. She also suggested he try pica-sulphate, a strong laxative, to help empty his bowels.

Early afternoon, I left Alan and visited mum. She was in good spirits and had been moved to a larger room on the ground floor. I put family photographs on her wall and gave her some chocolate eclairs - her favourite. She spoke of someone pouring hot water on her and calling in the police. These were the sort of things she had imagined in the past, so I didn't take it too seriously.

Back at the hospice, I was concerned when a nurse told me about an incident where Alan wasn't getting enough air from his ventilator machine. Alan was convinced someone had blocked up the intake valve. Carers denied anything was on or blocking the machine. I hoped this was not a sign that his breathing muscles were failing.

We watched the rest of the new drama. I felt irritable due to lack of sleep so left earlier than usual, fearing I would become impatient if I didn't get some proper rest. It was difficult to sleep, after reading more of *With the End in Mind*, so I sent text messages to people I hadn't spoken to in a while.

Sunday 28th April - Major incident with the non-invasive ventilator (NIV)
The day started badly. I couldn't stop crying and thinking about Alan's voice

disappearing. Frequent, open conversations had been a major part of our relationship, in particular, since he was diagnosed. Alan had a beautiful Sunderland accent and a large repertoire of affectionate things he said to me which I was going to miss. I wasn't sure how we would cope when his speech completely failed.

It took me till noon to get up. I couldn't face the world. Watching the London Marathon helped me feel less sorry for myself. I arrived at the hospice early afternoon.

Nurse Adam told me the pipe from Alan's NIV facemask had broken and, at one point, the NIV stopped working as they were wheeling Alan to the bathroom. Adam reported all the staff involved were shocked but got the situation under control quickly. I could only imagine the distress Alan had endured. Without an effective NIV Alan would die, which was why it was so important mask changeovers were handled efficiently and the battery in the machine was fully charged at all times, ready for when Alan was in transit. I was angry at myself for hiding away at home and being so selfish.

Friends from the golf club, Peter and Joy, came to visit Alan. Before I took them to room nine I explained they may not be able to understand Alan. There was a buzz in the air of the large foyer. People, who had been cycling 30, 70, or 100 kilometres for the benefit of the hospice, were enjoying cakes and drinks after their efforts. I read a text from Douglas to Alan, confirming he had completed the 106 kilometre Loch Ness cycle ride and that fundraising for MND Association was going better than planned.

Due to the incident with the ventilator earlier in the day, I retrained three of the carers and showed them how to use the Barbara book. With its list of pre-set requests, the book was going to be an invaluable tool. When any of us pointed to the requests, one after another, Alan would nod a "yes" when we reached the right one.

While Alan could still be understood, I asked, "How are you feeling Al?"

"I fear I am close to death," he sighed. "I'm worried what it will be like at the end, and how I will feel leaving you."

We agreed we needed to see Morgan, our psychologist, for a chat. "I also want to see Dr Nikki to better understand how I would be cared for at home if I got another infection," Alan requested, because he did not want to go back to hospital.

Monday 29th April - A crucial meetings with doctors

After making an effort to be positive, focus on Alan's needs, and telling myself I was going to be okay, I went into action mode when I got to the hospice. I organised meetings with Morgan and the doctor. I busied myself cleaning Alan's teeth, swabbing his mouth, and giving him a shave before his friend Malcolm arrived. At the tea station I had a chat with Lesley. Her husband was in the hospice having fought three lots of cancer!

Two of the hospice doctors asked to see me.

In the Family Room, I responded to their questions then shared my concerns about how we might manage Alan's wish to die at home, with the need for intensive support. Finally, I explained about mum and how hard it was coping with everything.

Around 2:30pm, Viv and John arrived. Within minutes a meeting started in room nine involving Alan, Viv, John and I, two doctors and two nurses. There was talk about reducing how much water Alan took orally, because of the risk of infection or pneumonia. A microbiologist was to be called in because Alan's oral thrush was not improving. Also, it was agreed to reduce the volume of glyco in his syringe driver.

Tuesday 30th April - Changes to drug prescription

The sun shone brightly as Viv showed me inside their new motorhome parked on our drive. I was pleased for Viv and John but grieved for the fact Alan and I could no longer travel.

At the hospice, with Viv's permission, I broke Scooter, the giant Easter chocolate rabbit, into pieces and shared them with the staff and volunteers throughout the hospice. "Will you take a video of the inside of the new motorhome when you get home, babe, so I can see it?" Alan requested. He might be becoming totally locked in, but Alan still had his wits!

Dr Andrew agreed with Alan to reduce the glyco to 700 micrograms, and increase the furosemide, which was being used to reduce water retention. For a while, Paul Whelan joined Viv, John and I in Alan's room. When a chaplain came to visit Alan, Viv and John said their goodbyes. I left around 10pm and spent the evening listening to classical music to help me relax.

Wednesday 1st May - Alan's legacy

A fitful night resulted in me only getting about five hours' sleep. Alan was very quiet. He'd had a bad night too. A physio was in his room and had set up a second NIV machine as a backup. Alan's voice was weak and garbled. Alan's friend David from Leeds left around 1:30pm following which Alan had a bath and a snooze.

Alan and I had a chat about his life's legacy. Always a modest man, he struggled to come up with any thoughts. "One legacy, Al, is you have given me the best thirteen years of my life." He blinked back his tears.

Two nurses repositioned Alan, to help reduce the wind that was building up in his bowels, while I did some paperwork near the tea station. Alyson, the hospice social worker, asked me in her warm Irish accent, "How are you doing?" On hearing about my recent meltdown, she told me I needed to look after myself. How do I do that when Alan needs me so much and then there is mum, the house etc?

As I walked Alan's nephews, Tom and Ben, from reception, I explained how much Alan had deteriorated - I didn't want them to be shocked. Simon Beacham arrived around 5pm so the three chaps entertained Alan while I drove to Sutton Coldfield to see Wendy. Her husband, Mel, was having similar challenges to Alan. I felt for her when she relayed the catalogue of issues she was having with carers.

My friend, Jo approved of the idea of us all leaving Alan's coffin at the church while we went on to the wake, rather than us all going over to the crematorium for twenty minutes and then to the wake. At a nearby Asda store, I finally managed to find peppermint cordial. It had been suggested as an aid for dealing with Alan's wind but had been hard to source.

Thursday 2nd May - Our Best Man volunteers for a key role at funeral

For the third time, I woke up to discover Alan's wedding ring had come off the chain around my neck, but the chain itself was still done up. Weird!

While at the Marie Curie Hospice, Alan's friend, Kevin, phoned me from Myton Hospice. Whoops, I had forgotten to let him know that Alan had moved. Pauline and Simon arrived around noon followed soon after by our Best Man, our nephew, Matthew.

I bumped into Morgan in one of the corridors and told her, "Alan has been more down lately - he's been thinking about his death."

With a heavy heart I added, "Also, I don't want to say anything to him, but I feel he would be better cared for at the hospice than at home."

"You two have always been honest with each other," she reminded me. "Alan would want to know your feelings."

She was right.

"Do you know why Alan wants to be at home?" she asked.

I didn't but I could guess.

I had to explain to Alan that social services could not meet with us until 17th May. I asked him how he felt about staying at the hospice till at least then. He was not happy. When he said he was getting bored I set him a challenge. "Maybe it's time you got to grips with using the Eyegaze communication tool?"

While I gave Pauline an arm massage, we discussed Alan's complex care needs. She thought it was best if Alan stayed at the hospice, because the care was excellent and available around the clock.

Alone with Matthew I mentioned, "I don't have anyone to give the eulogy at Alan's funeral." He volunteered without hesitation.

"I'm not getting enough air," Alan complained. The mask was fitted well, so I found a nurse and asked for a dose of oral morphine. One of the therapists gave Alan a soothing foot and head massage soon after Pauline and Simon left.

Friday 3rd May - Anger and frustration
If Alan made it home I decided Yvonne, the private carer who had been recommended to me, would be hired to supplement the state carers and give me more time to just be with Alan.

When I reached Alan he looked uncomfortable, his bed was a mess and the room looked different. He mumbled, "There's been issues with my masks and the call button system you rigged up didn't work." In anger, I hit the call button. Two carers arrived and finished off the wash they had started giving Alan an hour earlier.

After the team left, Alan and I tried to have a conversation. I was still angry at the staff and became frustrated because I couldn't understand what he was trying to say. Generally, I was fed up with our situation and felt distraught, because it was only going to get worse. I found some cycling on the TV for Alan to watch, while I went outside and gathered myself together. Two planned visitors texted to say they would be late. Sometimes well-planned days went like that.

While the nurse was topping up the medication in Alan's syringe driver I asked, "What happened before I arrived?"

"Alan became anxious about his breathing, so we gave him Oramorph, under doctor's orders, and left him to rest rather than continue with his wash." She added, "Communication became difficult. It would be easier if he used the Eyegaze device."

"Nice idea," I said, "but Eyegaze is impossible to use when he is being washed, or watching TV, because the device needs to be directly opposite his eyes."

Jo arrived with her new husband and was carrying a huge cheerful bouquet of flowers (which had to be donated to the staff, as they were not allowed in patient's rooms). After their visit, I walked the couple back to reception. "I am sorry we have not seen Alan sooner and were not able to invite you to the wedding," Jo sighed.

On his visit the doctor confirmed my suspicions. "Alan's breathing muscles are getting weaker - hence his voice is disappearing."

When nurse Adam came on duty I relayed the day's events. Before I left Alan, Adam and I checked and tested the call button system to make sure it worked properly.

Saturday 4th May – 'Talking' via technology
I woke with a headache, so stayed in bed until 8:30am. After some housework I set off to the hospice. Helen, Alan's niece, Richard and their two boys were already with Alan when I arrived.

Over lunch in the hospice café, I shared the plans for Alan's funeral with Helen. She knew Tom and Ben were being pallbearers and that Matthew was doing the eulogy. I asked her to consider reading a poem.

After lunch we set up Alan's Eyegaze device and he amazed his great nephews by 'talking' to them through it. Sounding like a Sunderland version of Professor Hawking, he asked "How are you?" They were amused when he responded to their questions. It didn't always work, due to operator error, resulting in laughter from us all. My feelings oscillated between joy at seeing him interact with his beloved family and heartache, because soon I would never hear his natural voice again.

I took the boys for a walk around the fairy garden so Helen and Richard could have private time with Alan. On the walk out of the hospice, Helen wept. "I will come again, soon, on my own," she sobbed as we hugged tightly.

Sunday 5th May - Simplifying Eyegaze
Alan didn't look comfortable when I arrived around lunchtime. I adjusted his pillows and set up the TV so he could watch the Tour de Yorkshire. On examining Alan's PEG site - which I did most days - it looked sore, but no one appeared concerned. He was drowsy due to the oral morphine he'd had earlier. I made some edits to the standard phrases we had set up in the Eyegaze device, to make the system easier for Alan to use.

At the tea station, I had a brief chat with Cathy, the lady from South Africa. "They have told me David is close to the end," she sobbed. I felt nervous, for her and myself. It was all getting too real. Alan asked for a sip of water but choked a lot while trying to drink it. Terrified he could choke to death, I decided I would only give water under his tongue using a syringe or feed him ice chips, in future.

Monday 6th May - Feeling totally useless
When I arrived at the hospice around 10am, Ian and Sue, parents of Jo from Leeds and Jo's sister Sam, were there with Sam's baby. Sam and I went for a short walk while Ian and Sue had private time with Alan. I was pleased Alan used Eyegaze a lot during their visit. Ski Gang friends, Bev and John, arrived at 2:30pm. I gave instructions, Alan was only to have ice chips if he got thirsty and left them while I met Teresa in Solihull.

Back at the hospice, Alan complained of issues with his mask. On examination I could see the strap was cutting into the top of his left ear and a pressure sore was coming up on his nose. A nurse told me these were common problems with ventilator masks, as we applied pressure relieving tape to the affected areas to reduce further damage.

Alan became emotional when we were watching TV because his voice was almost gone. Later, when I was giving him a shave, which had become one of my favourite jobs because I had to get really close to him, I began to feel totally useless and burst into tears. With difficulty Alan managed, "This is hard on you now."

My throat tightened. "I don't know what to say anymore, Al, or how to best help you."

At home, my mood was even lower. There was so much I needed to discuss with Alan. I wanted to talk about my fears of coping when he came home but was afraid to raise the matter, being at home meant so much to him. I felt unprepared for speaking with him, only via Eyegaze. Most of all, I wanted to tell him that I couldn't bear the thought of him dying.

Tuesday 7th May - Things getting worse

In the middle of the night, I woke up with a start. I thought I heard Alan calling me. Before I reached Alan at 11am I went for my bi-annual health screen. Despite all the pressures of late, surprisingly, my blood pressure was normal! Alan reported having slept well using a new style mask over his mouth and nose. He watched the news, while I sat in the corner writing up my journal.

"I am worried about the colour of Alan's saliva," the lady doctor said. "I will chase up the results of the mouth swabs." There was to be no change to Alan's current medicines, however, she thought Alan should start a short course of antidepressants. Alan declined to have his glyco dose reduced further.

Before Julie, our Macmillan nurse, came to see Alan, she and I had a chat about the challenges of caring for Alan at home. She explained that until social services responded regarding the care package, it would be difficult to make informed decisions. Additionally, she mentioned we may not be able to have the same care company, in which case, new carers would need to be trained. Neither Alan nor I had thought about that. Training up a fresh team of carers filled me with dread.

Our friends, Jo and Andy arrived. However, Alan was tired so was unable to use the Eyegaze machine effectively, which made conversation difficult. Later, alone with Alan, we listened to soft music and I held him for a long time while we both cried.

Wednesday 8th May - Another drug in the cocktail

Heavy rain was falling when I woke. I put more seed on the lawn, did the washing up and other chores, before going to the chemist. I briefly popped into the golf club, to see if I had missed any notices, then visited mum.

Tom, from the golf club, sent a text saying he had been unable to wake Alan when he arrived at 10am. Nurses had washed Alan and Tom stayed till 12:30pm. Bless him. Teresa and Phil were with Alan by the time I arrived. I trained them in using the Barbara book. They left at around 4pm with a hearty, "We will be back Saturday Alan, to watch the Sunderland game with you."

I met up with recently bereaved Dawn from the golf club. She had read out a tribute at her mum's funeral which convinced me I should speak at Alan's service. Dawn gave me hints on how to prepare properly for reading my tribute to Alan. We burst into giggles when she advised, "Clenching your bum cheeks will prevent crying!" Despite the laughter, we both cried a lot and had a huge hug before we said goodbye.

Work colleague, Kevin and Simon Beacham were at the hospice by the time I returned. When they had struggled to understand Alan wanted some ice chips, I realised I needed to give them, and all visitors, training in the use of the Barbara book.

After Kevin left, Simon gave Alan a shave and cleaned his teeth. It was always difficult deciding whether to invite people to help with care or not, as I didn't want to upset them, or Alan. In the main, people were willing to assist, and Alan always agreed. One of the nurses confirmed Alan had started his antidepressant drugs yesterday. Citalopram was now part of his cocktail.

Thursday 9th May - Deep and difficult conversations
More heavy rain fell while I read my journal entries from early November 2017 to September 2018. It was painful reading the period when only Alan and I knew what was going on - the last time our lives were private. Since diagnosis, everything had happened so fast. Since Alan went into hospital in December, our world had shrunk - we had become housebound and it was harder to have joy in our lives.

As I reflected, I realised we were now entering a new, probably final phase. It felt like I'd already lost Alan. Normal conversation about day-to-day things had gone. Dialogue nowadays consisted of me trying to understand Alan's needs, or me finding things to say to keep him cheerful. Trying to hold him had become awkward, because of the shape of his profile bed and the syringe drive and ventilator tubes. He even felt physically different when I did hold him - his bony shoulders a reminder of the toll MND had taken on his body.

As I wrote the entry for 8th May, I noted there were seventy-eight pages left - about thirty-nine days' worth. I calculated that our 5th wedding anniversary was thirty-six days away and Alan's sixty fifth birthday, forty-six days away. I hoped he would live to enjoy them.

At the hospice, Alan needed to be changed and washed, having passed a motion in his pad. The team cleaned him up ready for our meeting with the psychologist. Morgan tried to work out if Alan had accepted his situation, and if he had not, whether that was stopping him living In and enjoying the moment. He mumbled, "There are times when my mind goes to sad places."

Morgan asked, "How helpful is it when you drift into those thoughts?" Because Alan confirmed it was not helpful, it was agreed I had to signal to Alan if I thought he was not being 'present'.

Morgan explained, "Tiredness and weakness can make a person feel their demise is just around the corner, when it may not be."

Alan responded, "I am worried about how Hazel will cope after I die." We both admitted everything was hard now. It was tough trying to make the most of life, given our limited situation.

"You two are great at the human 'doing', but now is the time to be human 'beings'. All you need to do is be present, in the moment, with each other."

"I feel Hazel is withdrawing emotionally," Alan lamented.

"I have been trying to preserve my feelings because, I know, Alan could die any day," I admitted.

"Maybe Alan," Morgan began, "You could blink your eyes rapidly if you feel Hazel is not being present with you?"

Morgan's final question was telling: "What do you both specifically want out of the next few days?"

Alan went first. "I want things I cannot have," but he would not elaborate.

"I want more time holding Alan, and to lie with him on his bed, but it's difficult."

Before Morgan left I crouched down by Alan and she held his arm in place around my back. "You are always going to be with me in the future, Al, wherever I go. Even if it's places you don't want to go to!" I joked to try to ease the atmosphere.

Alan fell asleep after Morgan left, until a doctor arrived mid-afternoon. The usual medical things were checked - Alan's level of weakness (high), his outputs (pee and poo were regular), his skin (sore in places), his mouth (unpleasant), his breathing (difficult), etc. It could not have been a more different meeting to the beautiful one with Morgan.

"Do you want to know what's going on?" the doctor asked us. "Some people like to, and others don't." Then, "It's important you express who you want around you before and after you fall into unconsciousness, Alan." That statement shocked me.

Trying to say calm I explained, "Alan's sisters are relying on me to keep them informed if Alan's death is imminent. So, like it or not, we need to know what's going on."

As delicately as possible, the doctor explained, "Alan, you are entering end of life." I held my breath. "The nurses are in the best position to know when you are close to the end. I will pop by on Monday." That meant Alan would survive at least three more days, didn't it?

Alan wanted to watch TV. We had done enough 'talking'. We watched several episodes of *Game of Thrones*, holding hands the whole time. I gave Alan a shave and cleaned his teeth and organised for him to be repositioned before I told him I loved him and went home.

On the drive home I told myself I needed to get back to being the old Hazel - the one who tried to make Alan's life wonderful. I called my friend Katie, a musician who lived in Derbyshire. "How would you feel about visiting Alan on 14th June and playing your flute for him, as a wedding anniversary surprise?" She agreed without hesitation.

Friday 10th May - Alan less worried
My morning was spent at home sorting out washing, post, cleaning, etc. When I spoke to my friend Carol, to arrange for her and her husband to visit Alan, she made a good point. "You have coped with the last 18 months, so you will cope after Alan dies."

Alan looked and sounded well when I reached him just after lunch. To my relief, he announced, "I feel less worried today." I did his legs exercises for him and fed him some ice chips. Then we watched the last episode of series four of *Game of Thrones*. Four more to go - will Alan see them all?

Dr Andrew agreed with Alan not to change the glyco prescription. "I will ask a skin nurse to check your nose, because pressures from the NIV mask have caused the skin to break." When I bumped into Lesley in the corridor we exchanged phone numbers. I had grown close to her.

Around 9:30pm, I left Alan and walked to the nearby home of Penny, vice Lady Captain of my golf club. She poured me a large glass of wine.

Saturday 11th May - Sunderland's big game

My morning was spent in search of red and white balloons, to decorate Alan's room ready for the big match. Alan was awake, showered and wearing a smart red tee shirt when I arrived. He'd been visited during the morning by Brian, a man we knew with MND, who was on respite in the room next door. I popped in to see Brian, his wife Jenny and their daughter, and enlisted their granddaughter to help me blow up the balloons. I showed Jenny the Barbara book - just in case Brian's voice stopped.

My sister, Rowena arrived after lunch. Alan was tired so Ro and I strolled around the grounds, then I gave her an arm massage. She stayed a lot longer than I expected, which was nice, and told Alan, "You are a lovely brother-in-law."

Teresa and Phil arrived early evening, bringing Alan a red and white scarf. He was ready to support Sunderland against Portsmouth.

I had to leave around 8:30pm, for a MND Fundraising 60's night, organised by Simon and Rachel. Wearing a blue dress, to match the MND logo, during the interval I gave a brief update about Alan and thanked everyone for their support. Later, I found out Sunderland won the first leg of the playoffs 1-0.

Sunday 12th May - Not interested in going outside

It was a sunny morning, so I spent half an hour gardening and updating the neighbours before leaving for the hospice. Alan was resting quietly when I reached him. I changed his full night mask to the nose only version, cleaned his teeth and held a pee bottle for him. To enable him to see the sunshine on the lovely garden outside his room, I moved his bed and faced it towards the patio doors. He declined a spin around the grounds in the padded MND chair.

I left Simon, Rachel and Maddie with Alan, and popped into Brian's room. "How is Alan doing?" he asked.

When I started to cry while explaining the latest news, Brian apologised. "It's not your fault Brian. It's just the way it is, and I hate it."

Before going home, as always, I helped Alan with his teeth, changed over masks to the night one, set up the call button and generally checked he was comfortable. And then our usual farewells, "Love you Al."

"I love you too, babe. Thank you for looking after me."

Monday 13th May - Breakdown of communication

A strange beeping sound woke me. Initially, it looked like the battery on the bedside hands-free phone was low. Then I realised that nothing electrical in the bedroom was working. One of my neighbours confirmed his house was fine. With a bit of guidance from the 0800 utility company lady, hey presto, everything was back to normal.

I spent the rest of the morning tending the seeded lawn patches and sorting out mum's paperwork. The latter felt weird, because it was like dealing with the affairs of someone who had died.

Alan was in the middle of having a bed bath when I arrived at the hospice. Unlike the previous day, he agreed to go into the MND padded chair. As I pushed him out into to the garden, we were joined by Cathy and her husband David for a brief tour of the courtyard. Then Alan and I went through to the garden with all the arches. I couldn't get Alan in his chair over the door strip. Lesley, who was passing by, came to our rescue. Before returning to room nine I took Alan round to Brian's room for a chat with him and Jenny.

I ate a sandwich in the tranquil Marie Curie Garden, while Alan was being cleaned up. Jenny joined me, shortly followed by Fiona, our OT. It was one of my favourite places at the hospice. So calm.

Alan and I watched some *Game of Thrones* episodes until Dr Andrew arrived. A decision was made to stop the drug that was supposed to be improving Alan's oral thrush and to reduce the glyco dose. When Morgan visited, Alan gave the trip round the garden seven out of ten for impact on happiness.

While we were watching television Alan indicated he wanted something. His request was not in the pre-set items of the Barbara book, and I failed to understand him using the alphabet chart, so I fired up the Eyegaze machine. We both got frustrated when that didn't work either. I returned to the alphabet chart for another go, without success. It hurt that I could not fathom Alan's needs, so, I hit the call button for help.

The nurse arrived. Seeing my distress, she suggested I go and have a drink somewhere. In the café, I became more upset. Two strangers comforted me as I cried uncontrollably.

Back in Alan's room, nurse Adam had changed Alan's mask. Between us, we discovered Alan was trying to remind me about two birthdays that were coming up. Adam deserved a medal for his level of patience. Alan deserved to live forever for his big heartedness.

Tuesday 14th May - Hospice choir performance

Carol and Graham arrived. Once again I tried to get the Eyegaze technology working but it was hard work for Alan. Graham managed to find some cycling on Eurosport which Alan enjoyed. After they left, Alan slept during the afternoon until the nurse arrived to give medications.

At 5:45pm the two cyclists, Matt and Rob arrived. After an hour or so they left so nurses could put Alan into the padded MND chair. I wheeled him into the lobby for a performance by the hospice Daffodil choir. Alan appeared to enjoy the songs which included *You lift me up, Believe, My favourite things*, and *Tonight*. I noted that Jane, my bereavement counsellor was one of the singers. Maybe I could get a place in the choir?

Back in his room, Alan and I watched the last episode of season five of *Game of Thrones* and then went through the familiar bedtime routine.

Wednesday 15th May - Decision about lifesaving antibiotics

Just after I arrived at the hospice, Alan's cousin Kathleen, and her husband Michael, arrived from the Wirral.

After lunch, on the walk from reception to Alan's room, I briefed my brother Michael on what to expect, then introduced him to Alan's relatives. Alan was moved that before he left, my brother told him, "You are a special man."

At the monthly MND support meeting, there were at least three new attendees. It felt odd sitting there knowing Alan was residing in the hospice closer to death than any one of them.

At yet another review of Alan's various symptoms the doctor noted Alan's oral thrush was no better. The glyco prescription was to stay the same for fear of bringing on chest issues. Alan's ear had excess wax in it again. I mentioned that earlier that day a sizable lump of green sputum came out of Alan's mouth. The doctor asked me to keep reporting such incidents.

Alan agreed to receive antibiotics if he got another infection that was causing distress, but stressed, "I don't want antibiotics to prolong my life if the symptoms are not troublesome."

"There are other ways to manage symptoms in the event of the latter," the doctor assured us. I didn't like the decision, but I had to respect and accept it. Alan had been through enough.

We started series six of *Game of Thrones* before Simon Beacham arrived for his weekly catch up with Alan. Not long afterwards a therapist gave Alan's feet, arms and head a massage, while Simon and I took a walk around nearby Brueton Park. Simon confessed, "I am worried how I will react when Alan dies." Me too, I thought. We both agreed it would be good to continue these Wednesday sessions so we could support each other 'afterwards'.

Thursday 16th May - Sunderland football club doing their bit to cheer up Alan

Morgan asked, "Alan, is there anything you want to say to Hazel?" I wondered, does she think he will die soon and now is a good time for him to say what he might want to?

Using the alphabet page in the Barbara book, which took ages, he said, "I wish I could speak to her without the need for the Barbara book." Then, he agreed, he needed to make more effort using the Eyegaze.

When Pauline arrived she and I had a meeting with the hospice social worker in preparation for the forthcoming CHC. "You need to present the facts and find out what the options are," Alyson advised.

Pauline said, "Viv and I don't think it's fair that Hazel has to be the person who chooses the right course of action for Alan."

Alyson reassured her, "It will be a joint decision between all parties present."

Our friends, Steve and Jill from Surrey came to visit Alan.

At Shirley Golf Club Lady Captain's charity golf day, I gave a short speech. Several ladies participated in activities to raise funds for MND Association.

Pauline reported, "Alan slept for two hours, and we failed to set up the Eyegaze device."

Sunderland played Portsmouth in the second leg of play-offs. The match was a draw, but Sunderland qualified for the final on aggregate. Alan's wish to see Sunderland promoted might happen! Pauline and I left just after 10pm.

AUTHOR'S NOTE

It was a great shame we had not mastered the Eyegaze technology when Alan could still speak normally. The Barbara book was useful for the pre-loaded requests, but not for a conversation. We should have got to grips with the Eyegaze sooner. It's one of my greatest regrets.

Friday 17th May - Pivotal CHC meeting

Pauline and I arrived at the hospice at 10am, ready for the CHC meeting. The woman we were expecting had gone to our house by mistake. Eventually she arrived and asked, "How do you feel about Alan's care at Marie Curie Hospice and what do you want?" Pauline and I both stated the hospice had been excellent, and that Alan was probably better off there than anywhere else.

Alan slept through most of the meeting. We had to wake him to ascertain what he wanted. Given the disruption of moving him back home, and the fact that a new team of carers would need to be trained up, Alan decided, "I would rather stay at the hospice."

Once the long standard CHC review list was completed, the lady confirmed, "My recommendation will be that Alan stays at the hospice." I felt empty. It was like a death sentence had been handed down.

Around 4pm I left Pauline with Alan and took some time out. When I returned, Alan was awake. Viv was with Pauline, and they were using the alphabet board which helped them ascertain Alan wanted some ice chips.

Saturday 18th May - Sorting out possessions
Pauline, Viv and I did the five kilometre Coventry Park Run together. Alan had asked me to bring in his box of watches and cufflinks. He singled out two items for me and gave instructions regarding who should be offered the rest.

Mum was in the lounge of her nursing home when I arrived to drop off some of her clothes. She was singing *Somewhere Over the Rainbow,* so I joined in with the chorus. I chuckled when she stated, "I have given up all my boyfriends, and I need some money so I can give a loan to someone." I had learned not to take such comments seriously as her mind was not in today's world.

Back at the hospice, Alan, Viv and I watched the Cup Final at Wembley. Even though I had no appetite for football, it was nice relaxing with Alan. Next, the Eurovision song contest started. I created a method by which Alan could provide us with his score for each song. Viv and I also rated each one. This annual spectacle had kept Alan and I entertained many times in the past. Between the three of us we rated Norway the best, but Netherlands won.

Sunday 19th May - An unremarkable day
Viv and I arrived at the hospice around 10:45am ready for a visit from long standing friends, Chris and John, from Worcestershire. John gave Alan a hug and shared details of his own health issues before suggesting he and I play golf sometime.

Laura and I discussed the MND walk taking place on June 22nd. Cathy, the South African lady, and Jenny and I had a chat at the tea station. Brian would be going home soon.

Monday 20th May - Calmness

The wet room had not passed the building inspector's criteria, and needed to be corrected, if I was ever going to sell the house. The builders arrived to put in additional insulation to address the issue. Phil, one of the builders confirmed that his mum, who had MND, was no longer eating or talking. I choked up when I told him, "Alan will not be coming home from the hospice."

Viv and I gave Alan a shave and cleaned his teeth. When there was a private moment I asked Viv if she, Pauline, Helen, John or Simon would want to participate in the funeral service in some way. "I will ask John, but I think it will be too much for me, Helen and Pauline."

Lesley, Cathy, and Maureen (another lady with a husband in the hospice) decided we'd like to meet regularly in the hospice cafe, and agreed we needed a cheerful name for our emerging informal support group. My sparkly sandals inspired the name *The Glitter Girls*! I felt calmer than I had in a long time.

"I am proud to have you as my brother," were Viv's parting words to Alan, before I took her to the train station, tears rolling down her cheeks. When Dr Andrew arrived I raised my concerns about Alan's infrequent bladder activity. After an examination, Alan was offered a catheter, but he declined saying, "I prefer to see how things go in the next twenty-four hours."

Morgan dropped by in the afternoon and Alan confirmed there was nothing on his mind. She suggested, "You might want to let Hazel know what things you want around you from your home." Why didn't I think of that? Did I know it was allowed to bring in personal items?

Alan and I squeezed in an episode of *Game of Thrones*. Simon Beacham arrived at 6pm and helped me rinse Alan's mouth and clean Alan's teeth. Simon was a natural carer, not fazed by anything that Alan needed. Using the alphabet board, Alan asked Simon about his recent camping trip and enjoyed hearing all about it. It was nice to see Alan calm and more contented.

Tuesday 21st May - A death occurs

Alan's nephew, Matthew, arrived in the afternoon, and we took Alan for a spin in the padded MND chair. It was nice sitting in the sun by a fountain, while Matthew talked about his new job and what he'd done with Alan's financial gift. I'd arranged a surprise visitor for Alan, Vicky from his office. Once she had caught up with Alan, she and I went for a quick drink at a local pub.

Back at the hospice around 8pm Alan and I watched more *Game of Thrones*. While Alan was having his pad checked I overheard Cathy's son on the phone outside Alan's room, saying, "He is at peace now." My suspicions were confirmed. Cathy's husband had passed away.

I hugged the young man, "You were very brave to be with your dad at the end." He said he felt relieved. I immediately sent a text to Cathy offering her my sympathy.

Cathy tapped on our door a little later. We hugged. "I wasn't with him when he died but I've been by his side ever since." Her face was swollen from crying. My heart ached for her.

Wednesday 22nd May - Trying to connect with happy memories
As soon as I woke, I sent a text to Cathy. I was trying to imagine how she must be feeling. I pushed away thoughts that Alan could die next. The builders arrived and finished off the wet room.

Vicar Peter came to see Alan and prayed with us. As I walked with him back to the hospice foyer I spotted Cathy. I introduced him to her. He held her briefly then we all said the Lord's Prayer.

Alan struggled to cough up something from his airways. I hit the call button. Two nurses arrived and tried to clear Alan's throat. He looked distressed, so I grabbed the alphabet book and ascertained his chest rumbles had come back. A doctor checked Alan's chest. It was clear, so he wasn't concerned. I, on the other hand, worried something nasty was about to happen again. To calm down the atmosphere, good old *Game of Thrones* entertained us before I left around 9:30pm.

At home, I started to stow away the redundant slide sheets, slings and trolleys. It felt strange organising the collection of everything while Alan was still alive, but I knew it was wise to do it before the day came when I would be too emotional. Maybe getting the house back to pre MND days would help me resurrect happy memories?

Thursday 23rd May - Problems urinating
Helen, Alan's niece, visited Alan with her youngest son, Tom. I changed Alan's NIV mask and Helen helped me give Alan's mouth a wash. Tom liked having a plaster on his head to exactly match the one on his great uncle's head.

313

When Alan wanted to be repositioned, Helen, Tom and I went to the tea station and played games. It was nice to be around such a happy child having fun for a while. Alan slept for most of Helen's time with us. As I walked Helen away from Alan's room, Tom took my hand and gave me a big hug when we reached their car.

Brian was happy to be going home after his two-week respite break. I told the nurse giving Alan his medicines, "Alan has asked for a pee bottle three times, but nothing has been produced." The nurse did a bladder scan and then, with Alan's permission, fitted a catheter. Ouch! Alan was tired so I cleaned his teeth for him and left him around 8pm.

Friday 24th May - Neat way to relieve wind

When I arrived at the hospice, Alan was asleep. Before giving Alan his medicines at 4pm, nurse Adam withdrew three 60ml syringes of air from Alan's stomach via the PEG tube. I had never had to do that myself, but it was a great way of relieving wind!

Saturday 25th May - The innocence of children

My sister Rowena and her husband Steve, visited along with my great niece and nephew, Millie and Ollie. I left the grown-ups chatting and showed the children the fairy garden and the children's play area. These young children, like Tom the day before, were aware Alan was poorly but had no idea of the severity of the situation. Being around their innocence gave me a welcome break from all the intensity.

Viv and John arrived just after 3pm. Viv helped me clean Alan's teeth. We struggled to understand what Alan wanted to watch on TV. He and I both got frustrated using the Barbara book. Later, via the Barbara book we worked out Alan needed the bed pan. He didn't pass anything, but the nurse said she wasn't concerned because, "He had a large evacuation this morning." Good to know! I changed the dressings on Alan's nose and ear and gave him a face wash before Viv, John and I left around 9:30pm.

Sunday 26th May - Pneumonia brewing?

A man from a family who needed the riser chair in our lounge, called to collect it.

Viv brought to the hospice a 1936/7 Sunderland FC shirt which had been worn by a member of the family who was in the team! The fabric was stiff, and Alan's arms were floppy, making it a challenge to get him into it. Viv, Alan and Alan's nephew Tom watched Sunderland take on Charlton in the play-offs match at

Wembley. Disappointingly, at the very last minute Charlton scored a winning goal.

Minutes after Tom left, Alan's face went red and he became fretful. I hit the nurse call button. Alan's heart rate was up at 102! His blood pressure was up - 159/90! Temperature was 37.3C. Oh no!

The Sunderland shirt had to come off. Ice cubes, inside purple rubber gloves, were put under Alan's armpits. Alan indicated he wanted to go on a bedpan - his stomach looked distended. The carers got Alan into a sling and lifted him till he hovered over the bedpan. A large amount of wind came out, but nothing else.

Nurses gave Alan a five ml dose of Midazolam to relax him. I spotted something in his mouth, so I swapped his full-face NIV mask for the nose only version. Immediately, he began spitting out thick, green phlegm. I was shocked and worried because the last time he was like this he had pneumonia. As I rinsed out his mouth Alan became more settled, but he was exhausted. Alan started to drift off to sleep - so I quickly told him I loved him. He was unable to respond.

Monday 27th May - Bank holiday
Viv and John arrived, and Viv sat holding Alan's left hand, while I sat holding his right hand. He briefly opened his eyes. We chose our conversations carefully, just in case Alan could hear us. I suspected everyone was thinking the same as I was. Could he be about to die?

Alan needed eyedrops so I went into town with the prescription. I returned with the drops, and an "I love you" helium balloon. When Alan suddenly opened his eyes he was wide awake. Bizarre.

After Bev's visit, her tears fell as we walked down the corridor to reception. "I'm worried I may never see Alan again."

I tried to comfort her. "I know Bev. I'm praying he makes it to his sixty fifth birthday."

When Viv and John departed, we got stuck into series seven of *Game of Thrones*. Alan needed the suction machine to clear his airways before I cleaned his teeth.

Tuesday 28th May - Carter Castle - not the home it once was
Men arrived to take away all the hospital equipment. The dining room became an empty shell. The whole house felt strange - no longer the happy home it had once been.

A meeting took place at the retirement block where I still owned the flat I had bought for mum. Frustratingly, sixteen people could not decide on the colour of the carpeting for the hall and lounge. It was enough to put me off ever living in an apartment!

I swabbed Alan's mouth for him when I arrived. Nurse Andrew put in a new catheter because the balloon had deflated in the old one causing it to fall out. Watching the procedure always made me squirm. We finished the penultimate series of *Game of Thrones*.

Douglas, from the golf club, brought us interesting stories about cycling in Scotland, the world of Formula One and super yachts. The next visitor was Alan's former financial adviser. He was visibly shocked at how ill Alan was. Conversations with all visitors using the alphabet board was difficult.

Early evening, I caught up with Sue Garfitt, a member of Alan's Army who ran the Stratford-upon-Avon 10k. She mentioned a forthcoming trip to Jordan and Jerusalem and delicately asked me if I might be able to go with her. I apologised for not being able to make any commitments. By the time I arrived home I was exhausted, and a headache was brewing.

Wednesday 29th May - Last rites
Kevin, Sue and Tyler visited, followed by Vicar Peter. While Alan slept, I discussed Alan's funeral plans with Kevin and Sue. Less than five years since Kevin walked me down the aisle at my wedding, I asked him, "Would you accompany me to St Peter's church and walk with me down the aisle?"

We started watching series eight of *Game of Thrones*. Maureen told me Vicar Peter had given Ray last rites. She said she was feeling numb and unable to drive home. She didn't think Ray had long left.

Thursday 30th May - Paul standing in for Alan
My head was throbbing when I woke around 7am. Alan's wedding ring was in the bed. Again, it had become detached, even though the chain was still intact! I drove Alan's BMW to the garage for a service. The front tyre was illegal and had to be changed straight away. The almost worn out discs and pads would have to wait.

As I drove my youngest nephew, Conner, into the hospice car park, I prepared him for what to expect. Conner proved to be an excellent carer. He helped me with Alan's teeth cleaning, and easily picked up how to 'chat' with Alan using the Barbara book. At one point we asked Alan about his feelings. From the list in the book, he chose "Happy," "Fine," and "Frustrated."

When I asked Conner about his feelings, he burst into tears. I hugged him and took him for a long walk around the grounds. "You know you can talk to me any time about anything," I assured him. We popped into the Quiet Room and placed a pebble in the prayer bowl before I took him home.

Viv and John dropped me off at the Genting Arena. Paul Whelan was using Alan's ticket, as Alan was now too ill for date nights out. I helped Paul purchase some memorabilia and a beer. "You would make a wonderful carer," Paul joked. The two-hour Mark Knopfler concert included new material and popular songs like *Brothers in Arms* and *Local Hero*. It was difficult not to think of Alan, even when Paul made me laugh with his wit and sheer exuberance.

Friday 31st May - Treats for Ellie
My friend, Jo met me at a coffee shop in Solihull and provided much needed moral support before I went to the hospice.

Adrian and Alison chatted to Alan about Alison's recent volunteering trip to Africa. They picked my brains about their forthcoming trip to North Devon - my home county.

Impressively, Viv and John arrived at the hospice on their bikes. I showed them and Alan the videos I had taken of the concert and played some Dire Straits CDs to add to the atmosphere.

During my brother Michael's visit, Alan needed to go on the bedpan, so Viv, John and Michael said their goodbyes.

More *Game of Thrones* episodes were consumed. Losing ourselves in the fantasy world of Westeros was therapeutic for us both.

In the tea station area, I treated Ellie to nibbles and drinks ahead of her forthcoming twenty-sixth birthday.

I stayed at the hospice overnight.

JUNE 2019

Saturday 1st June - Who will be next?

Even though Alan slept well, with no mask issues, I woke up several times in the night. At 6am, two nurses gave Alan a bladder flush. Suddenly, the fire alarm went off. The nurse advised us to stay in the room. While the nurse investigated the situation, I gave Alan a hug and took a photograph of our clasped hands.

Panic over, I delivered a birthday card to Ellie in her mum's room. On the way I noticed Maureen's husband's room was empty. The nurse confirmed Ray had died peacefully in the night with Maureen by his side. Tears rolled down my cheeks. This was the second death associated with my new friends at the hospice.

Maureen appeared in the corridor. She had written a message to Ray on a stone that was going to become part of a hospice garden. We agreed to stay friends, and I invited her to come and visit Alan and I at any time.

Walking around the hospice grounds, in an attempt to get my emotions under control, I bumped into a stranger. "Are you okay or in need of a chat?" he kindly asked. I could not talk. He told me his wife was resting having had surgery to remove a brain tumour. "We don't have children," he confided, "and have always done everything together as a couple." I know how you feel, I thought.

Sunday 2nd June - Missed photo-opportunity

When I arrived at the hospice, Alan indicated he wanted a shower. Three nurses got him into his sling, hoisted him to his wet room while I helped move the ventilator. Unfortunately, after the bidet pan was removed from under the shower chair, Alan's bowels opened. A nurse had to clean up the floor before we could commence showering.

Alan smiled brightly as I rubbed shampoo into his scalp. "He looks so happy," a nurse said, "Do you want to take his photo?" Afraid he would become cold, I declined. Once he was back on his bed, dried, moisturised and dressed by the nurses, I gave Alan a shave, cleaned his teeth and put moisturiser on his face. He chose to wear a white tee shirt, which made him look angelic against his white bed sheets.

Viv and John arrived on their bikes and stayed a few hours. When Nurse Adam came in, I mentioned the blood I'd noticed in Alan's catheter tube. He suggested something might have been 'nicked internally' (Ouch!) and did a flush of the tube. I feared Alan's kidneys were failing and remained worried.

Over dinner, back at the house, Viv, John and I talked about all the things I needed to deal with in the future. I drank too much of the two bottles of red wine we opened.

Monday 3rd June - Uneventful day

For a change it was an uneventful day. Alan had been fully paralysed for a long time and I had got used to doing the myriad of things he needed help with - scratching him whenever he had an itch, feeding him ice chips, wiping his nose, moving his legs and arms when they became uncomfortable, etc.

Not being able to have a two-way conversation with him was something I didn't think I would ever get used to.

We finally finished the last series of *Game of Thrones* before I went home around 11pm.

Tuesday 4th June - What was Alan trying to say?

My playing partner, in a golf competition, was a lady who had been widowed in February. I played the first nine holes very badly because we spent most of the time chatting about our respective husbands.

Andy Gould was already at the hospice showing Alan pictures from bygone days of football when I arrived around 2:30pm. Alan loved hearing about my golf match and was impressed that I had come third overall after rallying on the last set of nine holes.

Andy took a picture of Alan and me (which is on the back cover of this book). Alan tried to say something. He became unusually frustrated, so it must have been important, but we could not fathom it between us. Nurse Adam confirmed, "The urine dip test showed no infection in the bladder, just a bit of blood."

With no more *Game of Thrones* left, we watched the first episode of *Chernobyl* before I washed Alan's face and told him I loved him. He looked right at me. MND had robbed him of his speech, but I suspected his look said, "Thank you for looking after me" and "Love you babe."

His beautiful, twinkly eyes were always one of his best features. Now they were his only means of communication.

Wednesday 5th June - Running out of time

I took my car to a local garage for its MOT. The receptionist drove me home so I could do household chores and admin. On my electric keyboard I started to compose a lullaby to play to Alan, on our 5th wedding anniversary, in nine days' time.

By 2pm, I was concerned I hadn't heard from the garage. When I called them, I was told the MOT machine has had issues. Luckily, I had arranged for Alan to have company during the afternoon. Malcolm called me when he left the hospice. "Nothing to report."

As the afternoon progressed, I became increasingly frustrated. At 5pm the garage called to say my car had failed the MOT and needed new tyres which were not in stock. Angrily, I told them to keep the car and jumped into Alan's BMW and rushed over to the hospice.

Simon Beacham had just arrived for his regular 6pm Wednesday visit and had to witness me giving Alan hugs and kisses. I felt guilty and stupid for not using Alan's car earlier, and hoped he had not been too worried about me.

Alan's urine bag was full, so I buzzed a nurse for assistance. Simon thought Alan looked sleepy and suggested he rest. I sensed Alan was struggling for air. Before I could change his mask, he needed a shave, which Simon and I managed between us. I washed Alan's face and applied moisturiser then fitted the full-face mask. Alan appeared agitated, so a nurse gave him Lorazepam, mentioning he had received a dose earlier in the day.

Alan appeared reluctant to have the full-face mask on, so I quickly changed it back to the nose mask. Suddenly he started to go pale. He moved his eyes to the far right and gave Simon a long look. Then he brought his eyes to the left and looked straight at me, locking onto my face. Simon and I tried to soothe him. Simon started to look worried.

I held Alan.

"Simon, get a nurse - I think he's slipping away," I said, trying not to panic.

As I stroked Alan's head, arms and hands, his breathing became shallow. I kept holding him and telling him how proud I was of him. I felt strangely calm.

The nurse who had given the Lorazepam just a few minutes earlier came back. She looked stunned on seeing Alan and quickly called for a senior nurse.

Within seconds, the nurses had checked Alan's pulse, lowered the head end of the bed, taken the support pillows from under his arms and had moved him to the right side of the bed. I wasn't sure what was happening. It all felt a bit surreal.

Then the senior nurse calmly told me, "We will take off his mask now, as he requested."

I wanted to be sure he would not struggle. "Is he at the end of his life now?" I whispered.

"It will be alright," the nurse said reassuringly, "You can get on the bed alongside Alan now."

There was a moment of awkwardness, as the nurses struggled to find the off switch on the ventilator. Then the room fell silent.

As I lay beside Alan I could hear and feel the air flow working beneath us but could not feel Alan breathing. His face relaxed and became pale. His skin began to cool.

My head next to his, I was shocked when suddenly air escaped from his lips, accompanied by a long, low sound. For a moment, I thought he might take a breath in and once again, defy death.

But he didn't.

I kept expecting, hoping, something of him would move. Maybe an eyelid would flicker, anything. But there was nothing.

It felt important to me to know the time. I looked up. It was 7pm - just under an hour since my arrival.

The next few minutes were suspended in a strange vortex. Eventually I heard Simon say, "Alan was a bit lost before you came into his life."

A minute or ten went by.

"You know Si, I think it was about this time thirteen years ago that Alan and I first spoke to each other."

More time went by.

Eventually Simon spoke. "I promised Alan I would look after you, so is there someone who can be with you tonight?"

Nurses told me I could stay as long as I wanted but I felt odd, and Alan looked terrible. I called my friend Teresa and without updating her asked, "Is it okay to pop over to your house?" Not long afterwards she sent a text offering to come to the hospice. I agreed.

For some weird reason, my teeth started to ache.

In the hospice reception, Teresa and I hugged. "He's gone," I managed.

A nurse saw me as we walked back to room nine. "We are all shocked he has gone so suddenly," she said, adding, "Alan has touched our hearts. We will never forget him." I took a deep breath, tears piercing their way into my eyes.

Teresa and I had some private time with Alan, in his eerily silent room. "I will stay with him while you call his sisters," Teresa offered softly.

I cannot remember what I said to Pauline and Viv, or, how they reacted.

When I returned, Teresa was talking to Alan saying he was an inspiration. Nurses slowly popped in one by one, each saying goodbye to Alan as if he was still alive. I found it odd. He was gone. I was bereft.

On my own with Alan, I could not believe how old he looked. The muscles had wasted away in his face – how had I not noticed that? I'd never seen a person die before. I wasn't sure if I was having a bad dream.

I kissed Alan's head, his eyes, his cheeks and lips.

I took a photograph of our clenched hands. His skin was as white as the sheets. I photographed his face, at peace, but empty of life. I placed his toy tiger onto his shoulder - to protect him - and took a final photograph. Why I took these pictures, I don't really know. Something drove me to do it. I think I was worried my memory might play tricks on me and I would not believe he had died without 'evidence'. Our life together had been captured in pictures at every stage. I could not miss this last chance to capture Alan.

Before leaving the hospice I went to the Quiet Room and placed a pebble in the bowl.

Show me Heaven played on the radio as I drove to Teresa's house.

Phil gave me a long hug. They both offered me food, but I had no appetite.

While Teresa was making up the spare bed, I tried to play my incomplete anniversary lullaby on Phil's piano. He played a beautiful Irish tune. The three of us talked about Alan and cried together, for hours.

Thursday 6th June - Millions of thoughts - lots of love
A million thoughts were rushing around my mind when I woke just after 3am. I felt terrible and angry about being prevented from reaching Alan sooner

yesterday. It would have been awful for him, not being able to say what he wanted to say, in his final moments. Why did I not think to drive Alan's car to the hospice, instead of waiting for mine? Maybe, subconsciously was I afraid Alan might die yesterday? I suddenly realised he must have held on to life all day until I got there. Maybe it was fate I was delayed so Simon would be with me? Like so many things in life and death, there were no answers.

There was no choice but to accept the things I couldn't change, but I kept asking myself could I have done more?

Staying patient had been tough when communication with Alan was difficult. It was hard being someone's carer twenty-four hours a day, and trying to make their life feel worthwhile, as well as running a home and all our affairs (and in the early days, working). Alan was always polite, and grateful for everything I did for him. I would have given my right arm to have saved his life.

All my teeth and my whole face hurt from crying. I couldn't sleep, so sent texts to lots of people including Julie, the Macmillan nurse and Fiona, our OT. I wrote a list of things I needed to do and put the light out at 4:30am.

When I got up, I sent a text to Pam, the Lady Captain. She would inform the whole club of my news. I had a phone call with my oldest friend, Jo, before having breakfast with Phil and Teresa.

In a daze, I took Alan's car to the BMW garage. En route, Michael Bolton was asking *How am I Supposed to Live Without You?* I don't know, Michael, I have the same question.

The funeral director took details from me, then told me, "We are dealing with two other 'clients' who have passed away, because of MND, this week!"

In response to my texts, Maureen called, and Stephanie from Doncaster replied with, "Alan has gone to look for James - his MND twin." There were lots of messages of condolence on my Facebook account and distressing telephone conversations with family members.

At the hospice, Leslie hugged me. She was visibly hurting. I wrote 'For my hero' on a memory pebble for the remembrance garden. The angels from the hospice team, Morgan, Fiona and Julie, sat with me for a while saying lovely things about Alan.

Suddenly, I became aware all the attention was now on me. Everyone was being wonderful, but my broken heart could not take It all in.

At home, there were hugs and tears when Viv, John and Pauline arrived. My sister Clare and my niece Melissa came to visit me. Everyone relayed stories about Alan. I wasn't sure if I could bear listening to them.

It occurred to me that I could see Alan one last time - at the funeral home - on the 14th of June - our fifth wedding anniversary and thirteen years since our blind date.

Phone calls came from Laura, our night sitter and friends, Carol, Angela and Jill. By chance, Vicar John turned up. I welcomed his presence. Pauline, Viv, and I went for a walk around the village. We dropped into St Peter's church, sat in silence for a while, and then lit a candle. At the vicarage next door, I let Vicar Peter know what had happened. We ate dinner at our local pub. Ironically, at the same table Alan and I and Jo and Andy had sat at in December 2018. So much had happened in just six months.

Friday 7th June - Haunted by a tragic look
In the night I was sick. A reaction to paracetamol I had taken for a headache. It was agreed with the funeral director and Vicar Peter that after the church service Alan's coffin would go to the crematorium for a private service with his family.

Our GP phoned. "I respected how Alan dealt with his illness," he said, and "How are you feeling?" Flowers arrived from Alan's work colleagues. Pauline, Viv and I went to Solihull to register Alan's death. We found a book in John Lewis that would be suitable for messages of condolence at the wake.

Back at the house, neighbours popped in and there were more telephone conversations with family members. During the evening, Pauline, Viv and I worked out an order of service. I couldn't stop thinking about Alan's face and the tragic look in his eyes as he died. What would he have said had he been able to speak? I would never know.

Saturday 8th June - Need to talk to Vicar John
It was raining as I checked my messages and emails. Jo and Andy brought flowers and niece Helen arrived, also with flowers. My sister, Rowena came with me to the fundraising event at Shirley Golf Club. All the lady members were wearing MND wristbands. Afterwards, we went to visit mum. She asked if I'd seen nan and grandad (who had died many years ago) but didn't ask about Alan. I chose not to update her.

I went to see Vicar John because I was struggling with some feelings. "Alan specifically told me to find someone new, but how could I love another when my love for Alan was so strong?"

John told me, "Real love is about giving. Alan doesn't feel sadness now and wants you to be happy." John's calmness was infectious as he continued, "Finding the right person is about using your head as well as your heart." And finally, "Sometimes you have to take a risk when looking for a new person, but you will love someone again."

Sunday 9th June - Procession of visitors

Lesley called to say Ellie's mum had died. It was now apparent Lesley would be the last one of *The Glitter Girls* to lose her loved one.

As the rain fell, Viv, Pauline and I went to the morning service at St Peter's church. Soon afterwards Viv's sons arrived followed by friends bringing gifts.

After Pauline, Viv, and John left, two ladies from Alan's office turned up, bringing more gifts. Vicky said, "When Alan told us about his illness, he said I will be in good hands with Hazel."

Christina told me, "I used to put a cup of black coffee out every day for Alan, after he'd stopped working with us. In his honour we have all only drunk black coffee since he died."

Later Val, with whom I used to lodge, popped by.

It was kind of so many people to care, but it felt a bit overwhelming. A strong desire to get away from everything washed over me. I started planning a trip in July to somewhere meaningful, where I could start dictating the book.

Monday 10th June - Final meeting with Morgan

More rain and more texts and emails offering support. At the hospice I had a chat with Paul Whelan who asked a lot of questions about how Alan's life ended. I delivered a box of various small devices to Fiona, in case they were suitable for somebody else.

Morgan smiled softly as I entered her room. "You were always in tune with Alan," she reminded me. "Alan just wanted you to be okay." She asked me what I needed.

After a moment to think I decided, "I need space and time to allow myself to process everything."

"I'm not going to worry about you, Hazel. You have the balance right. You will allow yourself to experience the feelings " I wasn't sure I had any balance at all. "I was impressed with you and Alan, because you always went away from my meetings and worked on the stuff we had discussed." I felt sad that we would not meet again. Her time at the hospice was ending.

"Thank you for helping us get through this, Morgan." You are an angel, I thought to myself.

After coffee in the café, Lesley and I walked to the fairy garden where I had placed a colourful windmill in May. For some strange reason I asked, "You will come here every day to check that it's okay, won't you Lesley?"

Arrangements for Alan's wake at Stonebridge Golf Club were finalised. The rest of the day was a blur of phone calls. Since Alan had passed away, I appeared to be operating on autopilot. I was busy being a human 'doer'. Morgan would not be pleased.

Tuesday 11th June - Invaluable help from my oldest friend.
Jo and I agreed to abandon our planned golf game - it would be no fun playing in the pouring rain. Instead, she came to the house. It was useful having the clear head of my oldest friend to help work out the people and businesses I needed to advise about Alan's death. My own head felt somewhat foggy.

Together, we considered what photos would be good for the Order of Service and reminisced about our days as single girls when we used to go on golfing and skiing holidays together. "I've been impressed how you've handled yourself, Hazel," Jo shared.

My niece Melissa, nephew Alex and his girlfriend Kayleigh also helped me select photographs when they arrived. From the Myton Hospice website, I purchased a red metal butterfly, and wrote a dedication about Alan on their Memory Wall.

AUTHOR'S NOTE
There is a lot to do after someone dies. Luckily helpful checklists exist on various websites and from hospices. 'Tell Us Once' is a free government service that allows you to report a death - they in turn notify all sorts of authorities, government departments and local social services.

gov.uk/after-a-death/organisations-you-need-to-contact-and-tell-us-once

Wednesday 12th June - No one comes close
Another rainy day. The carpet cleaning man did an excellent job of removing

the oil stains from the cream lounge carpets - erasing the reminders of the days Alan's wheelchair and riser recline chair had been at the house.

District nurse, Roz came and collected the unused medicines. It was sad saying goodbye to her as she was our first district nurse. It felt odd knowing I would no longer see all the health and care workers who had been part of our eighteen month journey. I suddenly felt very alone and disappointed I had not had a chance to thank them, before Alan was suddenly taken to Warwick Hospital.

The building inspector checked the wet room and voiced his concerns about fire safety. It all seemed a bit after the horse had bolted. My nephew, Martyn, met me at mum's flat to remove some furniture. Normal life had to continue, no matter how I felt.

Simon Beacham forwarded me an email from one of Alan's business contacts. It read: "I don't think I have met anyone in my entire life that comes close to being the gentleman that Alan was. Such a sad loss."

Thursday 13th June - A poor substitute
More rain. I counted fifty-three sympathy cards in the lounge and felt overwhelmed by all the love coming my way.

At my favourite beauty salon in Shirley, I caught up with Pookie, the owner, who had pampered me the day before my wedding and given me various treatments over many years. As she worked on my back, she said "I feel a strong sensation." Then minutes later, "You don't have to do this, caring for Alan, anymore." My heart cracked a little further.

At Teresa and Phil's house, I read out a draft of the tribute I proposed to share at Alan's funeral. Teresa gave me two red roses - for our forthcoming wedding anniversary - and a card, for me to put in Alan's coffin.

Simon Beacham helped me put the dining room table back into place. "I miss talking to Alan about my runs and achievements." I felt for him. He'd known Alan for many more years that I had. I was a poor substitute.

It was hard to sleep so I listened to the biography CD Alan had made at Myton Hospice. It was heart-breaking listening to Alan, struggling to breathe, while saying how much I meant to him. He loved me so completely, and I him. There would be no substitute for me.

Friday 14th June - One last look
The rain continued to fall as if the whole world was in mourning, on our 5th

wedding anniversary - thirteen years since our blind date. Vicar Peter tried to assure me by saying, "Alan is part of you " He asked questions about Alan's life and told me, "It's okay to get angry at God." I didn't feel angry at anyone. I just felt broken.

Clare and David arrived and took away photo books, music CDs, and the large canvas with a collage of photos from holidays I had with Alan. I knew I could rely on them to place them appropriately at the wake venue. Malcolm drove me to the Chapel of Rest. Waiting in reception, I felt strangely calm. Knowing I was near Alan made me feel safe.

Alan looked better than when I had last seen him. Unfortunately, the damage caused by the nose mask was impossible for the undertaker to disguise. I carefully placed an anniversary card from me, the card from Teresa and some family photographs around him. I folded the linen apron, embroidered with 'The Mr since 2014' I had bought him for our fourth wedding anniversary, and tucked it under his arm. His Sunderland supporters hat rested on his shoulder. A photo of Alan and I laughing went into his shirt breast pocket, over his heart. I stroked his hands and face, then kissed his forehead. He was colder than when I last touched him. I took another, last photograph, suddenly realising I didn't have a lock of his hair.

I collected Malcolm from reception. As we talked about seeing Alan again in the future, the lights flickered above Alan. Odd.

"Alan was laughing last time I saw him," Malcolm told me. This gave me great comfort as I was still tortured by not being able to get to Alan earlier on the day he passed away.

At a pub, Malcolm proclaimed, "All we have in life is hope." He was right. I felt a mixture of relief, tiredness and despair. I was glad I had managed to see Alan on our special date day, even though it meant leaving him one last time, forever.

Saturday 15th June - Reminders of Alan

It was a wet day. I tidied up the kitchen, thinking of the Saturdays when Alan made poached eggs on muffins. At the church, I met the lay preacher, Moira and her husband. They gently talked to me about the music and logistics of the funeral.

The words of *My Girl*, pricked at my heart at the annual Shirley Golf Club Captain's dinner. I can't do this, I thought, so went home.

Sunday 16th June - Video clips

The ongoing gloomy weather matched my mood. Since Alan died, I had kept the house silent - no radio, music, or TV. Some days I didn't get up till late.

Whilst in Tamworth, I went to see my nephew Darren and his wife Suzanne. Darren, being competent with technology, helped me pull together a collage of video clips of Alan to be shown at the wake. My emotions were all over the place.

Monday 17th June - Grateful Alan wasn't taken too quickly

In the hospice café, Lesley lamented all the families she had seen come and go in the nine months that her husband was an inpatient. Juliette told me, "The recliner chair we had from you and Alan was a great help... but Keith only lived twelve weeks with his liver and bowel cancer." Although Alan's eighteen months had been tough, I felt grateful he wasn't taken from me that quickly.

Tuesday 18th June - Kindness and perspective

When I woke, my throat was sore and I couldn't stop sneezing. Was I getting a cold or was it hay fever? I played golf with Penny who kindly invited me to visit her at her apartment in Portugal in July. One of the other lady players, a widow for seven years, spoke of never being able to move on from losing her husband. I ate most of a box of chocolates when I got home.

Wednesday 19th June - How to use my life for good?

At the hospice, I gave Lesley a card for her fifty fourth wedding anniversary. I also explained to nurse Adam how Alan died and provided details of the funeral arrangements. I briefly saw the social worker, Alyson and Jane, the bereavement counsellor. Then I went alone to the MND Support Meeting. Wendy and Mel were there, as was Paul Whelan, together with some familiar couples and one new couple. I donated the oversize mittens Alan's cousin had made, and the trousers with the front flap, to Paul. "You know I have rustproof shoulders, and you can call me any time," he kindly offered.

Putting on a brave face, I went on my first walk with the Knowle Ramblers. At the pub afterwards I ate belly pork, one of Alan's favourite dishes.

I spent the evening pondering. What things made me happy? What activities gave me most satisfaction? How was I going to fill my time effectively and use my life for good? I began to feel motivated about writing a book. I couldn't save Alan from MND, but I could help raise awareness of what it's like for ordinary people living with the disease. When I confessed to a friend I hadn't got a clue what to call the book, he suggested, "I haven't got a Scooby Doo what to call this book." I quite liked that. But no.

Thursday 20th June - Need to call Cruse
When I spoke to my GP about a painful ear, he picked up on my low mood. "You know it's okay to get help to fix a broken heart," and recommended I contact the charity Cruse Bereavement Support.

At the florist, I bought some cards for dedications and some roses. Back at the house Viv and John had already arrived, having been to the Chapel of Rest. They handed me an envelope containing a lock of Alan's hair. Pauline and Simon arrived at the same time as Simon Beacham. They had never met before. After Simon Beacham left, I didn't fancy going out to dinner with everyone, but I did.

AUTHOR'S NOTE
Cruse volunteers are trained in all types of bereavement - *cruse.org.uk*

Friday 21st June - Celebrating Alan's life
It was a sunny day. Under the blue sky a gentle breeze refreshed the air.

The funeral invitations asked people to wear bright colours rather than black. I wore a white and green full skirted halter neck dress, finished off with a black cardigan, black bag and black fascinator.

The words to the Christina Perri song I had considered having played at the funeral was whizzing through my brain.

"I have died every day waiting for you
Darling, don't be afraid
I have loved you for a thousand years
I'll love you for a thousand more."

It had been played at my nephew's wedding a few months earlier, but now made me feel low as it stubbornly weaved its way around my head.

An unexpected and very warm-hearted letter of sympathy arrived from Dr Mustafa, the consultant at Stoke Hospital ventilation unit.

Members of Alan's family started arriving. Firstly, niece Helen with Richard, then her brother Matthew with Suzanne. I began to feel a little overwhelmed, so retreated to the conservatory, trying to ignore the numbness I felt and the sensation of a heavy weight on my shoulders.

330

Just before 2pm, Michael, the funeral director, arrived. I gave him the dedication cards for the flowers, together with a framed photograph of Alan that Pauline and Viv had organised.

Michael slowly walked in front, as the hearse silently glided to the end of our drive.

Alan's family, my brother Kevin and I were driven to St Peter's Church in the car following Alan.

There was a short delay at the church because there were not enough seats for the 200 and more people who had come to pay their respects.

It was a surreal moment when Alan's nephews, Ben and Tom, along with the other pallbearers, lifted Alan's coffin onto their shoulders. I hoped he was not too heavy and admired them for having the emotional strength to undertake such a task. Just five years earlier, they had been the grooms at our wedding.

Kevin took my arm. We walked behind Vicar Peter. Behind us, Viv and Pauline. I couldn't make out what the vicar was chanting as we entered the church.

Familiar faces were at the ends of each pew, but my brain registered no one. I focused my mind on the words of the Pink Floyd song Alan had chosen, "I have become...comfortably numb."

After Vicar Peter said prayers, Alan's brother-in-law, John, read the poem *Weep Not*.

Nephew Matthew then spoke about Alan, ending his piece with, "Alan's life ended too soon." I felt myself gasp.

It took me several deep breaths to prepare myself for getting up and facing the congregation. I placed my red rose on the lectern, together with my notes. As I read out my tribute, I could hear sobs in the church. When I faltered, Vicar Peter put his hand on my shoulder. At the end, I turned towards Alan and laid my hand on his coffin. I kissed the rose and placed it carefully next to his photograph.

Back in my seat I felt something like an electric current race through my arms and legs. In the next moment people were singing the song I had chosen:

"Thank you for the days
Those endless days, those sacred days you gave me.

I'm thinking of the days
I won't forget a single day, believe me."

Vicar John talked of us only seeing the complex side of life. He asked us all to remember the other side was ordered and beautiful. He finished with "Alan's spirit has gone to a better place." My jaw clenched. I was welling up.

Simon Beacham read the poem *He's Gone*, before Vicar Peter led us in final prayers. Some people managed to sing the other song Alan had chosen, *I've Had the Time of my Life* but I could not get the words out.

Vicar Peter conducted the committal. "Now that his spirit has gone, there is no need for Alan's body."

The church bell tolled, and *Chariots of Fire* played as I followed Alan's coffin towards the door. Along the aisle I shook hands with a few people, including Alan's ex-wife. I nodded to other people as I tightly clutched the framed photograph of Alan close to my heart.

Outside people kept coming up to me as I was trying to watch Alan's coffin being placed back in the hearse. He was driven slowly away into the distance, Michael walking respectfully ahead of the vehicle. Vicar Peter was right, it was better for me this way. I had no need to go to the crematorium with Alan's family for the private service. My last memory of Alan was in our little village.

Jo and Andy drove me to the wake. My sister had done a good job of creating the tribute table at the venue. Above the chatter of guests, I could not hear Alan's voice coming from the video collage Darren had made, but it was nice watching Alan enjoying life.

After making a short speech, I invited Alan's eldest auntie to help me cut the cake Kevin and Sue had purchased. I invited everyone to join me in singing *Happy Birthday* to Alan. The room was full of love and joy. We had celebrated Alan's life, and his sixty fifth birthday in style. Alan would have loved it.

Several people came back to Carter Castle afterwards. I had a long chat with Simon Beacham and a cousin of Alan's. Before going to bed, I opened the gift my friend Jane had given me in the church grounds. It was a bracelet with two hearts linked together. It could not have been more appropriate.

PART 6 - LIFE AFTER ALAN

July 2019 - Getting started

"Why not start the story here?" said Jane, the bereavement counsellor at the Marie Curie Hospice. I had been telling her Alan wanted me to write our story but I didn't know how to begin.

After hearing how Alan died, gently Jane told me, "Even though you shared every heart-breaking moment of the last eighteen months with Alan, your subconscious mind will need to process the whole period." I gulped. The thought was horrible. "The book will probably help you," she reassured. "You also have to begin life again, Hazel."

I was sixty-two, a widow with no children. I had given up my job to care for Alan. All I had now was a blank canvas in front of me and no desire to paint. Jane mentioned, "Some people find your situation liberating. After caring for someone for so long, they feel released and relieved." I didn't feel either.

Jane confirmed, "Those that had loved deeply and had been loved so much, find it tougher." I'd had eleven and a half years of bliss, full of everything a good relationship could have. Then I had eighteen months doing my utmost to keep Alan's mindset strong as his body died bit by bit. More tough times lay ahead while I re-discovered and re-invented myself. I suddenly felt very alone.

And so, it began - life without the one person who knew me better than anyone on the planet. Without the person I had loved with all my heart, who had loved me like no one else.

In July, I took my two handwritten journals, the blue notebook and my laptop to Devon. Staying in a small, remote cottage with views over the rolling hills, not far from where I was born, I started writing this book.

Also in July, not long after Alan died, Ben and Claire named their new baby daughter, Mia Alana, in honour of her great uncle.

Later in 2019, I contacted the charity Cruse. From them I learned that grief has no time limit and that, when a person dies too soon, your relationship with them remains forever perfect. They never age. You never fall out. You never stop loving them, just because you cannot see them.

2020

Counselling from Cruse, Morgan and Jane at Marie Curie Hospice helped me put my thoughts in order. Without them, I have no idea how I would have coped in those early months.

I wished I had accessed psychological support for Alan and me much earlier, from the beginning of diagnosis. Indeed, I now feel this should be an automatic provision for every family from the day they receive a terminal diagnosis of any disease.

For some time, I wrote letters to Alan in my journal, telling him what I did every day. I was never able to talk to him, like I know some widows talk to their lost husbands.

In March, our country went into lockdown as gradually the world experienced the Covid pandemic. I spent the year doing my best to avoid the virus and writing this book, thinking all the time about Alan and how he wanted our story known.

Because everyone's life was affected by Covid, I didn't feel as alone as I did when caring for Alan. I did, however, feel different. Without exception, all the widows I knew had children and some had grandchildren too. I had neither. Most widows had been married many more years than we had, so had more happy memories to pull on.

Towards the end of the year I put Carter Castle on the market. It was too big to manage on my own and felt like a mausoleum. Try as I might, the distressing memories of Alan's illness overshadowed the happier memories from before the Mean Nasty Disease taught me that nothing in life can be taken for granted.

Sadly, Brian, who was diagnosed before Alan, died at home. Jenny and I were now fellow MND widows.

This poem I had found, acted as my mantra for most of the year.

BE UNAFRAID
We can do anything for just one day.
So, just for today, let us be unafraid of life,
and unafraid of death, which is the shadow of life,
unafraid to be happy,
to enjoy the beautiful,
to believe the best.
Just for today, let us live one day only,
forgetting yesterday and tomorrow,
and not trying to solve the whole problem of life at once.

2021

When Covid rules allowed, I tried to follow Alan's advice about being pampered and travelling. I scattered his ashes, according to his wishes and kept some in a pot we had purchased in Vietnam.

To help me look at life differently, I began an online practical philosophy course.

All the people I met with MND, and their family carers, humbled and inspired me. So, I became a volunteer campaigner for the MND Association, helping raise awareness and lobbying politicians.

Wendy's husband, Mel, died at home in March. He had developed the additional complication of frontotemporal dementia which made him very anxious, and even more dependent on Wendy.

On the anniversary of Alan's death, the Marie Curie Hospice posted my story as a blog on their website.

Marie's husband, Parmar, died at home in August. Parmar found it hard to accept help from external carers, meaning Marie had to step in, a lot.

It was too painful to look back when I drove away from Carter Castle for the last time. My new, smaller and more modern house was nearer the golf club and mum's care home.

2022 and beyond

The process of reading the draft of this book, triggered tough memories and difficult emotions. It possibly kept me stuck in my grief which, on occasions, was torture.

Editing the book, however, helped me realise I was blessed to have Alan to love and to be loved by him. He was full of grace and humility to the end. Also, I realised I was very lucky to be supported by so many friends, family, and live in an area where excellent professional help was available. Not every family is as fortunate.

It's impossible to thank everyone enough for the love and help that came our way, so I try to pay it forward, by being there for other carers going through similar battles and anyone in distress.

When I wasn't working on the book in 2022, I was travelling and turning my new house into a home.

Alan is in my thought almost every day. A pillow with a picture of his face on it, sits in a chair opposite mine. I hug it when I need to. His photographs are on the sideboard. The signet ring that was cut from Alan's finger has been turned into heart shaped earrings, helping me remember his loving words. I wear his wedding ring around my neck. In my handbag, there is a copy of the order of service from his funeral. It goes everywhere with me. I love the photographs and poems it contains.

Mum is still alive but is a shadow of her former self, due to her vascular dementia. She doesn't know about Alan dying or Covid or what's going on in the world, but she is safe and well cared for. Most times she knows who I am when I visit.

Wendy and Marie and I have been on holiday together a few times. We take an MND teddy with us, affectionately called MelAlanP (a mash up of our late husbands' names). People, who ask us about the teddy, are always moved by our story. I see Brian's wife, Jenny, occasionally. Stephanie in Doncaster is moving forward with her life but, tragically, James's mum died at the end of 2022.

I am still in touch with Lesley and Maureen, two of *The Glitter Girls* from the Marie Curie days. Cathy moved back to South Africa. Ellie and I are connected via Facebook.

Fiona, the OT from the Marie Curie Hospice, is a friend now. I have become a volunteer at the hospice which means I can help her with the MND Support Meetings and pass on my experience with MND to newly diagnosed families.

In June 2022, I donated a kidney to my brother, Kevin. I could not save Alan, but I could give a better life to Kevin. Sometimes I think I might write a book about that journey. Then, Alan's voice of reason kicks in, telling me to just get on with making sure my own 'life's good'.

For my work supporting people living with MND and, for making the kidney donation, I was shortlisted for the Inspirational Woman 2023 Award, from Warwickshire based Ladies First Professional Development Network. I didn't win it, but, to my surprise, the organisation gave me the Inspirational Author Award for 2023 for this book!

As part of my work as a campaigner, I attended the 20th anniversary dinner of the All Party Parliamentary Group for MND, held at the House of Lords.

Later in the year, Woman's Own magazine was the first publication to carry a story about my book.

Since Alan died, Christmas, Valentine's Day and the three significant days in June, (the 5th when Alan died, the 14th our blind date and wedding day, and his birthday on the 21st) have been tough. But I have followed Morgan's advice and arranged treats or done meaningful things on those days. On what would have been our 7th wedding anniversary, I went to The Welcombe Hotel in Stratford-upon-Avon with my friend, and fellow MND widow, Wendy. I wore my wedding tiara and strolled around the sunshine bathed grounds - just like I did with Alan in 2014.

To this day (in early 2023) certain triggers cause my grief to bubble up. I have learned that such feelings pass. Over time I have become calmer in myself and content with living alone. I fill the house with friends every so often, and love spending time with my family.

I feel Alan's spirit is with me when I am playing golf at Shirley. There is one hole, the 6th, where I often talk to him in my head. It doesn't always cure my rubbish shots but, recalling those days, when I used to video him as a beginner on that hole, makes me smile. When I go skiing I feel even closer to him - especially when I am high up amongst the mountain peaks.

I have travelled back to some of the countries Alan and I visited. It's been comforting, remembering our time there together. There are still places on our bucket list I have yet to reach but, I will make them happen. The list now includes places Alan had no desire to visit. I am lucky to have friends who wish to join me on such adventures.

Following Alan's instructions, just before the first lockdown I met a man who had tragically lost two wives - a double widower. He has become a great friend. His incredibly infectious positivity and carpe diem 'why not?' attitude have helped me move on with my life.

To finish, I have one final random thought:

If Alan were a book, I am sure his last words would be, "Thank you for reading me."

THE END

WHAT FAMILY AND FRIENDS SAY ABOUT ALAN

"Alan has been our brother for more than sixty years. We and our families have so many wonderful memories of him as children, teenagers, and adults that it is impossible to single any out. Alan's death has left a huge irreplaceable gap in our family. We think about him every day. Alan loved his family, and we loved him. Alan always had a great sense of humour, quick wit, a positive approach to life and great strength of character. We feel that all these attributes helped him to come to terms with and cope with living with MND.

To us he remained positive throughout, never felt sorry for himself, and in his own words, it would always be business as usual for as long as possible. When he was confined to a wheelchair and dependent on assisted breathing, he was still up for going to concerts, the pub, the cinema, restaurants, even the beach. Before he was diagnosed with MND, Alan was a very active person. Cycling, running, fell walking, skiing and golf were the sports in which he used to love taking part. It soon became apparent that these were beyond his capabilities as his body started to let him down.   Amazingly, he still maintained an interest in all the sports he loved: watching the Tour de France and other cycle races when he could no longer cycle, watching golf tournaments when he could no longer play, and enjoying Ski Sunday.

Totally selfless, he was always interested to hear about other people's sporting achievements and encouraging them to improve. Alan was always pleased to see any visitors, grateful and appreciative of the care given to him, and always took an interest in what everyone was doing, whether it was one of the carers, a golfing friend, or a member of the family. Lots of people called him "inspirational". He most certainly was and a very special person who loved life and who we are so proud to call our brother."
Pauline and Viv, Alan's sisters

"His USA cousins loved him dearly. He was very special to all of us."
Renee Kimberling, cousin

"I heard the phrase, ''You are lucky to be Alan's cousin'' numerous times as a teenage girl from my friends at school - they all loved Alan. I am lucky to have been his cousin and have many happy memories of long days on the beach, rain or shine, with Alan and his family. As an extended family we were all very close. Walking home from Sunday School through the park trying to avoid the keepers while we collected conkers and then sliding down a sandy bank and getting our Sunday clothes dirty are just a couple of things that I remember fondly. I was honoured to be asked by Viv to make the special gloves for Alan. Problem, what to use to make them warm and waterproof? The answer came with a visit to a

small company selling fabrics for outdoor clothing. A few samples later and the gloves were ready to post out. The thank you video Alan made even though speech was very difficult for him meant so much to me and shows how brave he was. Alan's last visit to our house was on a sunny but cool day, we sat in the garden with Hazel and Viv until he got cold and then went inside and talked about our families. That place in the garden is where I sit and often think about my special cousin Alan."
Christine, cousin

"I think about Alan and Hazel on most of my jogs and bike rides, because the privilege of becoming part of Alan's Army got me back off the sofa exercising again. When I'm struggling up a hill, or can't really be bothered to go out, their positive attitudes and strength inspire me to get on with it.

The memory of meeting Alan and Hazel for fish and chips in Whitby will always stay with me. I was feeling apprehensive but as soon as they entered the restaurant I knew, despite the tubes and wheelchair, it was still Alan. The most memorable comment came after we had eaten when Alan asked, "Will you join me in a glass of champagne, Lindsey?" It was a lovely couple of hours."
Lindsey, 2nd cousin

"Alan was a very thoughtful and caring man, always interested in the progress and development of his close and extended family. He lived life to the full, enjoying adventurous holidays and always ready to accept a challenge. He faced his greatest challenge when he was diagnosed with the cruel disease MND. He accepted his situation with grit and determination, and even humour, and achieved so much with the love and care of his wife Hazel. He was a shining example to us all in making the most of life in extreme adversity."
Kathleen, cousin

"In the twenty-seven years of knowing Alan as a business partner, close friend and confidante we never, I stress never, exchanged a bad or angry word between each other. We just understood each other and had what I would say was a unique relationship, one I haven't shared with anyone else, ever. This has left a huge gap in my everyday life and is why I miss him so much on a daily basis."
Simon Beacham, Alan's best friend and business partner

More tributes are available on *lifesgoodbook.co.uk*

WHAT'S AVAILABLE ON LIFESGOODBOOK.CO.UK?

For helpful tips and more information, go to my website:

lifesgoodbook.co.uk

There you will find the following, and more:

<u>Helpful Information</u>

- List of resources - an abundance of links to various helpful websites
- Tips for principal carers
- Tips for friends of a family affected by MND
- Tips for health care and social care professionals
- Alan's morning routine - in detail
- Alan's bedtime routine - in detail
- Barbara Book template
- List of medicines
- List of professionals involved in Alan's care
- Other books about living with MND
- Video's referred to in this book

<u>Personal information</u>

- Tributes to Alan
- Wedding day - Alan's speech in full
- Wedding day - Hazel's speech in full
- Wedding day - Readings and vows

ACKNOWLEDGEMENTS

Where to start? Firstly, I must acknowledge, the invaluable role played by our families, our friends, the teams of medical professionals and carers who looked after both Alan and me during his illness. Also, the many people who propped me up after Alan died. Your love has kept me going.

Regarding this book, thanks to those who encouraged me write it – in particular Fiona and Jane at Marie Curie and my friend, Angela. It felt like a mountain to climb at first, but it's been one of the most fulfilling things I have ever done.

Lesley Pyne, Tracey McAtamney, Anita Sharma-James and Carol Shaw - the experience and knowledge you shared about producing your own books was extremely helpful. My sincere thanks for the time you gave to me.

Thank you to Rohlig of Solihull for coming to rescue when I realise I would not be able to store several boxes full of books in my house or garage.

Several people pored over drafts of this book to correct my dreadful English and make invaluable suggestions. Thank you to you all, especially Vicki Dowd, Mike O'Brien, Carol Harvey, Pat Gardiner, Ian and Suzanne Hudson, Gill Speksnyder and Teresa Meredith.

Richard Todd and Rachel Hardy, you came to this project without knowing Alan. It's been brilliant having your assistance to set up the infrastructure necessary for handling book purchases and accounting. Your help with proofreading, and your kind testimonials are valued.

Professor Dame Pamela Shaw wrote the foreword during an extremely busy time in her schedule. Her generous comments gave me confidence that this was a viable and much needed book. I am extremely grateful for her input.

To ensure all sale proceeds could go to charity, several kind people contributed financially to the production of Life's Good. My sincere thanks to Zen Wealth Management and The W.E.D Charitable Trust. I am deeply grateful to an old friend of mine who very kindly made a substantial contribution following his friend's diagnosis of MND. Finally, one of Alan's friends made the largest contribution. Alan was proud of how you turned out. Thank you from both of us.

My eternal thanks go to Peter McNougher. Not only did you take on proofreading and editing, but you also came up with a beautiful book cover design, a great website, posters, banners and a Facebook page, at the same time as being an effective taskmaster. This book would not exist without you, and I would not be as sane.

Lastly, to my darling, departed, dearest true love, Alan.

Thank you for loving me and being so patient as I tried my best to care for you. You have been ever present in my heart and always will be.

I hope this book is a fitting legacy.
I also hope there is an afterlife.
It will be good to share it with you.

TWELVE FACTS ABOUT MND

- MND is a fatal, rapidly progressing disease that affects the brain and spinal cord.

- It attacks the nerves that control movement so muscles no longer work. MND does not usually affect the senses such as sight, sound and feeling, etc.

- It can leave people locked in a failing body, unable to move, talk and eventually breathe.

- Over 80% of people with MND will have communication difficulties, including for some, a complete loss of voice.

- It affects people from all communities.

- Around 35% of people with MND experience mild cognitive change, in other words, changes in thinking and behaviour. A further 15% of people show signs of frontotemporal dementia, which results in more pronounced behavioural change.

- It kills a third of people within a year and more than half within two years of diagnosis.

- A person's lifetime risk of developing MND is around 1 in 300.

- Six people per day are diagnosed with MND in the UK.

- It affects up to 5,000 adults in the UK at any one time.

- It kills six people per day in the UK, just under 2,200 per year.

- It has no cure.

QUOTATIONS ABOUT MOTOR NEURONE DISEASE

"Motor neurone disease (MND) is a devastating, fast-progressing, fatal illness that I have observed first-hand - and it is brutal. It affects an individual's ability to walk, talk, eat, drink, and breathe."
Eddie Redmayne, Patron of the MND Association since 2015. Portrayed Stephen Hawking in the film *The Theory of Everything*

"As you may understand, MND has been around for an awful long while. There's only one drug that came out thirty years ago and nothing has happened since. So, people with MND, they have no chance. The only drug that we have at the moment is your mind, your positivity - if you've got that then you're in a good shape."
Former Scottish rugby union international, Doddie Weir OBE, on Good Morning Britain, June 2020. Diagnosed with MND in 2017 aged forty-six. Died November 2022.

"It tries to rob you of your breath - but it can't sap your spirit."
Rob Burrows MBE, Former Leeds Rhino rugby league player. Diagnosed with MND in December 2019

"It's very difficult. Your body doesn't want to work anymore but your brain is functioning without problems. You start losing the ability to speak. Then the legs start to get wobbly. Then you can't lift your legs anymore and you start falling."
Former Rangers footballer Fernando Ricksen, video report by ITV News Scotland June 2019. Diagnosed with MND in 2013 aged thirty-six. Died September 2019

"I know that MND can have a devastating impact on a person's quality of everyday life and be a real struggle for patients and their loved ones. I would like to pay tribute and recognise the valuable contribution made by the family and friends of people with MND, many of whom dedicate countless hours to ensure the best possible care for the remaining life of the sufferer."
Saqib Bhatti MBE, MP Meriden

Professor Stephen Hawking overcame incredible obstacles and lived a brave and amazing life. He was diagnosed with motor neurone disease in 1963 at the age of twenty-one. He was given just two years to live. He lived to the age of 76.

When, at the Royal Institute, London, on 7th January 2016 (two years before he passed away) Professor Hawking said:

"Remember to look up at the stars and not down at your feet. Try to make sense of what you see and wonder about what makes the universe exist. Be curious. And, however difficult life may seem, there is always something you can do and succeed at. It matters that you don't just give up. ...It's also important not to become angry, no matter how difficult life may seem, because you can lose all hope if you can't laugh at yourself and life in general."

ideapod.com/stephen-hawking-beautiful-message-anyone-suffers-depression

MOTOR NEURONE DISEASE ASSOCIATON

The Motor Neurone Disease Association was founded in 1979 by a group of volunteers with experience of living with or caring for someone with MND. Since then, we have grown considerably with an ever increasing community of volunteers, supporters and staff, all sharing the same goal - to support people with MND and everyone who cares for them, now and in the future.

The Association provides support to people through our MND Care and Research Centre Network developed in partnership with the NHS. We also provide around £1.2m in support grants annually and each year responds to over around15,000 requests for information and support through our dedicated helpline.

Local support is provided by our network of 90 branches and groups, where people living with MND, their carers and families can access vital information and meet other members of the MND community. Working alongside our branch and group network are Area Support Co-ordinators, who work with a team of around 300 Association Visitors who, as volunteers, provide support to people with MND and their family and carers.

We are proud to take a leading role in the global fight against MND by funding ground-breaking research, facilitating collaboration, and raising vital awareness. At the end of May 2022, the MND Association had a research grants portfolio consisting of 88 grants with a total commitment of £16.2 million, involving 185 researchers.

We actively campaign and lobby the Government in London, the Welsh Assembly, the Northern Ireland Executive and local councils, to ensure the needs of people affected by MND are being met. We do this in collaboration with our network of 11,000 committed campaign volunteers and focus our efforts on those decision makers best placed to make the biggest difference to people with MND.

People with MND, their families and carers are at the heart of everything we do.

mndassociation.org

MARIE CURIE HOSPICE

Marie Curie is the UKs leading end of life charity. The charity provides essential nursing and hospice care for people with any terminal illness, a free support line and a wealth of information and support on all aspects of dying, death and bereavement. It is the largest charitable funder of palliative and end of life care research in the UK.

Marie Curie Nurses and Healthcare Assistants work night and day, in people's homes, providing hands-on care and emotional support. They help people living with a terminal illness to stay surrounded by the people they care about most, in the place they're comfortable.

The charity has nine hospices across the UK, which offer the reassurance of specialist care and support in a friendly, welcoming environment, both to people with a terminal illness and their loved ones.

Marie Curie is there to help with practical information and support on all aspects of life with terminal illness, dying and bereavement. Whether you need trusted information or to talk to someone, you can call them, chat to its staff online or visit the website - 0800 090 2309 *mariecurie.org.uk/help*

In addition, the charity provides a befriending service, Helper, which matches volunteers to people with terminal illness. Our volunteers provide support in the community, companionship and play a vital role in minimising social isolation. This service has also expanded with volunteers now supporting people throughout their stays in hospitals.

Last year the charity launched two new elements to its information and support service: Check-in and Chat and bereavement support. In the last year these services have been used over 6,000 times.

The charity also fights to ensure that people affected by terminal illness get the care and support they need so they can have the best possible experience at the end of life. Its campaigns have successfully changed legislation to improve the care provided to dying people and to make it easier for people with terminal illness to access the vital financial support they need.

mariecurie.org.uk

THE MYTON HOSPICES

At The Myton Hospices we believe that everyone matters for every single moment of their life; we focus on enhancing life when cure is no longer an option.

We have three hospices in Coventry, Rugby, and Warwick, and have the only inpatient beds in Coventry and Warwickshire. We care for people living with a wide range of terminal illnesses including Respiratory conditions, Heart conditions, Cancer, Organ failure and Neurological conditions.

As we look to the future, we want to ensure that everyone who needs our services is able to access them and we want to reach out to people earlier in their illness, to be alongside them from diagnosis to death. We are not only about end of life care, often people who have a terminal illness have a lot of living left to do and we want to support them to have the best possible quality of life, for as long as possible. When the time comes, we believe people have the right to a good, natural death, either in one of our inpatient beds or in their own home, with their loved ones supported.

We are a charity, and we have to raise over £9 million every year to continue providing our services free of charge. Just 20% of our funding comes from the NHS, we rely on donations and support from our local communities.

Last year we supported over 1,500 people and their families, in our hospices, via our patient and family support services, and in the community through Myton at Home.

If you would like more information, please go to *mytonhospice.org*

ABOUT THE AUTHOR

Born in 1957 in Lynton, North Devon, Hazel Carter is the eldest of five children. In 1962, her parents moved the family to the West Midlands.

Until she retired early in 2018 to care for her husband, Hazel had a successful career in the Financial Services industry, working at senior management and director level.

Unable to have children of her own, during her life Hazel has volunteered for various children's charities, including Action for Children, NYAS and National Children's Homes. In 2013, she went to Botswana to volunteer at three orphanages housing 500 orphans for a specialist UK charity called Project Volunteer.

Today, Hazel lives in a small village in the West Midlands. As a campaigner for MND Association, she gives talks to raise awareness of the impact MND has on people with the disease, and on the family members and friends who deliver physical care and emotional support twenty-four hours a day, seven days a week, behind the closed doors of their homes.

CONTACT HAZEL

If you want to contact Hazel about this book, or invite her to give a talk, she can be reached on *hazel@lifesgoodbook.co.uk* or via the website *lifesgoodbook.co.uk*